Crow and Walshaw's Manual of Clinical Procedures in Dogs, Cats, Rabbits, and Rodents

Fourth Edition

Crow and Walshaw's Manual of

Clinical Procedures in Dogs, Cats, Rabbits, and Rodents

Fourth Edition

Jennifer E. Boyle, RVT, VTS
Davis, California

With illustrations by **Cynthia Bronson Morton, Derek Fox, and Steve Oerding**

WILEY Blackwell

Editorial offices:
1606 Golden Aspen Drive, Suites 103 and 104, Ames, Iowa 50010, USA
The Atrium, Southern Gate, Chichester, West Sussex, PO19 8SQ, UK
9600 Garsington Road, Oxford, OX4 2DQ, UK

For details of our global editorial offices, for customer services and for information about how to apply for permission to reuse the copyright material in this book please see our website at www.wiley.com/wiley-blackwell.

Library of Congress Cataloging-in-Publication Data

Names: Boyle, Jennifer E., author. | Crow, Steven E. Manual of clinical procedures in dogs, cats, rabbits, and rodents
Title: Crow and Walshaw's manual of clinical procedures in dogs, cats, rabbits, and rodents / Jennifer E. Boyle ; with illustrations by Cynthia Bronson Morton, Derek Fox, and Steve Oerding.
Other titles: Manual of clinical procedures in dogs, cats, rabbits, and rodents
Description: Fourth edition. | Ames, Iowa : John Wiley & Sons, Inc., 2016. | Rev. ed. of: Manual of clinical procedures in dogs, cats, rabbits, and rodents / Steven E. Crow, Sally O. Walshaw, Jennifer E. Boyle. 3rd ed. 2009. | Includes bibliographical references and index.
Identifiers: LCCN 2015046811 | ISBN 9781118985700 (pbk.)
Subjects: LCSH: Dogs–Diseases–Handbooks, manuals, etc. | Cats–Diseases–Handbooks, manuals, etc. | Rabbits–Diseases–Handbooks, manuals, etc. | Veterinary clinical pathology. | MESH: Dog Diseases | Cat Diseases | Rabbits | Rodent Diseases
Classification: LCC SF991 .C76 2016 | NLM SF 991 | DDC 636.089–dc23 LC record available at http://lccn.loc.gov/2015046811

A catalogue record for this book is available from the British Library.

Wiley also publishes its books in a variety of electronic formats. Some content that appears in print may not be available in electronic books.

Cover images courtesy of the author.

Set in 10/12pt ITC New Baskerville Std by Aptara Inc., New Delhi, India
Printed and bound in Singapore by Markono Print Media Pte Ltd

1 2016

Contents

Preface

Crow and Walshaw's Manual of Clinical Procedures in Dogs, Cats, Rabbits, and Rodents is intended as a textbook for veterinary technology and veterinary medical students, as well as a useful clinical tool for new veterinarians and veterinary technicians in small animal practice or laboratory animal care facilities. As in the previous editions, the text is organized by procedure, with each technique described in detail using a step-by-step approach. The *Manual* may be used as a clinical handbook in addition to being a teaching instrument. Features that make this manual most useful are the rationale/amplification segments, which answer the reader's how and why questions, and the illustrations, which show exactly how to physically manage the patient, equipment, and assistants. In addition to the illustrations, a number of color photographs have been added to this edition to better elucidate certain procedures.

Veterinary medicine continues to be an ever changing and progressive profession. For this reason, many procedures in this edition have been revised from previous versions to include the most current techniques. You will also notice that some chapters have been removed entirely, either because the procedures have become obsolete or they have advanced beyond the scope of this book. This edition includes new chapters on Blood Pressure Measurement, Arterial Catheter Placement and Sampling, and Cardiopulmonary Resuscitation.

The safety of personnel and patients in the veterinary workplace continues to be a high priority for employers, employees, and the general public. Chapter 1, Restraint of Dogs and Cats, is as timely today as in the first edition. Today, many entering veterinary students have very little practical experience in holding and working with animals in a clinical or laboratory setting. Chapters 36 through 38 focus on safe and effective methods of restraint of rabbits and other small mammals. Adequate restraint of animals by trained employees is vital in providing humane care for these small animals. In addition, knowing how to handle animals is essential for the safety of veterinary health care team members and animal owners. Throughout the *Manual* we describe proper disposal of medical waste. Careful use and disposal of sharp items is encouraged. It is our hope that proper knowledge of the clinical procedures in the *Manual* will enhance workplace safety as well as contribute to animal health.

We recommend that the reader use the *Manual* in the following ways:

- While this textbook is for veterinary technicians as well as veterinarians, be advised that there are some procedures that are particularly invasive or fall under the category of "surgery" and therefore *must* be performed by a veterinarian. Chapters/procedures that are exclusively for veterinarians will be noted as such at the beginning of the chapter. Please refer to your local veterinary medical board regulations regarding what procedures licensed technicians and laypersons are authorized to perform in your state/province.
- When first learning a procedure, the entire chapter or segment should be studied, including purposes, indications, contraindications, possible complications, equipment needed, restraint and positioning, and preparations. This background is essential if proper application of each procedure is to be achieved.
- Careful attention to comments in the rationale/amplification sections will help the operator avoid common errors of omission or commission.
- For subsequent cases, the reader may use the technical action guidelines in a cookbook fashion; however, periodic review of other sections of the procedure/description is recommended.
- Careful attention should be paid to Notes that appear in italics throughout the *Manual*.
- To ensure proper positioning of needles, catheters, and hands, the reader must attempt to duplicate the orientation shown in the line drawings.

If these guidelines are followed, we are confident that the user of the *Manual* can become proficient in a wide variety of diagnostic and therapeutic techniques.

The greatness of a nation and its moral progress can be judged by the way its animals are treated.

GANDHI

Acknowledgments

The author would like to express her gratitude to the following individuals for their assistance and/or helpful comments during the preparation of this edition of the text.

Clare Knightly, RVT, VTS (Anesthesia)
Steven Epstein, DVM, DACVECC
Paul D. Pion, DVM, DACVIM (Cardiology)
Tony Johnson, DVM, DACVECC
Laura Territo, RVT, VTS (ECC)
Michele Gaspar, DVM, DABVP (Feline), MA
Goldorado Veterinary Hospital, Cameron Park CA

About the Companion Website

This book is accompanied by a companion website:

www.wiley.com/go/boyle/manual4e

The website includes:

- Supplementary interactive multiple choice questions and answers
- PowerPoints of all figures from the book for downloading

The password for the site is the last word in the caption for Figure 27-3.

Part I

Routine Clinical Procedures

The procedures described in this section are those commonly performed in small animal practices or laboratory animal facilities. Busy veterinary practitioners are likely to employ these techniques one or more times daily. Proficiency in these procedures will allow veterinarians and technicians to perform their duties more efficiently.

Many readers will have considerable experience with these routine procedures; however, attention to indications, contraindications, and preparations should help even the most experienced clinician to select and apply these techniques more appropriately.

Experience enables you to recognize a mistake when you make it again.

FRANKLIN P JONES

Chapter 1

Restraint of Dogs and Cats

Don't be impatient with your patients.
CARL OSBORNE

Restraint is the restriction of an animal's activity by verbal, physical, or pharmacologic means so that the animal is prevented from injuring itself or others.

NOTE: *Restraining a dog or cat forcibly is dangerous to both the handler and the animal. Most privately owned dogs and cats can be handled safely and humanely with gentle and minimal physical restraint; however, we strongly recommend the use of pharmacologic agents to assist in proper restraint for:*

- *procedures that are painful*
- *procedures that require holding an animal in a position that compromises its respiration*
- *severely frightened or aggressive animals*

Purposes

1. To facilitate physical examination, including ophthalmic and rectal examinations
2. To administer oral, injectable, and topical materials
3. To apply bandages
4. To perform certain procedures (e.g. urinary catheterization)
5. To prevent self-mutilation (Elizabethan collar)

Complications

1. Dyspnea
2. Hyperthermia
3. Tissue trauma (e.g. muscle strain)
4. Stress

Crow and Walshaw's Manual of Clinical Procedures in Dogs, Cats, Rabbits, and Rodents, Fourth Edition. Edited by Jennifer E. Boyle. Published 2016 by John Wiley & Sons, Inc.
Companion Website: www.wiley.com/go/boyle/manual4e

Equipment Needed

- Strips of gauze or cloth, 100–150 cm in length, 2–5 cm in width; or commercially available nylon or plastic muzzles
- Elizabethan collar of appropriate size

VERBAL RESTRAINT

Procedure

Technical Action	Rationale/Amplification
1. In general, begin with the least severe restraint technique and proceed to more severe methods if necessary.	**1.** The amount of restraint needed will depend on the environment, the animal's behavior, and the degree of discomfort caused by the procedure.
2. Speak to the dog or cat when approaching it.	**2.** Speaking to the animal initially in a calm, soothing voice helps to prevent startling it. This is especially important if the animal is blind or is looking in another direction.
3. Use the animal's name.	**3.** Pet animals are usually conditioned to respond to their names.
4. If necessary, speak firmly to the animal.	**4.** Say "no" in a sharp, clear tone of voice. Verbal restraint can be a useful adjunct to the physical restraint of pet animals.
5. *Assistant*: Stand on opposite side of animal from person performing procedure.	**5.** The intended site for treatment or examination must be easily accessible.

PHYSICAL RESTRAINT WITH DOG IN STANDING POSITION (FIG. 1-1)

Procedure

Technical Action	Rationale/Amplification
1. Place one arm under dog's neck so that forearm holds dog's head securely.	**1.** The dog's head should be positioned so that it is virtually impossible for the dog to bite either the person restraining it or the person performing the procedure.
2. Place other arm underneath dog's abdomen or thorax.	**2.** An arm underneath the dog's abdomen will prevent the dog from sitting down during the procedure.

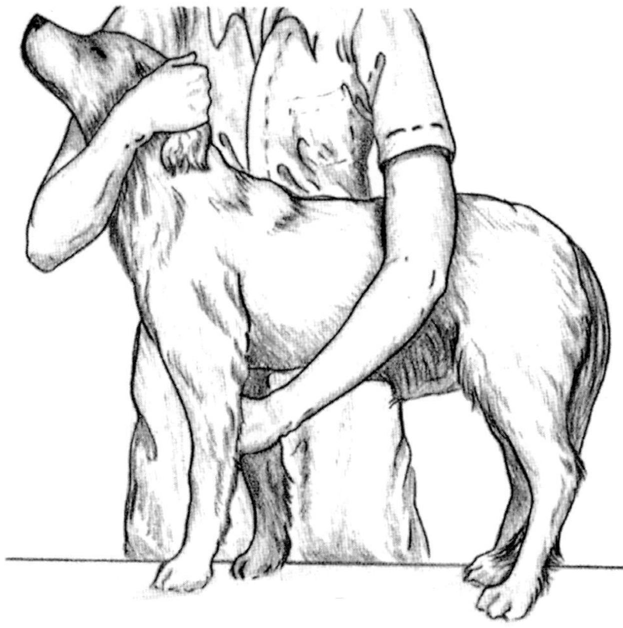

Figure 1-1 Restraint with dog in standing position.

Technical Action	Rationale/Amplification
3. Pull dog close to chest of person performing restraint.	3. The restrainer has more control of the animal's movement if the animal is held closely.

PHYSICAL RESTRAINT WITH DOG SITTING OR IN STERNAL RECUMBENCY (FIG. 1-2)

Procedure

Technical Action	Rationale/Amplification
1. Place one arm under dog's neck so that the forearm holds dog's head securely.	1. Adequate restraint of the dog's head is important for all procedures.
2. Place other arm around dog's hindquarters.	2. An arm underneath or around dog's hindquarters will prevent it from standing up or lying down during the procedure.
3. Pull dog close to chest of person performing restraint.	3. The restrainer has more control of the animal's movement if the animal is held closely.

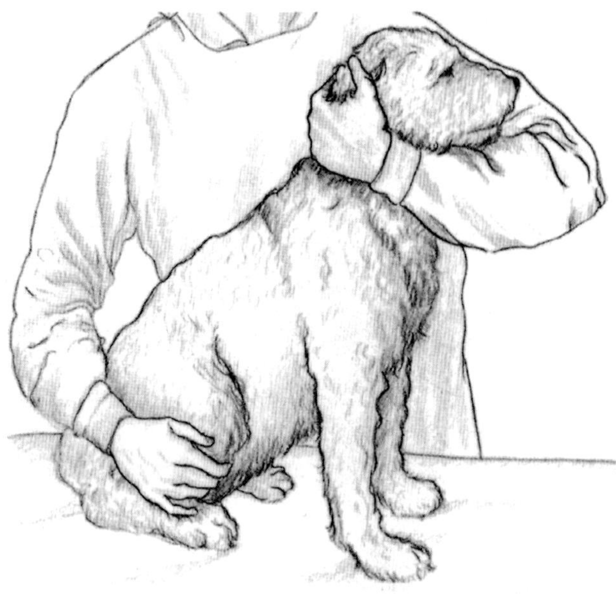

Figure 1-2 Restraint with dog in sitting position.

PHYSICAL RESTRAINT WITH DOG IN LATERAL RECUMBENCY (FIG. 1-3)

Procedure

Technical Action

1. With the dog in standing position, reach across dog's back and take hold of both forelegs in one hand and both hind legs in other hand.
2. Place index finger of each hand between the two legs being held.
3. Gradually lift dog's legs off table (or floor) and allow its back to slowly slide against your body to a position of lateral recumbency.
4. To immobilize head, exert pressure on side of dog's neck with forearm.
5. Hold legs proximal to carpus and tarsus, if possible.

Rationale/Amplification

1. If the dog is a giant breed, it will suffice to reach across the dog's back and take hold of the foreleg and the hind leg that are closer to the person doing the restraint.
2. Placing the index finger between the legs ensures a good grip if the dog tries to move its legs.
3. The dog should be shifted from a standing position to lateral recumbency gently and gradually.
4. Adequate restraint of the dog's head is important for all procedures.
5. Holding the animal in this manner provides better control of the legs.

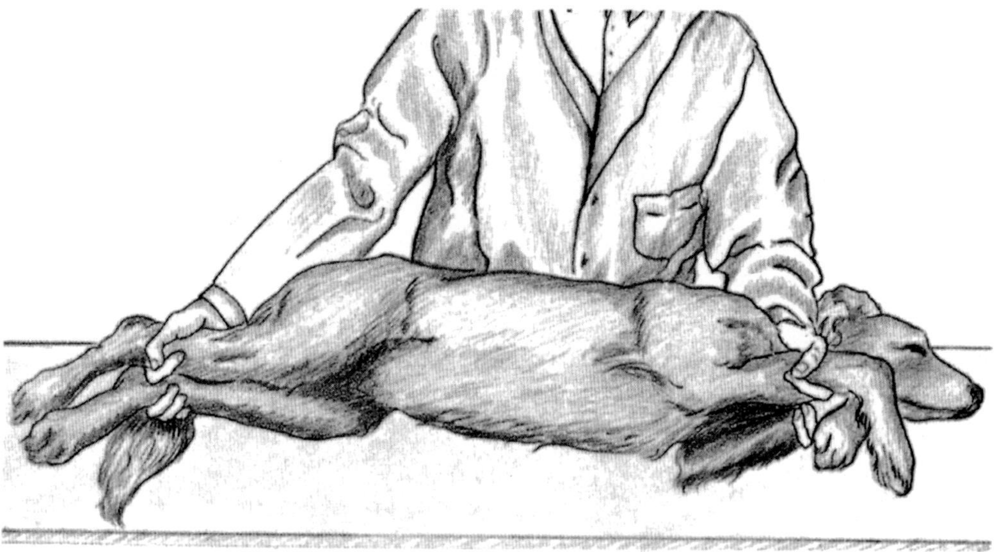

Figure 1-3 Restraint with dog in lateral recumbency.

USE OF A MUZZLE ON THE DOG (FIG. 1-4 AND 1-5)

Procedure

Technical Action	Rationale/Amplification
1. Place commercial muzzle of appropriate size on dog (Fig. 1-4). Alternatively, cut strip of gauze or cloth approximately 125 cm in length for a 40–50-lb. dog.	1. Use of sturdy or double-thickness gauze is recommended for large dogs. A weak or poorly made muzzle leads to a false sense of security and the possibility of one's being bitten by the dog. Gauze muzzles can be used in aggressive dogs, allowing the basket muzzle (Fig. 1-5C) to be placed with minimal risk of injury to handler. Commercially available muzzles should be disinfected between uses in order to avoid disease transmission.
2. Before approaching animal, make loop with one half of a square knot so that diameter of loop is about twice the diameter of dog's snout.	2. Preparation of the muzzle in advance helps to ensure rapid placement and minimizes the length of time the operator's hands must be near the dog's mouth.
3. Slip loop over dog's nose and mouth with the half square knot on dorsal surface of dog's snout (Fig. 1-5A), then tighten quickly by pulling on ends (Fig. 1-5B).	3. The hands should be kept as far away from the dog's mouth as possible while the muzzle is applied. Placing a muzzle on a fractious dog requires at least two people; one person holds the

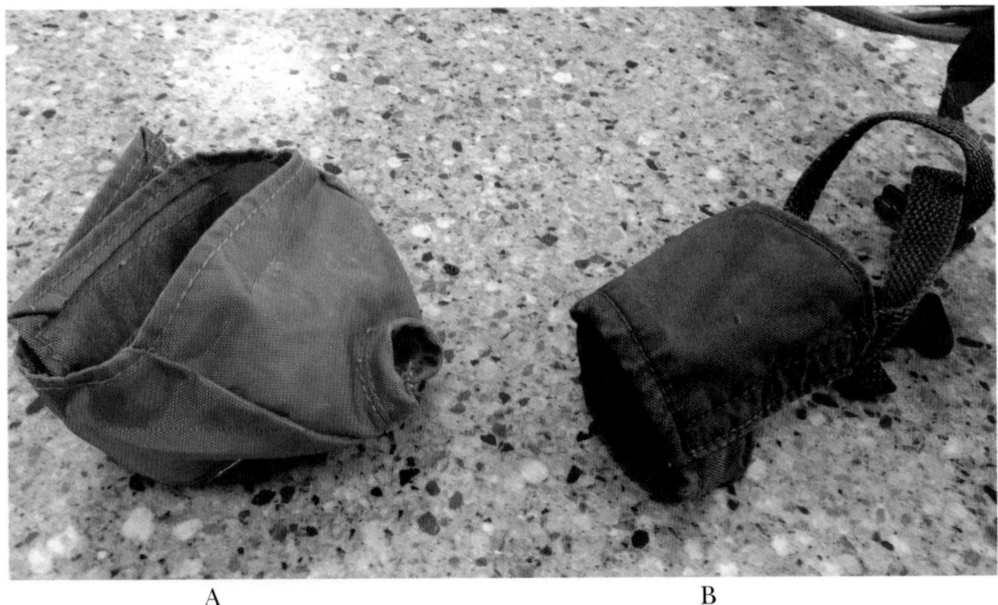

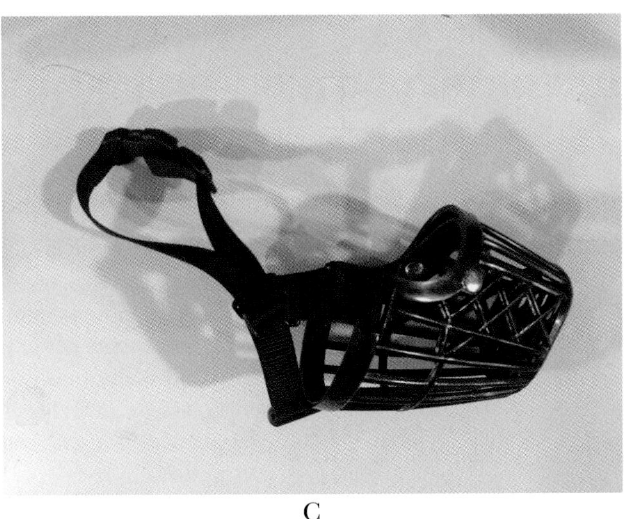

Figure 1-4 Commercial muzzles (A) Nylon cat muzzle and (B) Nylon dog muzzle (C) Basket muzzle.

Technical Action	Rationale/Amplification
	leash and distracts the dog while the other applies the muzzle.
4. Cross (but do not tie) free ends of muzzle under dog's lower jaw (Fig. 1-5C).	**4.** Each step of this procedure must be done quickly if the animal is fractious. If the ends are crossed but not tied under the mandible,

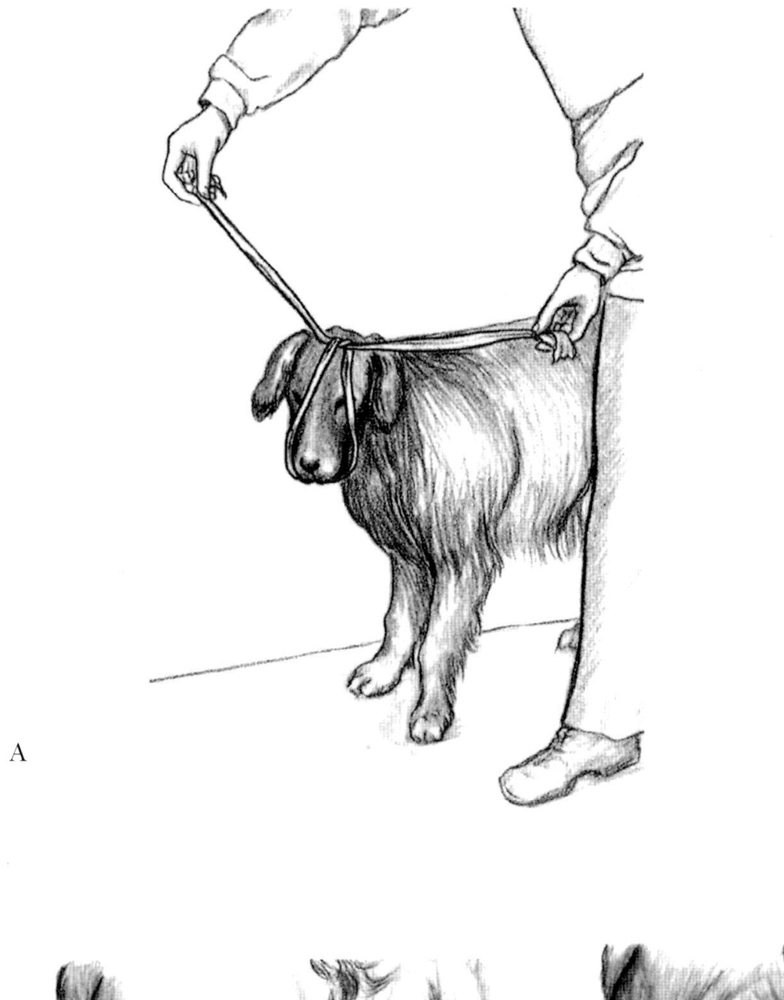

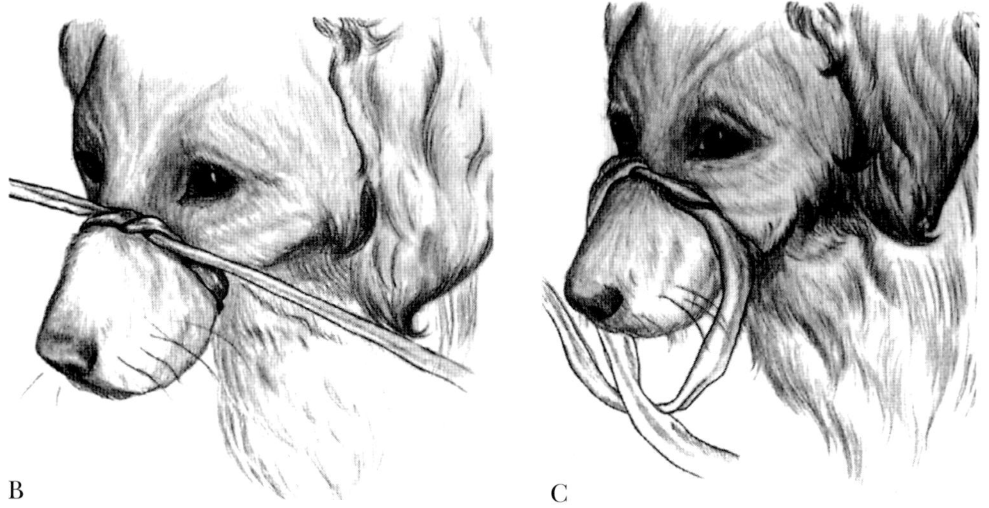

Figure 1-5 (A, B, C, D, and E) Applying muzzle to dog.

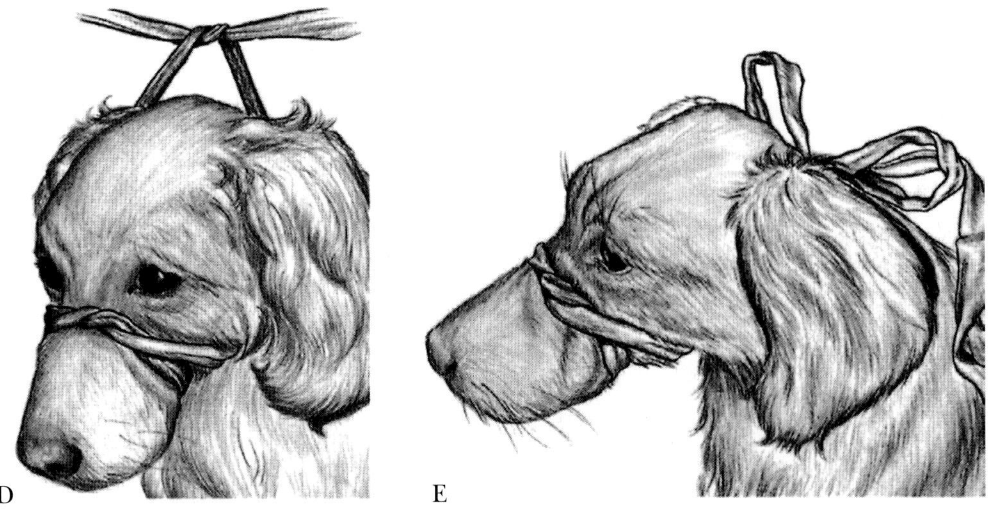

Figure 1-5 *Continued*

Technical Action	Rationale/Amplification
	the muzzle can be removed quickly in case of emergency (see No. 6 below).
5. Bring ends of muzzle up behind dog's ears (Fig. 1-5D) and tie in a bow (Fig. 1-5E).	**5.** The bow should be placed directly behind the dog's ears and tied tightly. The dog will be able to open its mouth if the muzzle is tied loosely.
6. To remove muzzle quickly from a fractious dog, untie bow and pull on one end of muzzle material.	**6.** A muzzle prevents panting and must be used judiciously in heavy-coated animals or in warm environments. A muzzle should be removed immediately if an animal has difficulty breathing or starts to vomit.

USE OF ELIZABETHAN COLLAR (FIG. 1-6)

Procedure

Technical Action	Rationale/Amplification
1. Select or make an Elizabethan collar of appropriate size and strength for the animal.	**1.** In general, Elizabethan collars should be made of tough, flexible materials like plastic rather than easily torn substances like cardboard. Ideal length is approximately 2–3 cm longer than the animal's snout, with the base of the collar pushed caudally against the shoulders.

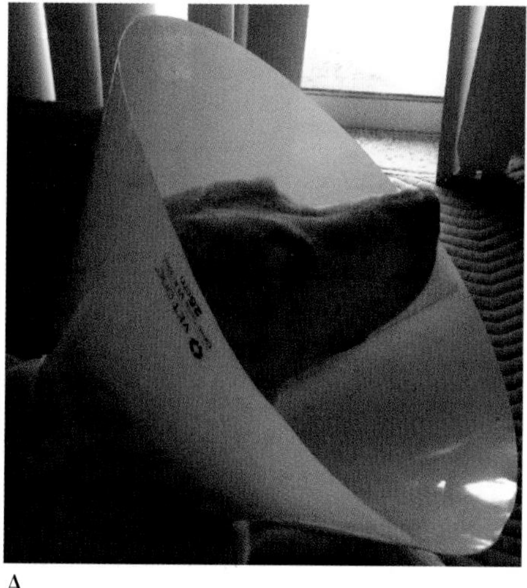

A

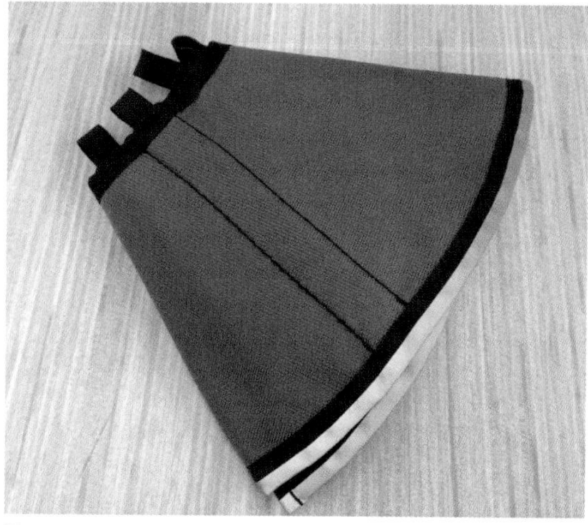

B

Figure 1-6 Commercial Elizabethan collars (A) Plastic (B) Soft.

Technical Action

2. Place Elizabethan collar on neck of fractious dog or cat to prevent animal from biting while it is being handled or to prevent the animal from biting or licking itself.

Rationale/Amplification

2. Some advantages of the Elizabethan collar as a restraint device are that the animal can pant with the collar in place; the collar can be left on the animal when it is returned to a hospital kennel, facilitating later removal of the animal for further treatments; the collar is reasonably well tolerated by most animals.

Technical Action

3. To ensure that collar will remain on animal, use prefabricated attachment loops.

Rationale/Amplification

3. Most collars are sturdy, reusable, and easily cleaned. Several companies supply a variety of sizes of Elizabethan collars, and most of these can be cut to size for animals that fall between the standard sizes.

PHYSICAL RESTRAINT WITH CAT IN LATERAL RECUMBENCY (FIG. 1-7)

Procedure

Technical Action

1. Clip curved end of cat's claws if it must be restrained for lengthy or uncomfortable procedure or if it is fractious (Chapter 11).

Rationale/Amplification

1. Restraining a cat can be more difficult than restraining a dog because cats: a) can move very quickly; b) are agile and strong; c) may use their

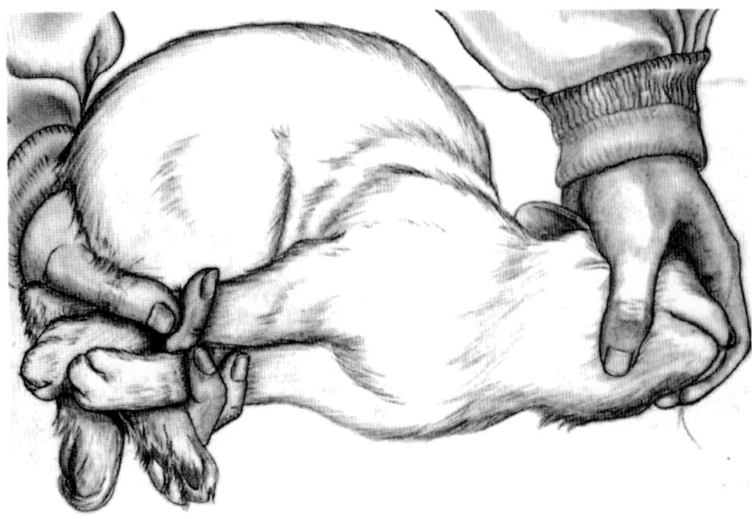

Figure 1-7 Restraint with cat in lateral recumbency.

Technical Action

Rationale/Amplification

claws as well as their teeth to defend themselves; d) are small animals that can be injured by indiscriminate use of force.

2. With cat in standing position, reach across cat's back and take hold of both forelegs in one hand and both hind legs in other hand.

3. Gradually pull cat's legs off table and allow its back to slide against your body to a position of lateral recumbency.

3. The cat should be shifted from a standing position to lateral recumbency gently.

4. After placing cat in lateral recumbency, use one hand to hold all four legs (Fig. 1-7).

4. If necessary, separate strips of 1-inch wide adhesive tape can be used to bind together the front legs and the hind legs, respectively.

5. Place other hand so that palm of hand surrounds the top of cat's head and cat's jaws are held closed by fingers and thumb (Fig. 1-7).

5. Placing an Elizabethan collar on a fractious cat before beginning the restraint procedure eliminates the necessity of holding the cat's mouth closed with one hand while holding all four legs with the other hand. A cat's small size and great agility make immobilization of its head with the restrainer's forearm virtually impossible.

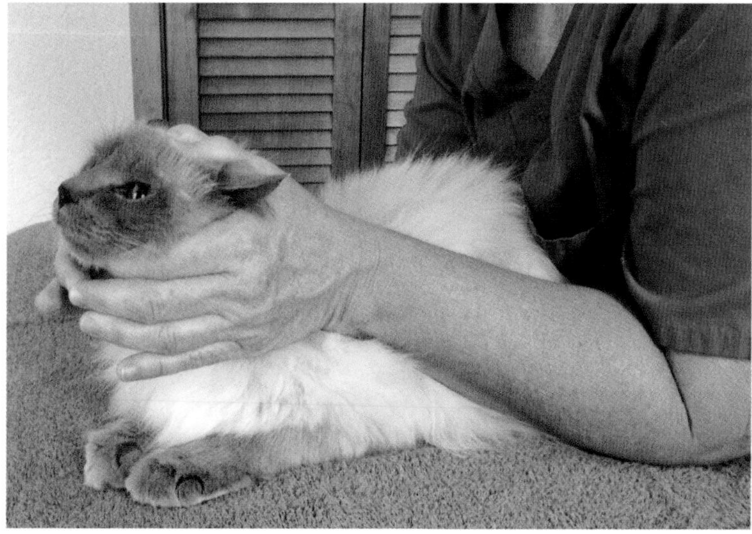

Figure 1-8 Restraint with cat in sternal recumbency.

PHYSICAL RESTRAINT WITH CAT IN STERNAL RECUMBENCY (FIG. 1-8)

Procedure

Technical Action	Rationale/Amplification
1. Apply gentle, firm pressure to cat's back to encourage it to assume position of sternal recumbency.	1. Sternal recumbency is a position to which few cats object.
2. Place one forearm against each side of cat's body with cat's head facing away from restrainer.	
3. Immobilize cat's head using both hands.	3. The person doing the procedure can approach from the side or from the cat's rear so as to remain out of reach of the front claws, should the cat attempt to strike.

PHYSICAL RESTRAINT OF MODERATELY FRACTIOUS CAT (FIG. 1-9)

Procedure

Technical Action	Rationale/Amplification
1. Close all doors and windows of the room.	1. If the cat gets away from the restrainer, it will not escape from the building.

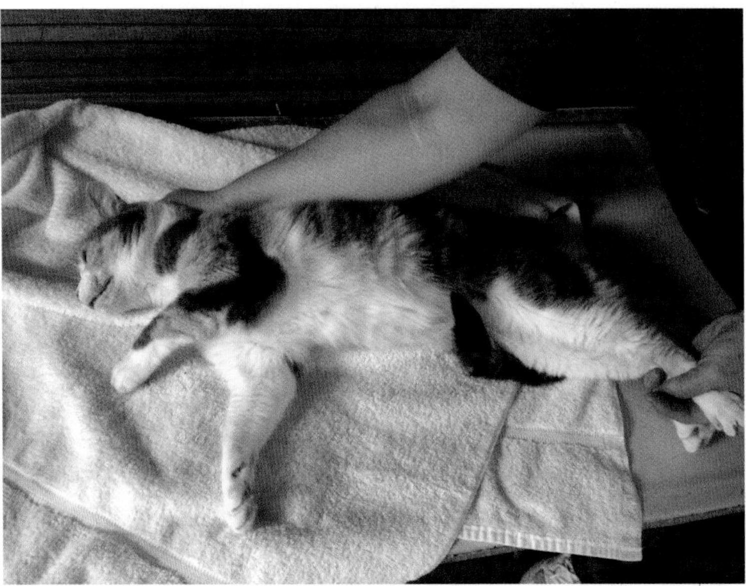

Figure 1-9 Restraint of moderately fractious cat.

Technical Action	Rationale/Amplification
2. Take scruff of cat's neck in one hand.	**2.** It is important to grasp as much of the loose skin as possible along the cranial portion of the cat's neck, beginning between its ears. Otherwise the cat may be able to turn its head around and bite.
3. Wrap fingers of other hand around and through cat's hind legs.	
4. Gently stretch the cat out by separating your hands.	**4.** A cat restrained in this manner may be held in lateral recumbency or in vertical position. Most fractious cats will raise strong vocal protests to this procedure. The necessary procedure should be done quickly. If the restrainer begins to lose control of the cat, he or she should alert other people involved in the procedure, then let go of the cat with both hands at the same time.

NOTE: *An alternate method of restraint for a moderately fractious cat is to grasp the zygomatic arches with thumb and fingers of one hand while resting the top of the cat's head against the palm of the same hand. Meanwhile, an assistant wraps a thick terrycloth towel snuggly around the cat's neck and torso, being sure to enclose all 4 legs in the towel. The cloth is wrapped around several times before folding over the bottom end. The body of the cat can then be held under the arm of the person restraining the head. This form of restraint is particularly useful for drawing blood from or inserting a catheter into the jugular vein or for administering oral medications.*

Vicious dogs and cats require special restraint techniques, for example rabies poles and pharmacologic agents. Such procedures carry significant risks for animals and persons involved.

PHARMACOLOGIC RESTRAINT OF DOGS AND CATS

Complications

1. Respiratory distress
2. Anaphylactic reaction
3. Excessive or inadequate sedation
4. Cardiac arrhythmias
5. Hypotension
6. Vomiting

Equipment Needed

- Sterile syringes and needles of appropriate size
- Elizabethan collar and/or muzzle
- Oral or injectable pharmacologic agents appropriate for patient and procedures planned

Procedure

Technical Action	Rationale/Amplification
1. Weigh animal.	1. All chemical restraint drugs must be dosed carefully to avoid improper dosage.
2. Review animal's history and perform complete physical examination prior to administering any drugs, if possible.	2. Choice of the appropriate drug or drugs requires careful attention to detail, including drug interactions, contraindications and complications, and the health status of the animal. If the animal is fractious and may injure itself or personnel, examination may not be appropriate.
3. *Assistant:* Using minimal but adequate physical restraint, hold the animal so that the drug or medication may be administered orally or by intravenous, subcutaneous, or intramuscular injection.	3. Follow principles and techniques described in the previous sections of this chapter.

Technical Action	Rationale/Amplification
4. Observe animal until adequate sedation is obtained.	**4.** Untoward reactions to chemical restraint agents may include vomiting, hypotension, seizures, and respiratory distress. If any of these signs are noted, immediate examination and treatment by a veterinarian is required.
5. When procedure(s) are completed, administer reversal agent, when available.	**5.** An advantage of narcotic and α-1 agonist drugs is the availability of antidotes to reverse or minimize excessive or prolonged sedation.

Bibliography

Anderson RS, Edney ATB: Practical Animal Handling. Oxford, England, Pergamon Press, 1994

Aspinall, V: Clinical Procedures in Veterinary Nursing. 3rd edition. Oxford, England, Elsevier, 2014

Lane DR, Cooper B: Veterinary Nursing (Formerly Jones's Animal Nursing, 5th edition). Oxford, England, Pergamon Press, 1994

McCurnin DM, Poffenbarger EM: Small Animal Physical Diagnosis and Clinical Procedures. Philadelphia, WB Saunders, 1991

Wolz G: Personal Communication, 1982

Chapter 2

Venous Blood Collection

It is impossible for anyone to begin to learn what he thinks he already knows.
EPICTETUS

ROUTINE VENIPUNCTURE

Routine venipuncture is the placement of a needle into a vein.

Purposes

1. To obtain a sample of venous blood for routine clinical pathology tests, for example, complete blood count (CBC) and serum chemistry determinations
2. To administer medications, fluids, blood, and certain test substances

Complications

1. Minor hemorrhage
2. Subcutaneous hematoma formation
3. Vascular trauma
4. Thrombophlebitis

Equipment Needed

- Cotton
- 70% alcohol or other skin disinfectant
- 3-mL, 6-mL, or 12-mL syringe, Vacutainer®* holder, or 21- gauge to 23-gauge butterfly catheter

* Becton-Dickinson Co., Rutherford, NJ.

Crow and Walshaw's Manual of Clinical Procedures in Dogs, Cats, Rabbits, and Rodents, Fourth Edition. Edited by Jennifer E. Boyle. Published 2016 by John Wiley & Sons, Inc.
Companion Website: www.wiley.com/go/boyle/manual4e

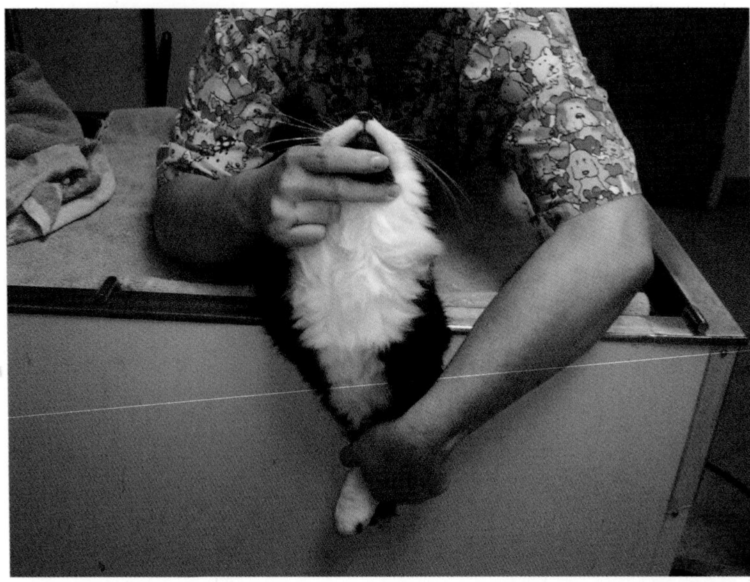

Figure 2-1 Restraint for jugular venipuncture.

- 20-gauge to 22-gauge, 1-inch hypodermic needle
- Blood collection tubes, with or without anticoagulant, depending on laboratory tests to be performed
- Adhesive tape, 1 inch wide

Restraint and Positioning

Routine blood collection in dogs and cats generally requires two persons: one obtains the blood sample while the other restrains the animal. For an uncooperative dog, muzzling may be necessary. An Elizabethan collar is useful for the restraint of an uncooperative cat or brachycephalic dog. A puppy or kitten may relax for blood collection from the jugular vein if grasped by the skin at the back of its neck.

Position for Collection from Jugular Vein

1. Place animal in sternal recumbency on table.
2. With one hand, grasp animal's front legs at carpal joints and pull front legs off edge of table.
3. With other hand, extend animal's neck by grasping its muzzle and directing its nostrils toward ceiling (Fig. 2-1).

Alternate positions: Restrain animal in lateral recumbency with neck extended and front legs pulled caudally (Fig. 2-2). Large dogs can be restrained in a sitting position on the floor (Fig. 2-3).

NOTE: *Whenever possible, obtain blood samples by jugular venipuncture.*

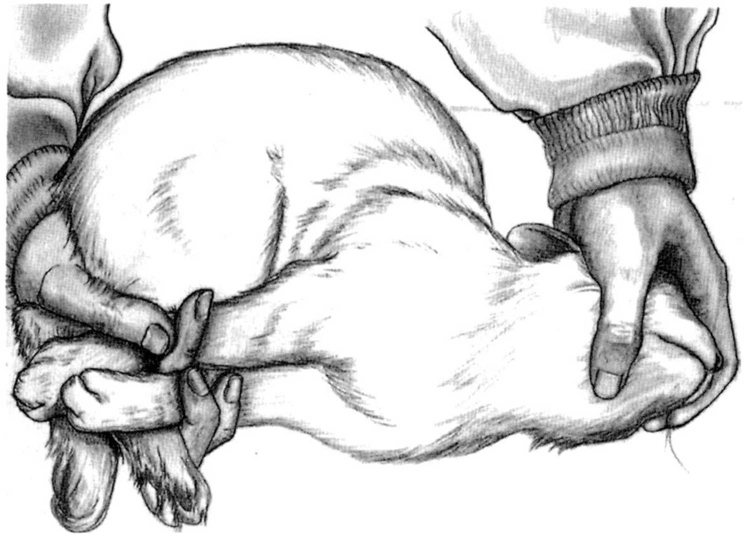

Figure 2-2 Restraint for jugular venipuncture with animal in lateral recumbency.

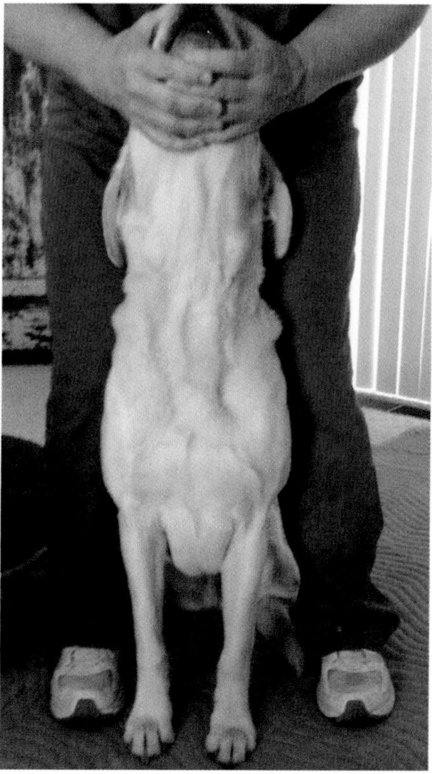

Figure 2-3 Restraint for jugular venipuncture with dog in sitting position.

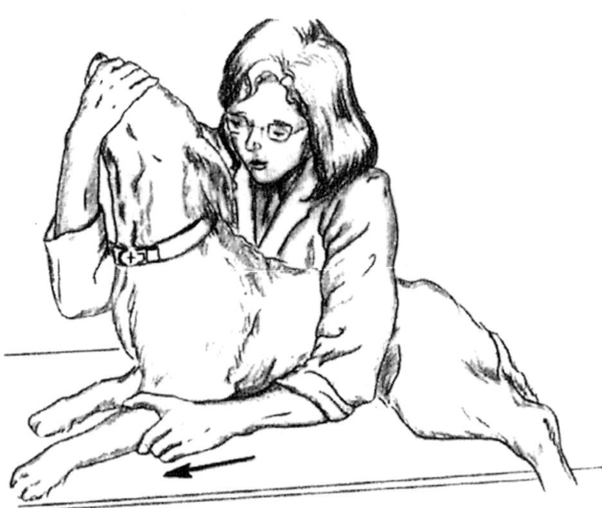

Figure 2-4 Restraint of dog for cephalic venipuncture.

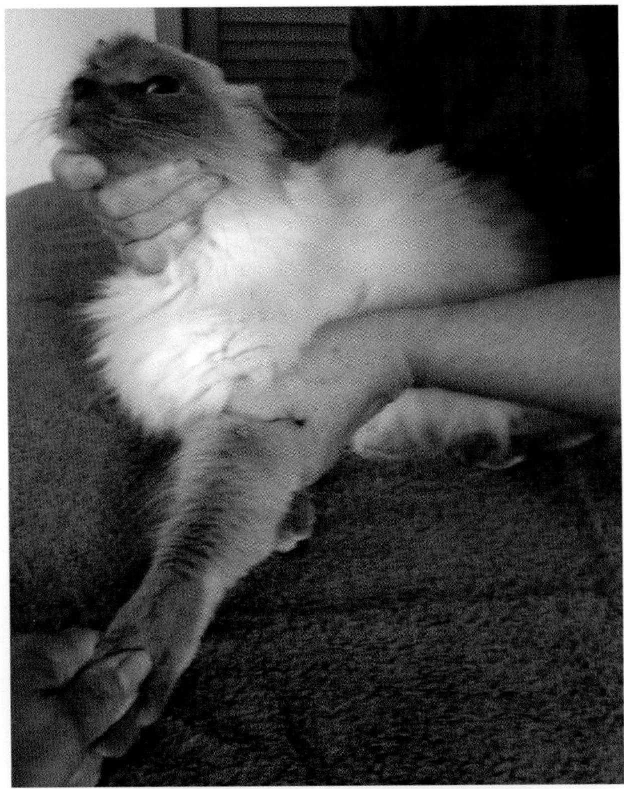

Figure 2-5 Restraint of cat for cephalic venipuncture.

Position for Collection from Cephalic Vein (Figs. 2-4 and 2-5)

1. Place animal in sitting position or sternal recumbency.
2. Extend animal's front leg by placing fingers of one hand behind animal's elbow.
3. Compress cephalic vein with thumb and stabilize vein on dorsal surface of front leg by stretching skin slightly.

Position for Collection from Lateral Saphenous Vein (Recurrent Tarsal Vein) (Fig. 2-6)

1. Place animal in lateral recumbency.
2. Extend stifle and compress vein by firmly grasping animal's distal thigh or proximal tibial segment.

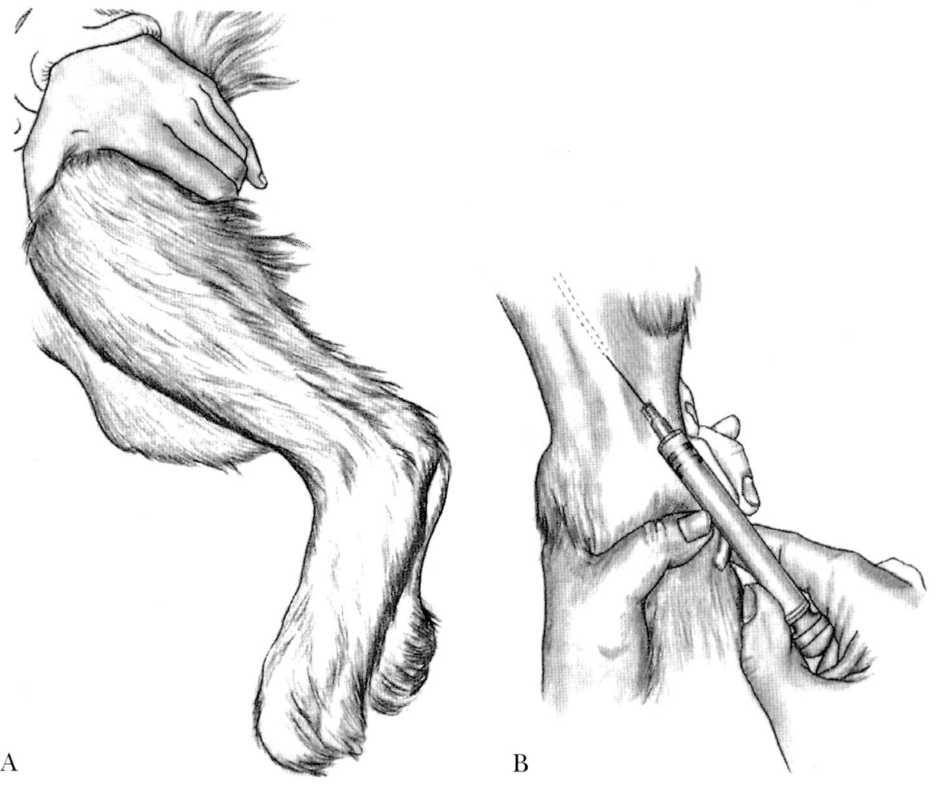

Figure 2-6 Lateral saphenous venipuncture (A and B).

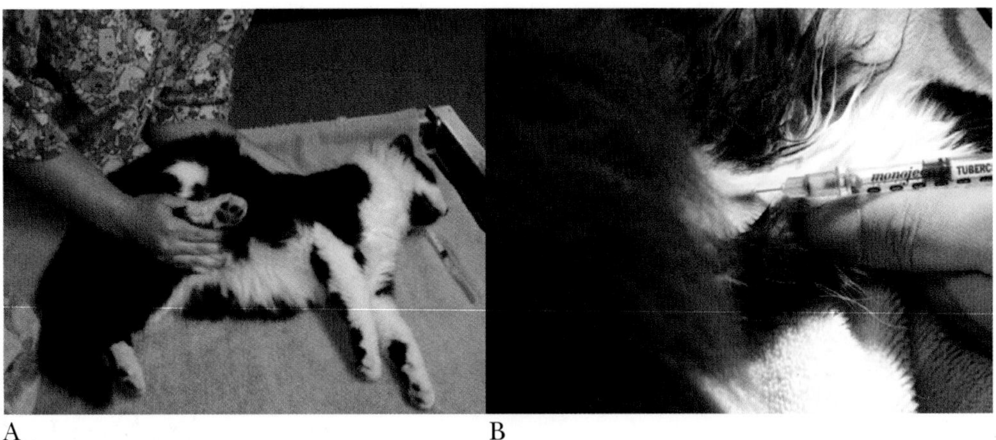

A B

Figure 2-7 (A) Restraint for medial saphenous venipuncture (B) Medial saphenous venipuncture.

Position for Collection from Medial Saphenous Vein (Fig. 2-7)

1. Place animal in lateral recumbency.
2. Extend opposing stifle and compress vein by firmly pressing on animal's upper inner thigh (inguinal area).

Position for Collection from Femoral Vein (Fig. 2-8)

1. Place animal in lateral recumbency.
2. With one hand, abduct uppermost hind leg to permit access to medial aspect of other hind leg.
3. With other hand, compress femoral vein on medial side of upper thigh with thumb.

NOTE: *An additional person may be needed to restrain the head and forelegs of the animal for this procedure.*

Procedure

Technical Action	Rationale/Amplification
1. Prepare bandage for cephalic, lateral saphenous, or medial saphenous vein from dry cotton ball and 1-inch wide adhesive tape. Fold over tab at one end of adhesive strip.	1. Bandaging peripheral veins following venipuncture minimizes hemorrhage and hematoma formation. Folding over the end of the adhesive tape facilitates removal of the bandage later.

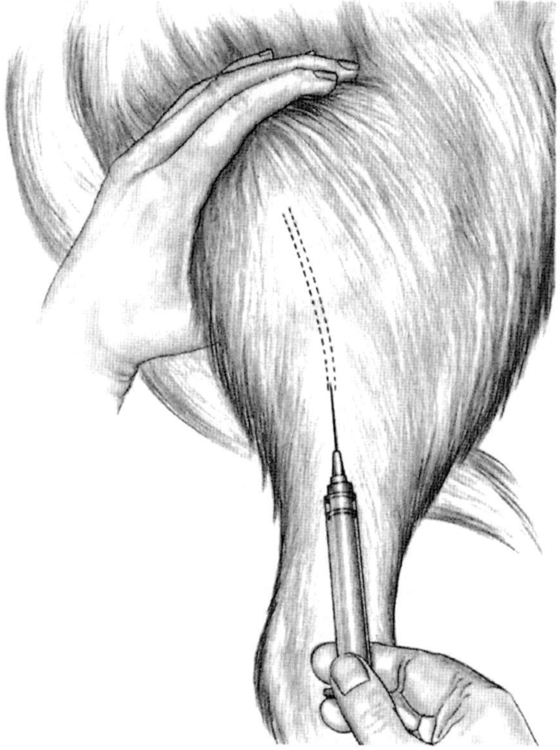

Figure 2-8 Femoral venipuncture.

Technical Action	Rationale/Amplification
2. Swab area of vein with cotton moistened with 70% alcohol or other skin disinfectant.	**2.** Skin disinfectant removes surface debris and moistens hair, making vein easier to see.
3. Distend vein with blood ("raise vein") by compressing vein closer to heart than venipuncture site.	**3.** The restrainer distends the vein for cephalic, saphenous, and femoral venipuncture, while the person performing venipuncture holds the leg at metacarpal/metatarsal region with one hand. The person performing jugular venipuncture distends the jugular vein with one hand by pressing firmly with thumb or fingertips on lower neck near thoracic inlet (Fig. 2-9).
4. Clip hair from area if vein cannot be seen or palpated.	**4.** All veins are difficult to see and palpate in obese animals. In emergency situations, a cut-down procedure may be necessary to expose

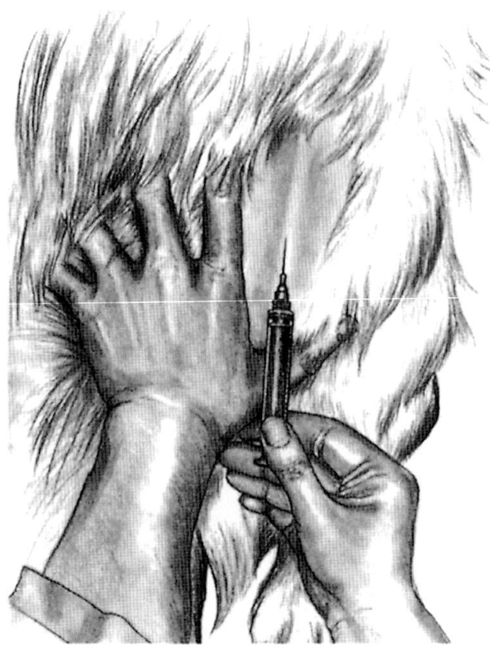

Figure 2-9 Distending jugular vein.

Technical Action	Rationale/Amplification
	the vein. The jugular vein is preferred for blood collection in cats and toy breed dogs because of the small size of leg veins. Hair clipping should be avoided whenever possible if the animal is exhibited regularly.
5. Select appropriate venipuncture equipment for vein and animal.	**5.** Use of appropriate equipment will help to minimize trauma to the vein. A 22-gauge needle is suitable for animals weighing up to 60 lb.; a 20-gauge needle may be used for dogs over 60 lb. in weight. The Vacutainer® system should not be used on small veins because the vacuum in the blood collection tube may cause collapse of a small vein.
6. Inspect venipuncture equipment for flaws.	**6.** Discard any needles with barbed ends. If needle and syringe are to be used, firmly attach the needle to the syringe and move the syringe plunger back and forth several times to determine that it moves freely.

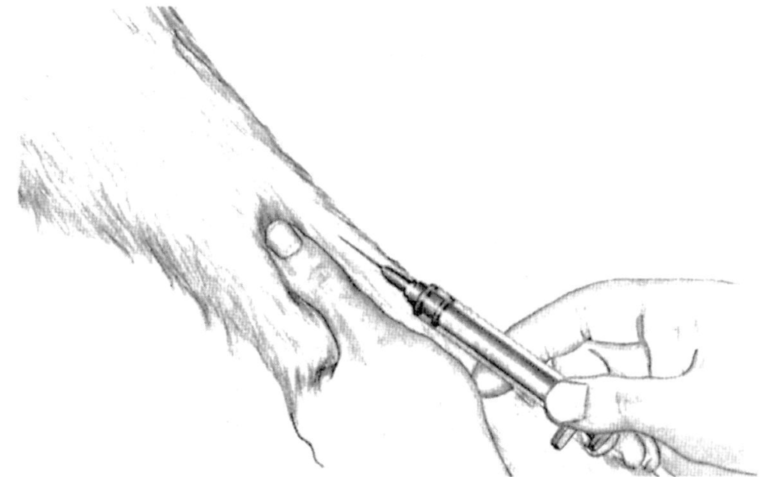

Figure 2-10 Introducing needle into vein.

Technical Action	Rationale/Amplification
7. Hold syringe barrel, butterfly catheter, or Vacutainer® system so that needle bevel is up. Insert needle at approximately 30-degree angle with skin so that distal 1–1.5 cm of needle is threaded into vein (Fig. 2-10).	**7.** Usually the needle can be inserted through the skin and directly into the vein with one motion. Appearance of a few drops of blood in the needle hub or at the distal end of the Vacutainer® needle is evidence of successful venipuncture.
8. If vein rolls to either side, insert needle under skin lateral to vein, then puncture vein.	**8.** Rolling of the blood vessel under the skin is a common problem in certain breeds (e.g. Dachshund), and with certain veins (i.e. the lateral saphenous vein).
9. Aspirate blood by withdrawing syringe plunger. If Vacutainer® system is used, force blood collection tube stopper onto distal end of needle after one or two drops of blood have appeared.	**9.** A needle inserted into the cephalic vein can be stabilized by holding the syringe or Vacutainer® holder in place with the thumb and wrapping the fingers around the animal's leg until collection is completed (Fig. 2-11A). If blood flow stops suddenly during collection, rotate the needle slightly within the vein, thereby positioning the bevel in the main stream of blood flow. For cephalic, lateral saphenous, medial saphenous, or femoral venipuncture, the animal's foot may be gently squeezed

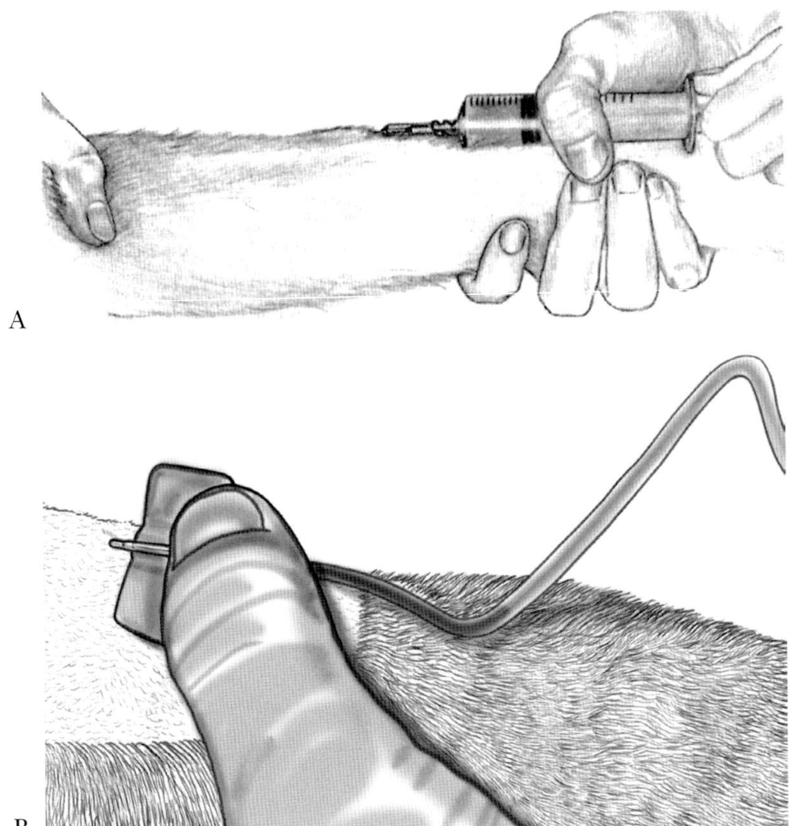

Figure 2-11 (A) Stabilizing syringe during blood collection. (B) Collecting blood using a butterfly catheter.

Technical Action	Rationale/Amplification
	to stimulate venous blood return. Alternatively, a butterfly catheter may be used for blood collection (Fig. 2-11B). Refer to Chapter 4 for insertion technique.
10. Release (or ask restrainer to release) distending pressure on vein.	**10.** The distending pressure on the vein should be released before the needle is removed from the vein to minimize hemorrhage from the venipuncture site.
11. Remove needle from vein and immediately apply pressure to venipuncture site with dry cotton ball.	**11.** Pressure on the venipuncture site immediately after needle removal will decrease the possibility of hemorrhage.

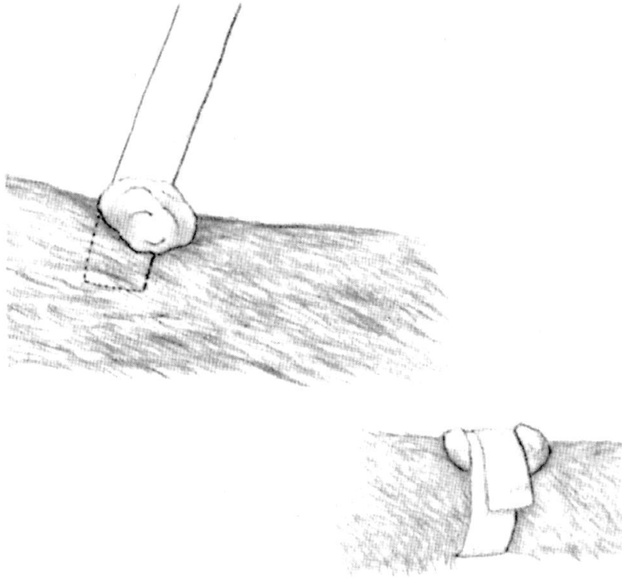

Figure 2-12 Bandaging venipuncture site after removal of needle or catheter.

Technical Action

12. Apply previously prepared bandage with some compression to cephalic, lateral saphenous, or medial saphenous venipuncture site (Fig. 2-12). Hold firm pressure on jugular or femoral venipuncture site for at least 60 seconds.

Rationale/Amplification

12. Bandaging to prevent hemorrhage and subcutaneous hematoma formation is especially important in seriously ill animal patients because repeated venipuncture for diagnostic and therapeutic procedures may be necessary.

13. Place blood promptly into appropriate collection tube(s) by allowing sample to flow into tube. When using anticoagulant coated tubes, invert blood sample gently several times to mix sample with anticoagulant.

13. Hemolysis of the blood sample or clotting of the blood in the syringe or anticoagulant tube can be prevented by careful handling of the sample after collection. Avoid forcefully squirting the blood through the needle into the collection tube. Vigorous shaking of a blood sample in an anticoagulant tube is more likely to result in hemolysis than is gentle inversion of the tube several times.

14. Remove bandage from animal's leg vein in 30–60 minutes.

BLOOD COLLECTION FOR COAGULATION STUDIES

Coagulation studies are performed on venous blood.

Complications, Equipment Needed, Restraint, and Positioning

These are the same as for routine venipuncture, except that a Vacutainer® holder and two tubes or a butterfly catheter and two syringes are required for each blood sample collected.

Procedure

Technical Action	Rationale/Amplification
1. Follow procedure for **Routine Venipuncture** using a Vacutainer® holder or a butterfly catheter (Nos. 1 to 9).	**1.** The Vacutainer® system is best for obtaining blood for coagulation studies from the jugular vein.
2. Aspirate 1 mL of blood into first syringe or insert first tube in Vacutainer® holder. Leaving catheter or holder in vein, detach and retain first syringe or tube. Attach second syringe to needle or insert second tube in holder and collect sufficient blood for laboratory tests.	**2.** The butterfly catheter prevents excessive blood loss and potential contamination of sample. The tube or syringe can be used for other tests, if needed.
3. Follow procedure for aspirating blood, handling sample, and care of vein in **Routine Venipuncture** (Nos. 10 to 14).	**3.** The two-syringe technique minimizes the amount of tissue thromboplastin in the final sample. Tissue thromboplastin released by venipuncture can alter the results of coagulation studies.
4. Obtain control samples by repeating entire procedure on normal animal.	**4.** A control specimen should be collected each time coagulation studies are to be performed.
5. If any problems occur during collection, discard sample and obtain a new sample from a different site or at a later time.	**5.** Blood collection problems that could affect the accuracy of coagulation studies include failure to collect a sufficient amount of blood and traumatic puncture of the skin.

COLLECTION OF BLOOD FOR TRANSFUSION

Transfusion collection is the obtaining of blood from a donor for use in treating a recipient.

Complications

1. Hemorrhage
2. Subcutaneous hematoma formation
3. Fibrosis of jugular vein

Equipment Needed

- Cotton
- Clipper with No. 40 blade
- Skin preparation material:
  - 2% chlorhexidine scrub
  - 70% alcohol
  - Sterile gauze sponges (2 inch × 2 inch)
- Drugs for sedation or anesthesia if necessary
- Bandaging material
  - Sterile gauze sponges
  - Antimicrobial ointment
  - Gauze bandage
  - Adhesive tape (2 inches wide)
- Collection apparatus for canine blood
  - Commercial plastic blood collection bag containing anticoagulant (e.g. citrate phosphate dextrose adenine; CPDA) with accompanying needle and tubing
- Collection apparatus for feline blood
  - 60-mL syringe containing 7 mL of CPDA (for collecting 53 mL of feline blood)
  - 18-gauge needle or 21-gauge winged infusion set

Restraint and Positioning

Sedation or administration of anesthetic may be needed because the animal must remain relatively immobile throughout the 5–15-minute collection procedure to minimize trauma to the jugular vein.

A dog should be restrained in sternal or lateral recumbency on a table for collection from the jugular vein (Fig. 2-1). Large dogs can be restrained in a sitting position on the floor (Fig. 2-3).

A cat should be restrained in lateral recumbency with its head held slightly lower than its body over the edge of the table and with the cat's nose turned toward the ceiling. In this position, the cat's jugular vein is easily visualized and stabilized for venipuncture.

Procedure

Technical Action	Rationale/Amplification
1. Clip hair from ventral neck area.	1. Good visualization of the jugular vein helps prevent traumatic venipuncture.

Technical Action	Rationale/Amplification
2. Prepare skin of ventral neck area, using 2% chlorhexidine and alcohol.	**2.** Strict attention to asepsis is important to decrease the possibility of thrombophlebitis and subsequent fibrosis of the donor animal's jugular vein.
3. Distend jugular vein with blood as for routine venipuncture (Fig. 2-9).	
4. Insert needle (with bevel up) into jugular vein.	**4.** The needle hub may be taped loosely to the animal's neck during collection, using 1-inch wide adhesive tape.
5. Collect sample, gently agitating collection container several times during collection.	**5.** Gentle agitation of the blood collection container ensures mixing of the blood with the anticoagulant.
6. Release distending pressure on vein if it has been necessary to maintain distending pressure throughout collection.	**6.** The distending pressure on the vein should be released before the needle is removed from the vein to minimize hemorrhage from the venipuncture site.
7. Remove needle from vein and immediately hold pressure with dry cotton ball on venipuncture site for at least 1 minute.	
8. Apply sterile bandage to neck area directly over venipuncture site.	**8.** Firm pressure for at least 1 minute, followed by bandaging of the neck area for at least 24 hours after transfusion collection, will help to prevent hemorrhage, subcutaneous hematoma formation, and thrombophlebitis.

Bibliography

Bistner SI, Ford RB: Kirk and Bistner's Handbook of Veterinary Procedures & Emergency Treatment, 8th edition. Philadelphia, WB Saunders, 2006

Brunner LS, Suddarth DS: The Lippincott Manual of Nursing Practice, 3rd edition. Philadelphia, JB Lippincott, 1982

Burkitt J, Davis H: Advanced Monitoring and Procedures for Small Animal Emergency and Critical Care. Oxford, England, Wiley-Blackwell, 2012

Dial SM: Hematology, chemistry profile, and urinalysis for pediatric patients. Comp Contin Educ for Prac Vet 14(2): 305–308, 1992

Intravartolo C: Blood transfusions in dogs and cats. Comp Contin Educ for AHT 2(6): 302–308, 1981

Pichler ME, Turnwald GH: Blood transfusion in the dog and cat, Part I. Physiology, collection, storage, and indications for whole blood therapy. Comp Contin Educ for Prac Vet 7(1): 64–71, 1985

Schall WD, Perman V: Diseases of the red blood cells. In Ettinger SJ (ed.): Textbook of Veterinary Internal Medicine, Vol. 2. Philadelphia, WB Saunders, 1975

Chapter 3

Injection Techniques

Well done is better than well said.
BENJAMIN FRANKLIN

There are five major routes by which injections can be given: intravenous (within a vein), intramuscular (within a muscle), subcutaneous (under the skin), intraperitoneal (within the peritoneal cavity), and intradermal (within the skin).

Purposes

To administer fluids, pharmacologic agents, biologic preparations, and certain test substances.

NOTE: *The injection route that has been determined by the manufacturer to be the most effective and the safest usually is indicated on the product label. Certain materials must be administered intravenously because they will cause tissue necrosis if given outside the vascular system. Most suspensions (cloudy-appearing liquids) should not be given by the intravenous or intraperitoneal routes. An exception to this would be the anesthetic Propofol, which should be given IV. When no information is given regarding appropriate routes of administration, refer to guidelines in Table 3-1.*

Complications

1. Irritation, necrosis, or infection at injection site
2. Allergic reaction to material injected
3. Nerve damage (mainly a complication of intramuscular injections)
4. Damage to abdominal viscera and peritonitis (a complication of intraperitoneal injections)

Crow and Walshaw's Manual of Clinical Procedures in Dogs, Cats, Rabbits, and Rodents, Fourth Edition. Edited by Jennifer E. Boyle. Published 2016 by John Wiley & Sons, Inc.
Companion Website: www.wiley.com/go/boyle/manual4e

TABLE 3-1 Recommended routes of injection.

Prescribed Agent	Possible Route(s)
Biologic preparations, (e.g. vaccines)	Subcutaneous, intramuscular
Pharmacologic agents, (e.g. antibiotics, tranquilizers)	Intravenous, intramuscular, subcutaneous, intraperitoneal
Local anesthetic agents	Intradermal, subcutaneous
Fluids	Intravenous, subcutaneous, intraperitoneal
Certain test substances	Intravenous, intramuscular, intradermal
Dialysis solutions	Intraperitoneal

Equipment Needed

- Cotton
- 70% alcohol or other skin disinfectant
- Sterile syringe of appropriate size
- Sterile needle of appropriate size
- Adhesive tape, 1 inch wide (for cephalic or saphenous vein injections)
- Clipper with No. 40 blade (for intradermal and some intravenous injections)

Restraint and Positioning

The degree of restraint required depends on the temperament of the animal and the route of injection. It is helpful to have an assistant restrain the animal, although this may not be necessary for subcutaneous injections in tractable animals. The animal should be positioned so that the intended injection site is accessible (See Chapter 1).

PREPARATION FOR INJECTIONS

Procedure

Technical Action	Rationale/Amplification
1. Check medication with regard to "The Five Rights": right patient, right drug, right dose, right route, right time and frequency. Also check expiration date and examine medication for presence of foreign material.	1. It is important to take measures to prevent errors in medication administration.
2. Wash hands.	2. Washing hands between patients is important in controlling communicable diseases in a hospital.
3. Select appropriate needle size.	3. Use of appropriate needle size will help to minimize trauma to the tissues. For intravenous, intramuscular, subcutaneous, and intraperitoneal injections, use 22-gauge needle for animals weighing

Technical Action	Rationale/Amplification
	up to 60 lb. and 20-gauge or 22-gauge needle for dogs over 60 lb. For intradermal injections, use 25-gauge or 27-gauge needle.
4. Aseptically attach sterile needle to sterile syringe.	**4.** Syringe size will be dictated by volume of material to be injected, for example, a tuberculin syringe is routinely used for intradermal injections.
5. Use cotton moistened with 70% alcohol to swab rubber stopper of bottle containing material to be injected.	**5.** Cleaning the rubber stopper removes any dust or other contaminants.
6. Remove needle cover and aspirate into syringe a volume of air equal to that of material to be injected. Inject this air into bottle.	**6.** Pressurizing multiple-dose vials with air facilitates withdrawal of material to be injected.
7. Insert needle through center of bottle stopper.	**7.** Careful insertion of needle into bottle stopper minimizes needle damage.
8. Invert bottle and position needle bevel within liquid in bottle. Hold apparatus with needle end pointed toward ceiling.	**8.** Proper needle position will minimize air bubble aspiration into syringe.
9. Withdraw syringe plunger to aspirate desired amount of medication and, if possible, an additional 0.5 to 1 mL.	
10. While holding bottle and needle/syringe in vertical position, tap on syringe to force any air bubbles in syringe to rise toward needle hub.	**10.** Removing air bubbles from the syringe eliminates the risk of air embolism when the material is injected. Large air bubbles displace liquid material and could cause inaccurate dosing.
11. Push syringe plunger back to desired amount of medication, thereby forcing any air bubbles back into bottle.	**11.** It is safer to remove air bubbles this way than to contaminate the room and its occupants with potentially hazardous materials from the bottle (e.g. chemotherapeutic agents).
12. Remove needle from bottle. Slide needle loosely into needle cover using one hand only to prevent needle stick injury.	**12.** Needle contamination must be avoided to minimize causing iatrogenic infection. Cytotoxic substances for treating cancer and potent anesthetic agents are examples of hazardous materials that could be accidentally injected when recapping a needle.

NOTE: *Steps 5 through 11 are unnecessary if using ampoules. An ampoule is opened by fracturing the glass, and then the contents are drawn directly into the needle and attached syringe.*

INTRAVENOUS INJECTION

Procedure

Technical Action	Rationale/Amplification
1. Prepare for injection.	**1.** See **Preparation for Injections.**
2. Place animal in appropriate position for intravenous injection into jugular, cephalic, lateral saphenous, or femoral vein.	**2.** See Chapter 2.
3. Follow procedure described for blood collection (Chapter 2, Procedure: Nos. 1 to 4).	**3.** Prepare bandage, disinfect venipuncture site, distend vein with blood, and clip hair (if necessary).
4. Hold syringe barrel so that needle bevel is up. Insert needle at approximately 30-degree angle with skin.	**4.** If vessel rolls, insert needle under skin lateral to the vein, then puncture the vein. Appearance of a few drops of blood in the needle hub is evidence of successful venipuncture.
5. Advance needle until at least half of needle is within vein.	**5.** When syringe plunger is withdrawn, blood should flow quickly into syringe.
6. Release (or ask assistant to release) distending pressure on vein.	**6.** The distending pressure must be released to allow the injected material to flow easily into the circulation.
7. Aspirate small amount of blood into needle hub.	**7.** A rapid flow of blood into the syringe is assurance of proper needle placement.
8. Inject material at moderate rate into vein. Stabilize needle inserted into cephalic vein by holding syringe barrel with thumb while wrapping fingers around animal's leg (see Chapter 2 Fig. 2-11).	**8.** When a volume greater than 5 mL or when any irritating substance is injected intravenously, it is advisable to check needle placement within the vein by aspirating blood into the syringe several times during the injection.
9. Remove needle from vein and immediately apply pressure with dry cotton ball to venipuncture site.	**9.** Pressure on the venipuncture site immediately following needle removal will decrease the possibility of hemorrhage and perivascular leakage of the injected material.
10. Apply previously prepared bandage with some compression to cephalic, saphenous, or femoral venipuncture site. Hold firm pressure on jugular venipuncture site for at least 60 seconds.	**10.** Bandaging to prevent hemorrhage or subcutaneous hematoma formation is especially important in seriously ill animal patients because repeated venipuncture for diagnostic and therapeutic procedures may be necessary.

Technical Action

11. Note on animal's medical record that medication was given.

Rationale/Amplification

11. Note date, time, medication, serial/lot number, dosage, route, initials of persons administering medication, and comments.

12. Remove bandage from animal's leg in 30–60 minutes.

INTRAMUSCULAR INJECTION

Procedure

Technical Action

1. Prepare for injection.

2. Place animal in lateral recumbency or in sitting or standing position.

Rationale/Amplification

1. See **Preparation for Injections**

2. Intramuscular injections are given in the quadriceps muscle group or anterior thigh, lumbodorsal muscles on either side of lumbar vertebrae, or triceps muscles, posterior to humerus in front leg (Fig. 3-1). All three of the recommended muscle groups can be used when the animal is sitting, standing, or recumbent. The hamstring muscle group (semitendinosus, semimembranosus) should be avoided if at all possible because of the risk of sciatic nerve injury.

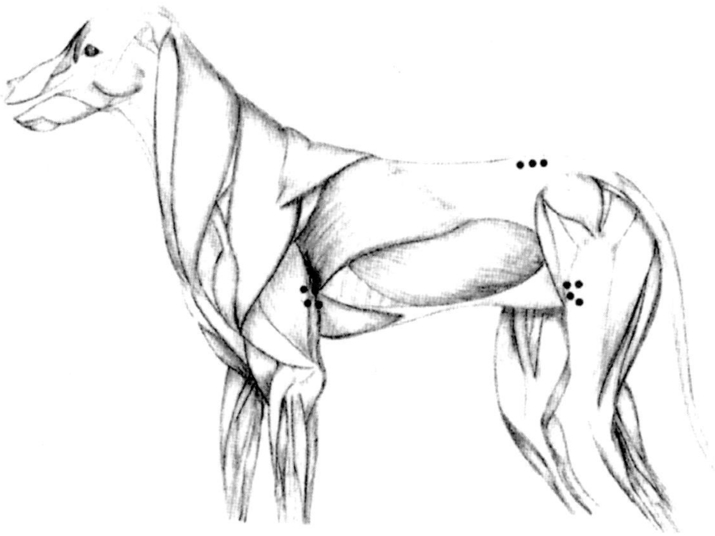

Figure 3-1 Muscle groups suitable for intramuscular injection.

Technical Action	Rationale/Amplification
3. Restrain animal as needed.	**3.** Intramuscular injections can be painful.
4. Swab skin over intended injection site with cotton moistened with 70% alcohol or other skin disinfectant.	**4.** A disinfectant removes surface debris from the skin and hair.
5. Insert needle through skin into muscle at approximately 45-degree to 90-degree angle (Fig. 3-2).	**5.** Quick insertion of the needle through muscle tissue is less painful than slow advancement of the needle.
6. Before injecting, pull back on syringe plunger. If blood enters syringe, select a different injection site in another muscle or a different part of same muscle.	**6.** The presence of blood in the syringe indicates that a blood vessel has been entered. Some agents, approved for intramuscular use only, may cause severe allergic reactions and even death if given intravascularly.
7. If no blood is aspirated into syringe, inject material at moderate rate into muscle.	**7.** The maximum volume that should be injected intramuscularly at any one site is 2 mL in the cat and 3–5 mL in the dog. Muscle tissue is dense and cannot accommodate large volumes of injectable material.

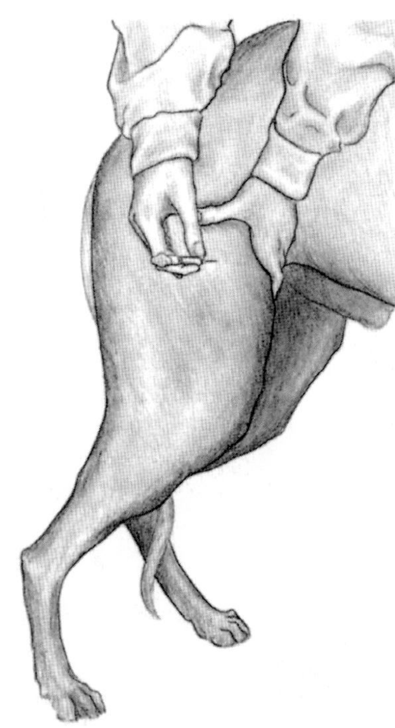

Figure 3-2 Placement of needle for intramuscular injection into quadriceps.

Technical Action	Rationale/Amplification
8. Remove needle from muscle and gently massage muscle.	**8.** Massaging the muscle after injection aids in dispersal of the injected material and decreases pain.
9. Note in animal's medical record that medication was given.	**9.** Note date, time, medication, serial/lot number, dosage, route, initials, and comments. It is important to note the injection site so that the available sites can be rotated during subsequent intramuscular injections.

SUBCUTANEOUS INJECTION

Procedure

Technical Action	Rationale/Amplification
1. Prepare for injection.	**1.** See **Preparation for Injections.**
2. Place animal in sternal recumbency, or in standing or sitting position.	**2.** Most cats and dogs tolerate subcutaneous injections quite well so that minimal restraint is required.
3. Pick up fold of skin over animal's neck or back by pinching skin between thumb and fingers.	**3.** Cats and dogs have freely movable skin along the dorsal portion of the neck and back.
4. Swab skin over intended injection site with cotton moistened with 70% alcohol or other skin disinfectant.	**4.** A disinfectant removes surface debris from the skin and hair.
5. Insert needle to its hub through skin fold into subcutaneous tissue space (Fig. 3-3).	**5.** The needle should slide easily under the skin. If resistance is met, the needle may be positioned intradermally or intramuscularly and should be redirected.
6. Before injecting, pull back on syringe plunger and observe if any blood enters syringe. If blood enters syringe, select a different injection site.	**6.** The presence of blood in the syringe indicates that a blood vessel has been entered. Some agents, approved for subcutaneous use only, may cause severe allergic reactions and even death if given intravascularly.
7. If no blood can be aspirated into syringe, inject material at moderate rate under skin (Fig. 3-4).	**7.** The dorsal subcutaneous tissue of dogs and cats can accommodate relatively large volumes of fluid, from 30 mL to 50 mL at one site.
8. Remove needle from skin and massage injection area.	**8.** Massaging the injection site aids in dispersal of the injected material.
9. Note in animal's medical record that medication was given.	**9.** Note date, time, medication, serial/lot number, dosage, route, initials, and comments.

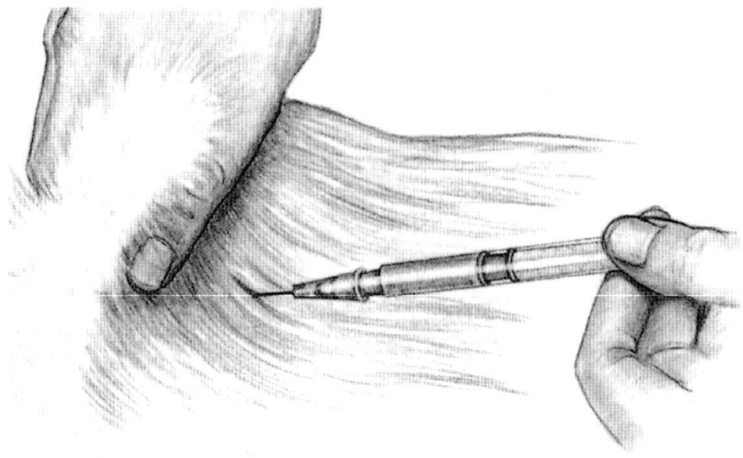

Figure 3-3 Placement of needle for subcutaneous injection.

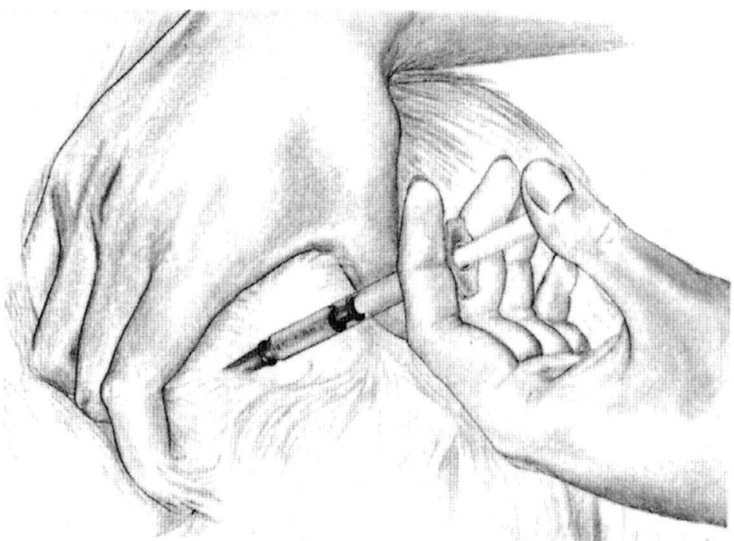

Figure 3-4 Subcutaneous injection.

INTRAPERITONEAL INJECTION

Procedure

Technical Action	Rationale/Amplification
1. Prepare for injection.	1. See **Preparation for Injections.**
2. Select an appropriate gauge and length needle.	2. The needle used for intraperitoneal injections should be 3–5 cm in length. An over-the-needle intravenous

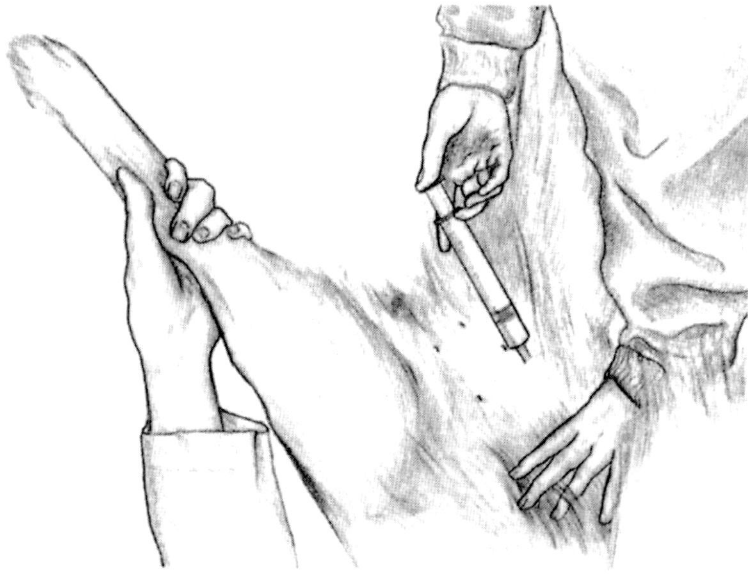

Figure 3-5 Intraperitoneal injection.

Technical Action | **Rationale/Amplification**

catheter may be used instead of a needle for this procedure.

3. Palpate abdomen to determine whether urinary bladder is empty.
   - If the animal's bladder is empty, the possibility of inadvertently puncturing this organ is markedly reduced. If the bladder is distended, allow the animal to urinate or empty bladder by catheterization.
4. Place animal in dorsal or lateral recumbency.
   - Depending on the animal's size and temperament, one or two assistants will be needed to restrain the animal.
5. Swab skin over intended injection site with cotton moistened with 70% alcohol or other skin disinfectant.
   - A disinfectant removes surface debris from the skin and hair.
6. Elevate animal's hindquarters approximately 10–15 cm higher than front quarters.
   - Elevation of the hindquarters allows most of the viscera to move anterior to the intended injection site.
7. Insert needle at a point midway between umbilicus and pubis just lateral to linea alba (Fig. 3-5).
   - Direct needle toward pubis into abdomen.
8. Before injecting, pull back on syringe plunger and observe for blood, urine, or intestinal contents entering syringe.
   - The presence of blood, urine, or intestinal contents in the syringe indicates that the needle is positioned incorrectly within the peritoneal cavity or that there is abdominal disease or injury.

Technical Action	Rationale/Amplification
9. If blood, urine, or intestinal contents are not aspirated into syringe, inject material at moderate rate into peritoneal cavity.	**9.** The peritoneal cavity of dogs and cats can accommodate relatively large volumes of fluid (e.g. up to 5 liters in a large dog). Intraperitoneal fluid administration can be a lifesaving procedure in tiny hypovolemic animals, such as seriously ill neonates.
10. Remove needle from abdomen.	
11. Note in animal's medical record that medication was given.	**11.** Note date, time, medication, serial/lot number, dosage, route, initials and comments.

INTRADERMAL INJECTION

Procedure

Technical Action	Rationale/Amplification
1. Prepare for injection.	**1.** See **Preparation for Injections**
2. Clip hair from intended injection site.	**2.** For a single injection, clip about a 10-cm square area on lateral abdomen or thorax. For intradermal skin testing, clip a large area on the thorax or abdomen. Clipping should be done in an area that is free of skin lesions. Gentle use of the clippers is essential to avoid trauma to the skin.
3. Avoid use of soaps or disinfectants on skin where intradermal skin test injections will be made.	**3.** Such agents may cause local allergic reactions that will mask test results.
4. For intradermal skin testing, place animal in lateral recumbency.	
5. Mark skin beneath each intended injection site with felt-tip pen.	**5.** Marking ensures even spacing of injections and facilitates recording of test results.
6. Hold syringe barrel with needle bevel up at approximately 10-degree angle with skin.	
7. Stretch skin between thumb and forefinger of one hand and insert needle within epidermis until bevel is completely enclosed within skin layers (Fig. 3-6).	**7.** It is not necessary to insert the needle to its hub when giving an intradermal injection.

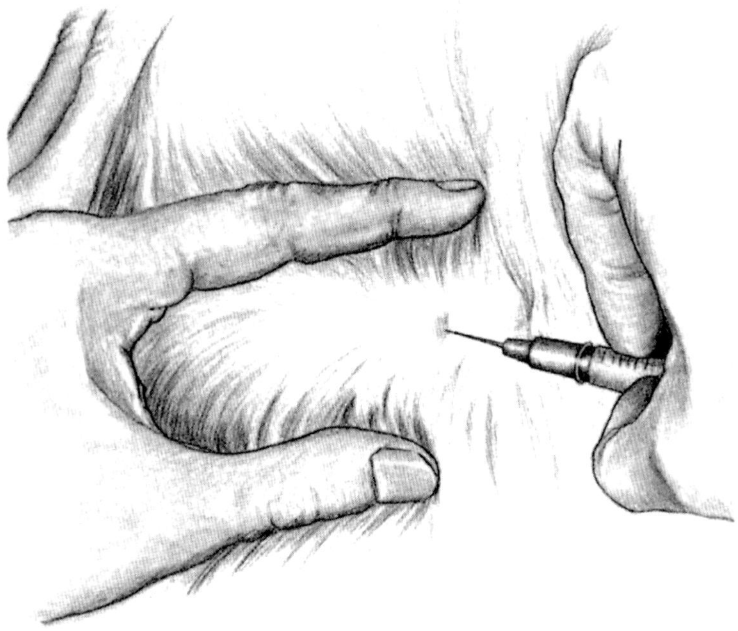

Figure 3-6 Inserting needle intradermally.

Technical Action	Rationale/Amplification
8. Check for correct placement of needle intradermally by lifting up on tip of needle.	**8.** The metal of the needle should be just visible through the epidermis if the needle is positioned properly.
9. Inject 0.05–0.1 mL intradermally (Fig. 3-7); then remove needle from skin.	**9.** A small intradermal bleb of fluid should be present at the injection site.
10. For intradermal infiltration of local anesthetic agent, place animal in position that affords access to area to be injected.	**10.** Local anesthesia may be used for excision of small benign skin lesions and suturing of small wounds.
11. Clip hair from area to be infiltrated with local anesthetic and prepare skin, using 2% chlorhexidine scrub and 70% alcohol (Chapter 16, Skin Preparation).	
12. Inject local anesthetic intradermally, repeating Nos. 6–8.	**12.** The volume of local anesthetic used will depend on the size and location of the lesion.

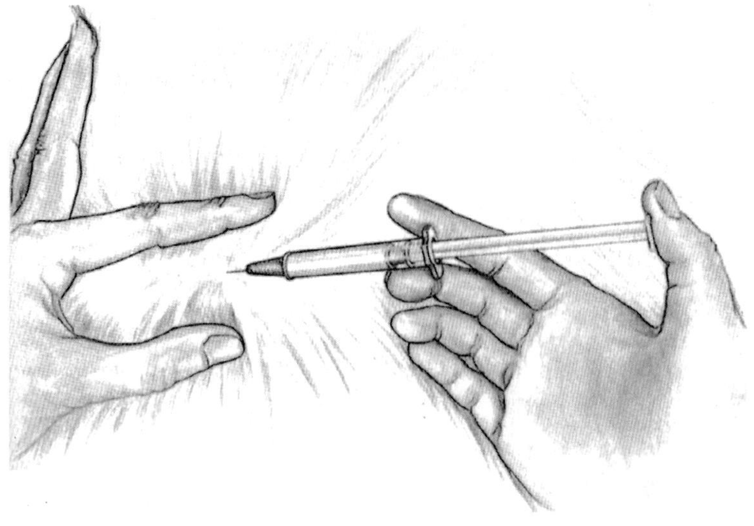

Figure 3-7 Intradermal injection.

Bibliography

Bistner SI, Ford RB: Kirk and Bistner's Handbook of Veterinary Procedures & Emergency Treatment, 6th edition. Philadelphia, WB Saunders, 1995

Boothe DM, Tannert K: Surgical considerations for drug and fluid therapy in the pediatric patient. Comp Contin Educ for Prac Vet 14(3): 313–329, 1992

Brunner LS, Suddarth DS: The Lippincott Manual of Nursing Practice, 3rd edition. Philadelphia, JB Lippincott, 1982

CDC: Guideline for Prevention of Surgical Site Infection. www.cdc.gov/ncidod/dhqp/gl_surgicalsite.html, 1999

Kirk RW, Bistner SI: Handbook of Veterinary Procedures and Emergency Treatment, 4th edition. Philadelphia, WB Saunders, 1985

O'Grady NP et al.: Guidelines for the prevention of intravascular catheter-related infections. MMWR 51(RR10):1–26. www.cdc.gov/mmwr/preview/mmwrhtml/rr5110a1.htm, 2002

Pratt PW (ed): Medical Nursing for Animal Health Technicians. Santa Barbara, American Veterinary Publications, 1985

Chapter 4

Placement and Care of Intravenous Catheters

The recollection of quality remains long after the price has been forgotten.
BENJAMIN FRANKLIN

Intravenous catheterization is the placement of a hollow device, a catheter, into a vein.

Purposes

1. To administer fluids, medications, anesthetic agents, blood components, and certain test substances
2. For blood sampling
3. To measure central venous pressure
4. To provide ready access to the circulatory system for anticipated metabolic emergencies (e.g. seizures, hypoglycemia, and shock)

Complications

1. Occlusion, malpositioning, and breakage of the catheter
2. Thrombophlebitis
3. Extravasation and resultant infiltration of subcutaneous tissues
4. Infection
5. Hemorrhage and subcutaneous hematoma formation
6. Pyrogenic reaction
7. Circulatory overload
8. Air embolism
9. Allergic reaction

Crow and Walshaw's Manual of Clinical Procedures in Dogs, Cats, Rabbits, and Rodents, Fourth Edition. Edited by Jennifer E. Boyle. Published 2016 by John Wiley & Sons, Inc.
Companion Website: www.wiley.com/go/boyle/manual4e

Equipment Needed

Clipper with No. 40 blade
- Skin preparation materials
  - 2% chlorhexidine scrub
  - 70% alcohol
  - Sterile gauze sponges (2 inch × 2 inch)
- Bandaging material
  - Sterile gauze sponges (and/or sterile bandaid)
  - Gauze bandage
  - Adhesive tape (½ inch, 1 inch, and 2 inch)
- Syringe containing 1 mL of heparinized saline (500 IU sodium heparin in 250 mL of normal saline)

Note: *There have been studies done in human medicine in recent years that argue that there is no significant difference between 0.9% sodium chloride and heparin flushing solutions in the ability to prevent catheter occlusion, as well as concerns in pediatric medicine of overuse of heparin solutions. Given these findings, 0.9% sodium chloride may be the preferred flushing solution for short-term use central venous catheter maintenance.*

- Injection cap
- T-port (if necessary)
- Fluid administration set (if necessary)
- Extension tubing (if necessary)
- Intravenous catheter(s)
  - Winged infusion set ("butterfly")
  - Over-the-needle catheter ("needle inside")
  - Through-the-needle catheter ("needle outside")
  - Through-the-needle catheter with break-away needle ("needle outside")
  - Multiple lumen intravenous catheter

Restraint and Positioning

There are five veins in both dogs and cats that are accessible for intravenous catheterization: jugular, cephalic, lateral saphenous (recurrent tarsal), medial saphenous, and femoral. The jugular is the vein of choice for administration of hypertonic solutions, long-term fluid administration, and central venous pressure measurement.

Adequate restraint is important throughout the procedure to ensure aseptic placement of the catheter and proper bandaging of the catheterization site. The position used depends on the vein selected for catheterization (see Chapter 2).

PREPARATION FOR INTRAVENOUS CATHETERIZATION

Procedure

Technical Action	Rationale/Amplification
1. Wash hands.	1. Every precaution must be taken to reduce the chance of causing iatrogenic infection.

TABLE 4-1 Recommended intravenous catheter sizes for routine use in dogs and cats.

Animal	Vein	Catheter Type	Size
Cat	Cephalic	Over-the-needle	20 gauge, 1 ½ inches
	Femoral	Over-the-needle	20 gauge, 1 ½ inches
	Jugular	Through-the-needle	19 gauge, 8 inches
Dog	Cephalic	Through-the-needle	19 gauge, 8 or 12 inches
		Over-the-needle	18 or 20 gauge, 1½ inches
	Lateral saphenous	Through-the-needle	19 gauge, 8 or 12 inches
		Over-the-needle	18 or 20 gauge, 1½ inches
	Jugular (≤30 kg)	Through-the-needle	19 gauge, 8 or 12 inches
	Jugular (>30 kg)	Through-the-needle	16 gauge, 12 inches

Technical Action	Rationale/Amplification
2. Clip hair over a wide area around insertion site.	**2.** Good visualization of the vein aids in atraumatic venipuncture. Clipping of hair is a necessary part of skin preparation. Be sure to clip adequately below where the catheter will be placed to avoid dragging the sterile catheter through hair.
3. Prepare clipped area as for surgery.	**3.** Use 2% chlorhexidine scrub and 70% alcohol (see Chapter 16).
4. Select intravenous catheter of appropriate diameter and length (Table 4-1).	**4.** Factors influencing catheter selection include size and location of vein and the reason for catheterization. To minimize thrombophlebitis, use the smallest diameter catheter that will allow the infusion rate required for the animal's needs.
5. Inspect catheter for flaws.	**5.** Discard any catheter with a barbed needle, frayed tip, or immobile parts.

INSERTION OF WINGED INFUSION SET ("BUTTERFLY")

Procedure

Technical Action	Rationale/Amplification
1. Prepare for catheterization.	**1.** See **Preparation For Intravenous Catheterization**. The relatively short needle on the winged infusion set limits its use, for the most part, to cephalic, saphenous, and femoral veins.

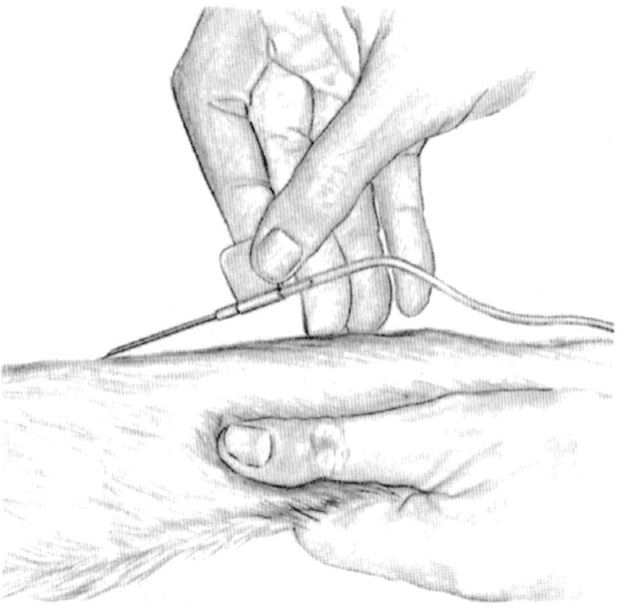

Figure 4-1 Inserting winged intravenous infusion set.

Technical Action	Rationale/Amplification
2. Distend (or ask assistant to distend) vein with blood.	**2.** See Chapter 2, Procedure: No. 3.
3. Hold winged infusion set so that bevel of needle is up, while squeezing wings of set together between thumb and index finger (Fig. 4-1).	**3.** In general, insertion of a needle into a vein with its bevel up helps to minimize trauma to the wall of the vein.
4. Insert needle (with bevel up) at approximately 30-degree angle with skin.	**4.** A flash of blood should appear in the plastic tubing near the proximal end of the needle.
5. Advance needle into vein.	**5.** Inadvertent puncturing of the opposite wall of the vein usually can be avoided by lifting the wings slightly while threading the needle into the vein.
6. Release (or ask assistant to release) distending pressure on vein.	
7. Attach injection cap, syringe, or fluid infusion set, and begin administration of prescribed fluid or agent.	**7.** Starting the infusion helps to anchor the needle in the vein and prevent backflow of blood. In general, winged infusion sets are suitable in animals only for short-term administration of pharmacologic agents or for fluid administration during anesthesia. An injection cap is not required under these circumstances.

Technical Action

8. Hold infusion set in place by applying adhesive tape parallel to needle on each wing, then across entire apparatus and encircling leg.

Rationale/Amplification

8. The tape serves to hold the needle in place.

Technical Action

9. Make loop in tubing and tape this loop to animal.

Rationale/Amplification

9. If the animal moves, the butterfly needle can easily become dislodged or puncture the opposite wall of the vein. A loop in the tubing prevents traction on the needle when the leg and infusion set are moved.

Technical Action

10. Repeatedly check position of butterfly needle within vein by aspiration of blood into a syringe or by lowering fluid bottle below animal's body level.

Rationale/Amplification

10. Frequent checking of correct needle placement is advisable when irritating substances are being administered through a winged infusion set. This catheter is not meant as a long-term catheter. Never leave the patient unattended when using a butterfly catheter for fluid or medication administration.

Technical Action

11. Remove needle from vein and immediately apply pressure to venipuncture site with dry cotton ball.

Rationale/Amplification

11. Pressure on the venipuncture site and bandaging of the site following needle removal will decrease the possibility of hemorrhage and subcutaneous hematoma formation.

Technical Action

12. Apply previously prepared bandage with gentle compression to cephalic, saphenous, or femoral venipuncture site (Chapter 2, Fig. 2-9). Maintain firm pressure on jugular venipuncture site for at least 60 seconds.

Rationale/Amplification

12. Bandaging to prevent hemorrhage and subcutaneous hematoma formation is especially important in seriously ill animal patients because repeated venipuncture for diagnostic and therapeutic procedures may be necessary.

Technical Action

13. Remove bandage from animal's leg vein in 30–60 minutes.

INSERTION OF OVER-THE-NEEDLE CATHETER ("NEEDLE INSIDE")

Procedure

Technical Action

1. Prepare for catheterization.

Rationale/Amplification

1. See **Preparation For Intravenous Catheterization**. Over-the-needle catheters are not recommended for use in the jugular vein. The short

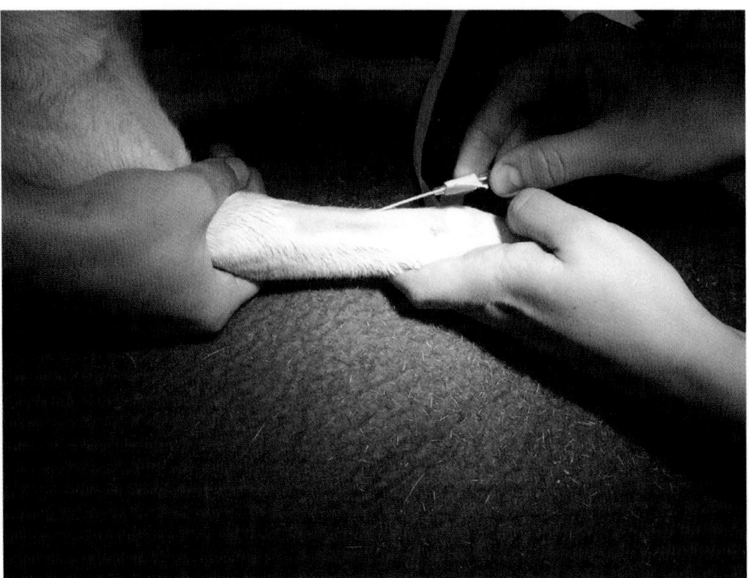

Figure 4-2 Inserting over-the-needle intravenous catheter.

Technical Action	Rationale/Amplification
	length of these catheters impedes securing them in the neck. Also it is difficult to puncture the thicker skin in the neck area with an over-the-needle catheter.
2. Place sufficient length of ½-inch adhesive tape around catheter hub to encircle animal's leg.	**2.** This tape will serve to anchor the catheter firmly to the leg once it has been placed in the vein.
3. Distend (or ask assistant to distend) vein with blood.	**3.** See Chapter 2, Procedure: No. 3.
4. Insert needle and catheter into vein with needle bevel up (Fig. 4-2).	**4.** Rapid flow of blood into the hub of the needle indicates successful venipuncture.
5. Advance needle into vein until at least 1.5 cm is within vein.	**5.** The catheter is slightly shorter than the needle in an over-the-needle catheter. Entry of the catheter into the vein is ensured by placing a sufficient portion of the needle within the lumen of the vein.
6. Hold needle in place and slowly advance only catheter farther into vein until catheter hub is at point of skin puncture (Fig. 4-3). If catheter will not thread easily, remove entire	**6.** Once the advancing of the catheter has begun, the metal needle must not be reinserted through the catheter because the needle could cut the catheter.

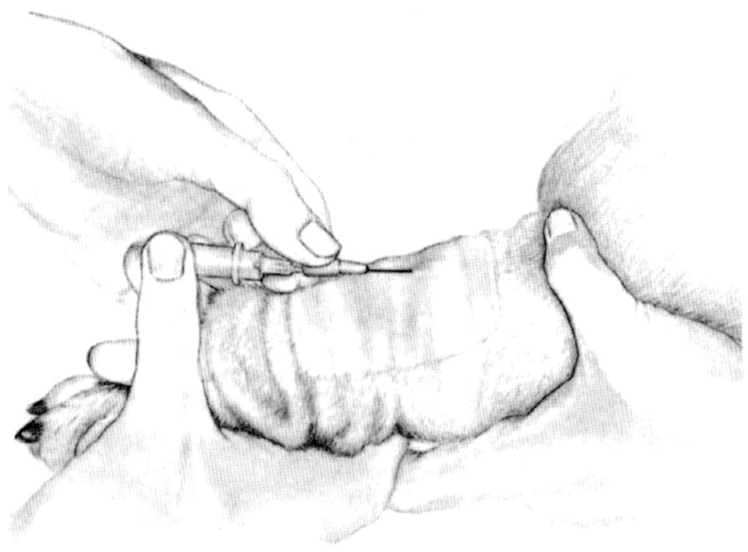

Figure 4-3 Advancing over-the-needle intravenous catheter.

Technical Action	Rationale/Amplification
apparatus, place a temporary bandage over venipuncture site, and attempt catheterization in another vein or at a more proximal part of same vein.	
7. Hold catheter hub and withdraw needle from catheter.	**7.** The catheter can be removed inadvertently if it is not held in place while the needle is withdrawn.
8. Place injection cap or T-port on catheter (Fig. 4-4).	**8.** An injection cap provides a sterile seal to the intravenous catheter. A T-port should be placed on the catheter for continuous fluid administration (Fig. 4-5).
9. Wrap adhesive tape strip attached to catheter hub around animal's leg.	**9.** This tape anchors the catheter to the leg. Firm anchoring of the catheter prevents trauma to the vein caused by excessive movement of the catheter.
10. Flush catheter with heparinized saline.	**10.** Heparinized saline will keep the catheter patent while the bandage is placed on the leg.
11. Cleanse venipuncture site of any blood with cotton.	**11.** Blood is a good culture medium for bacterial growth. Removal of any blood extravasated during the procedure will help to decrease the possibility of infection.

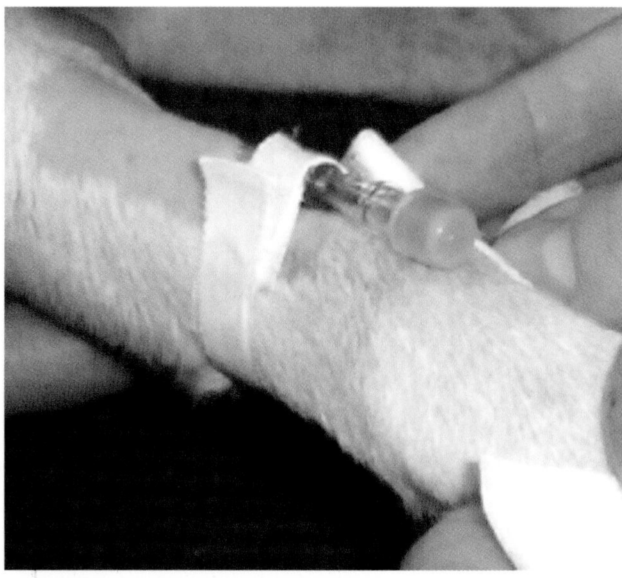

Figure 4-4 Injection cap on intravenous catheter.

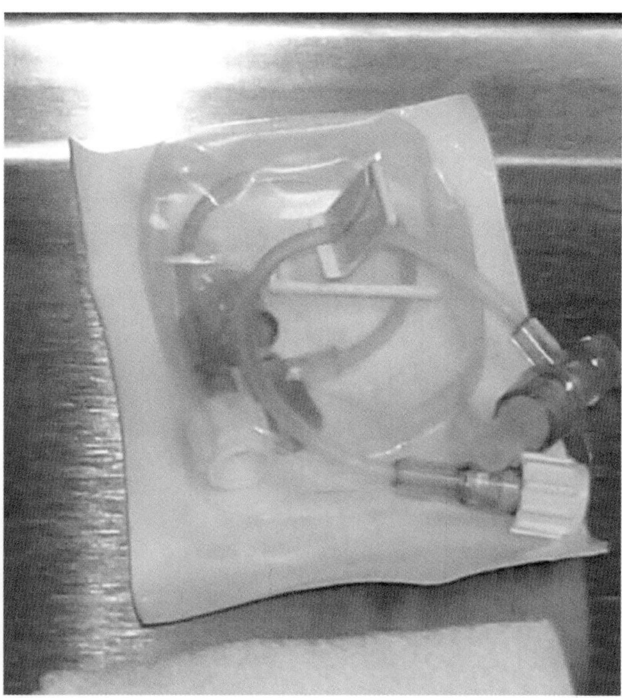

Figure 4-5 T-port.

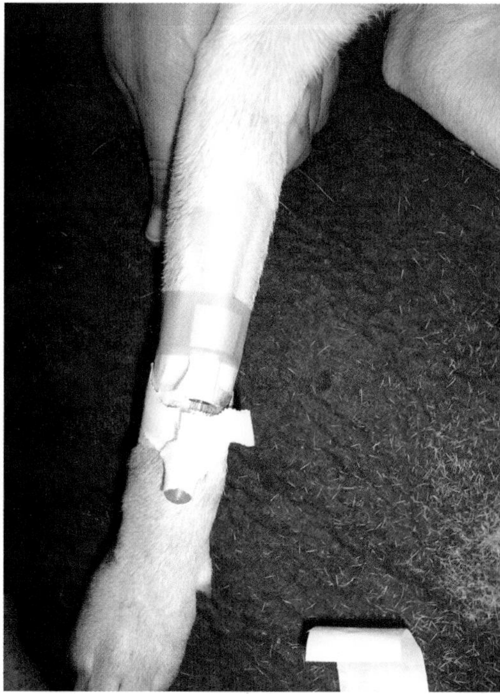

Figure 4-6 Covering catheter insertion point with sterile Band-aid®.

Technical Action	Rationale/Amplification
12. Place sterile gauze sponge or Band-aid® over insertion site (Fig. 4-6).	**12.** The CDC has determined that the most effective way to prevent catheter-related infections is to avoid multiuse antimicrobial ointment. A sterile gauze sponge or sterile Band-aid® should be aseptically placed over the catheter insertion site.
13. Bandage area above and below the catheter using gauze bandaging material and adhesive tape, leaving only injection cap exposed (Fig. 4-7).	**13.** Bandaging of the leg with gauze helps to prevent contamination of the catheter insertion site and resulting infection. Care should be taken to avoid bandaging too tight and causing swelling of foot.
14. Flush catheter with heparinized saline every 8–12 hours when not in continuous use.	**14.** The heparinized saline will keep the catheter patent.
15. Remove bandage and inspect leg every 24 hours, or immediately if animal gives evidence of pain in catheterized leg, or if intravenous infusion cannot be administered easily.	**15.** The bandage should be changed immediately if it becomes wet or soiled. The bandage should be changed and the leg inspected for swelling, pain, redness, or increased

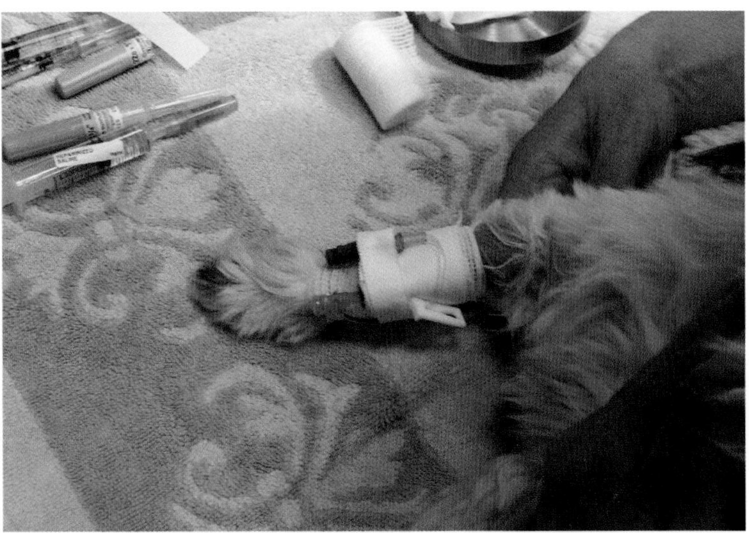

Figure 4-7 Intravenous catheter wrap with T-port

Technical Action	Rationale/Amplification
	skin temperature every 24 hours. Such signs may indicate one or more of the following complications: infiltration of subcutaneous tissues due to catheter moving out of the vein, thrombophlebitis, or infection. If any of these signs are present, the catheter should be removed and the catheter tip should be submitted for bacteriologic culture.
16. If continuous intravenous fluid administration is maintained, a T-port should be placed on catheter to help avoid contamination of fluid line (Fig. 4-7). Change fluid administration set every 24–72 hours.	**16.** Utilizing a T-port allows for venous access while preventing contamination by disconnection and reconnection of fluid line. A needle should never be inserted into the injection cap for the purpose of long-term fluid administration. Changing the fluid administration apparatus helps to prevent the infusion of microorganisms originating within the apparatus itself.
17. When catheter is removed, immediately apply pressure to catheterization site with dry cotton ball. Then apply previously prepared bandage.	**17.** Pressure on the venipuncture site and bandaging of the site following catheter removal will decrease the possibility of hemorrhage and subcutaneous hematoma formation.

INSERTION OF THROUGH-THE-NEEDLE CATHETER

Procedure

Technical Action	Rationale/Amplification
1. Prepare for catheterization.	1. See **Preparation For Intravenous Catheterization**. Examine the apparatus carefully to determine that the catheter moves easily within the needle.
2. Distend (or ask assistant to distend) vein with blood.	2. See Chapter 2, Procedure: No. 3.
3. Insert needle (with catheter withdrawn inside needle) into vein with needle bevel up (Fig. 4-8).	3. Because of the length of this type of catheter 20 or 30 cm, it should be inserted close to the carpus if the cephalic vein is used. A through-the-needle catheter is inserted downward into the jugular vein toward the thoracic inlet (Fig. 4-9). It may be easier, especially in the neck area, to insert the needle through the skin before venipuncture is attempted.
4. Advance needle into vein until at least 1.5 cm is within vein.	4. Venipuncture is confirmed when a flash of blood is seen in the catheter. Entry of the catheter into the vein is ensured by placing a sufficient portion of the needle within the lumen before the catheter is threaded.

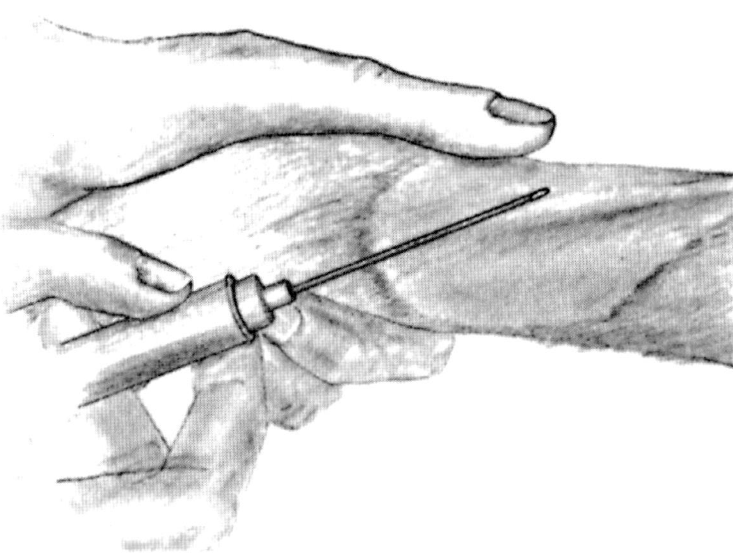

Figure 4-8 Inserting through-the-needle intravenous catheter into cephalic vein.

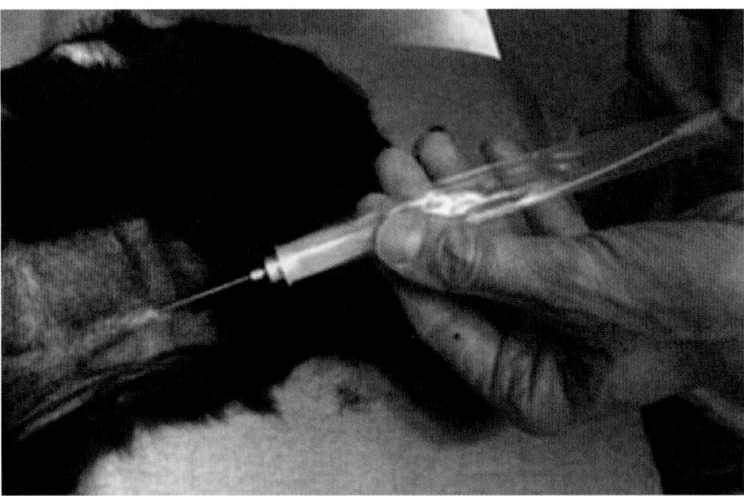

Figure 4-9 Inserting through-the-needle intravenous catheter into jugular vein. With permission from: Advanced Monitoring and Procedures for Small Animal Emergency and Critical Care, Burkitt Creedon J and Davis H. Catheterization of Venous Compartment. p. 58, Copyright Wiley-Blackwell (2012).

Technical Action	Rationale/Amplification
5. Hold needle firmly with one hand and thread catheter into vein by pushing catheter hub within plastic sleeve (Fig. 4-10A) until catheter hub has been advanced into needle hub (Fig. 4-10B).	**5.** Occasionally the animal's leg or neck must be flexed or extended to allow the catheter to advance as far as possible into the vein.
6. Disconnect plastic sleeve from needle (Fig. 4-11).	**6.** It is sometimes necessary to hold the needle hub with a forceps to prevent excessive needle motion and possible laceration of the vein.
7. Withdraw needle from skin and remove wire stylet.	**7.** The function of the wire stylet is to add rigidity to the catheter while it is being advanced into the vein.
8. Place injection cap or T-port on catheter.	**8.** An injection cap provides a sterile seal to the catheter. A T-port should be placed on the catheter for continuous fluid administration to allow for venous access while preventing contamination by disconnection and reconnection of the fluid line.
9. Flush catheter with heparinized saline.	**9.** The heparinized saline will keep the catheter patent while the catheterization site is bandaged.
10. Place needle guard over point at which catheter emerges from tip of needle (Fig. 4-12) and snap it shut.	**10.** The needle guard protects the catheter from being severed by the needle.

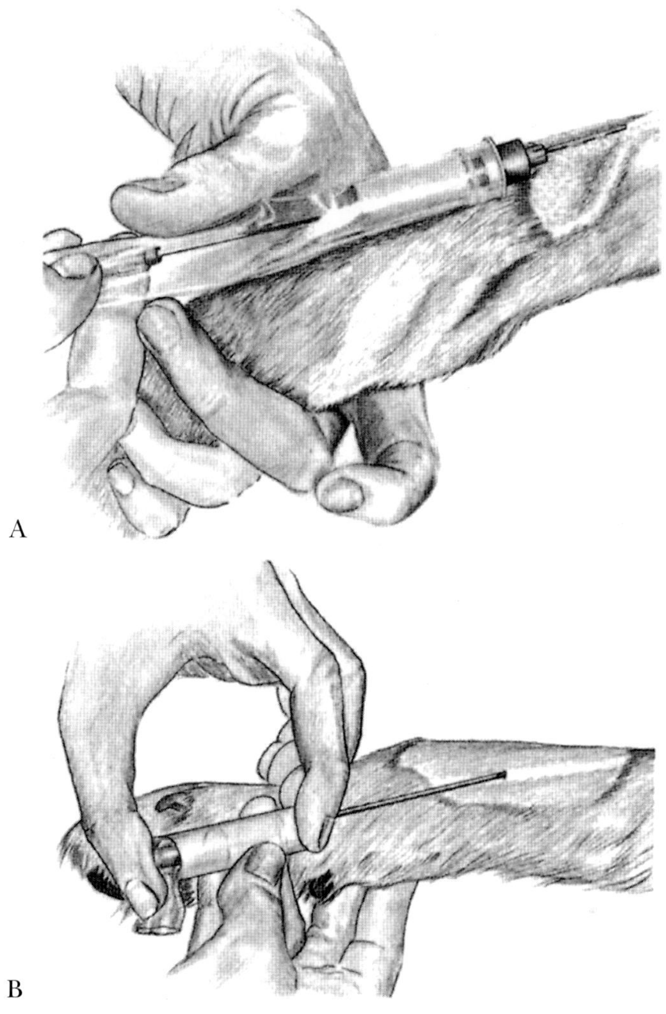

Figure 4-10 (A) Advancing through-the-needle intravenous catheter inside plastic sleeve, and (B) Catheter hub fully advanced into needle hub.

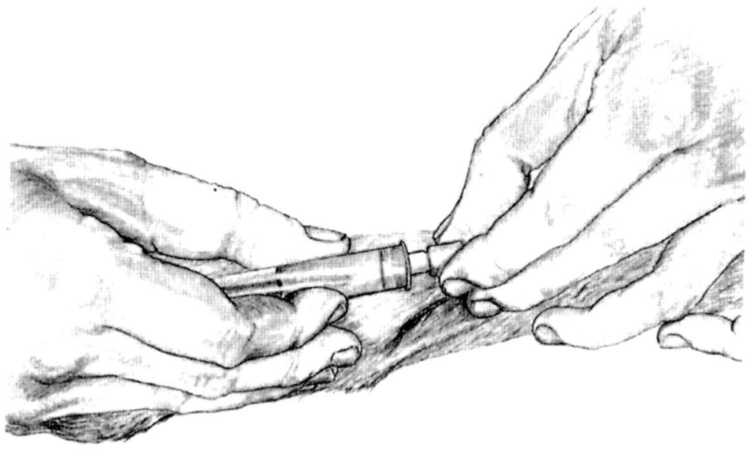

Figure 4-11 Disconnecting plastic sleeve from needle hub.

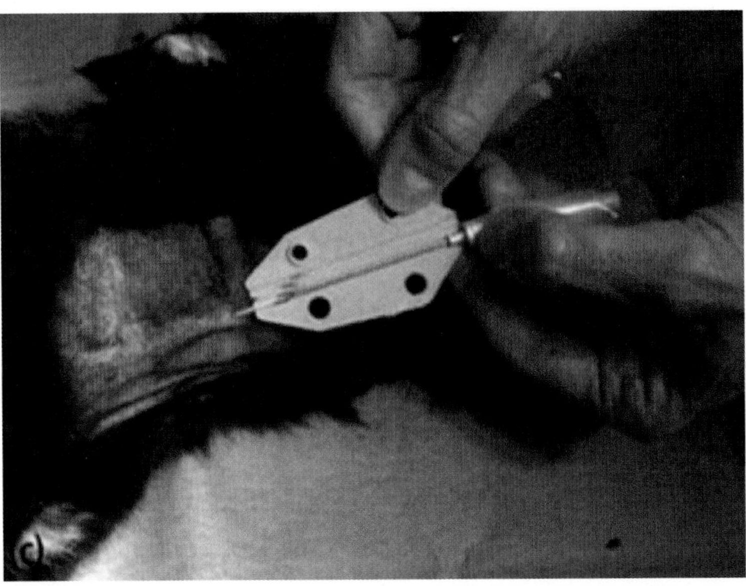

Figure 4-12 Placing needle guard on through-the-needle intravenous catheter. With permission from: Advanced Monitoring and Procedures for Small Animal Emergency and Critical Care, Burkitt Creedon J and Davis H. Catheterization of Venous Compartment. p. 58, Copyright Wiley-Blackwell (2012).

Technical Action	Rationale/Amplification
11. Double back external portion of catheter to facilitate bandaging (Fig. 4-13).	**11.** Be careful not to kink the catheter.
12. Follow complete bandage procedures previously described for bandaging, care, and removal of catheter (Fig. 4-14). (See Insertion of Over-The-Needle Catheter, Nos. 11 to 17.)	
13. If hypertonic fluids are to be administered, radiograph thorax to check catheter position within jugular vein.	**13.** It is important to make sure that the catheter is properly positioned (e.g. not folded back on itself or positioned in a small vein such as the internal thoracic vein). Hypertonic solutions should be given only in large veins, where the volume of blood will decrease the possibility of thrombophlebitis.

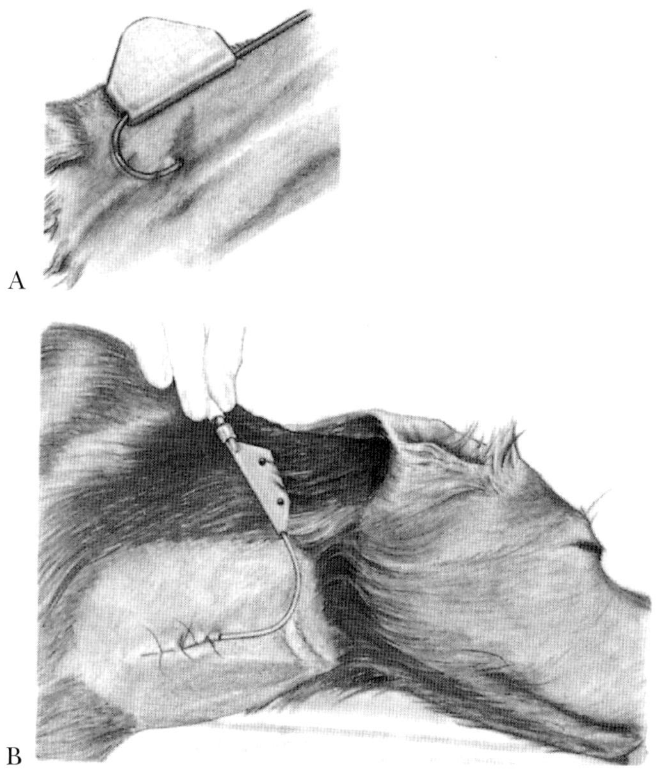

Figure 4-13 Positioning external portion of through-the-needle intravenous catheter prior to bandaging: (A) leg and (B) neck.

INSERTION OF INTRAVENOUS CATHETER WITH BREAK-AWAY NEEDLE

Additional Equipment Needed

- Small sterile drape
- Surgeon's gloves
- Sterile scissors (if placing catheter in jugular vein)
- Suture material (for suturing catheter flange to skin)

Procedure

Technical Action	Rationale/Amplification
1. Prepare for catheterization.	1. An intravenous catheter with a break-away needle is especially useful for the jugular and lateral saphenous veins in the dog and for the jugular and medial saphenous veins in the cat.

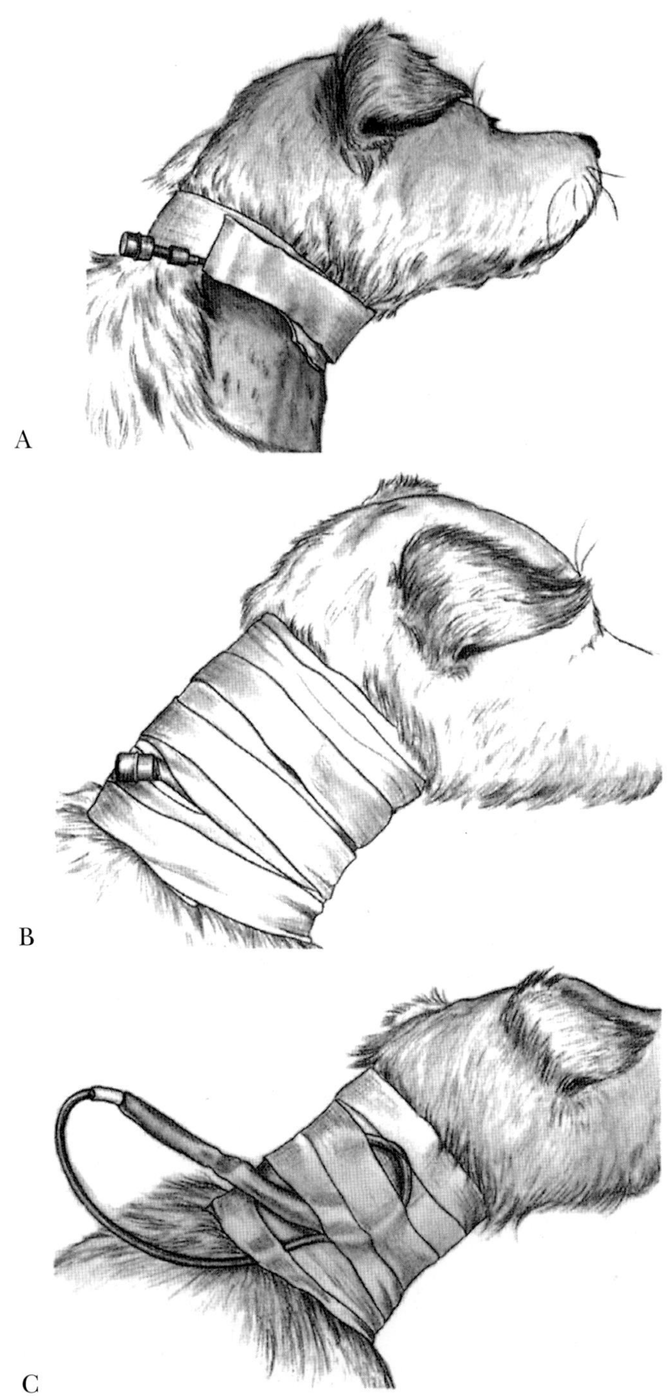

Figure 4-14 Bandaging intravenous through-the-needle catheter in jugular vein (A, B, C).

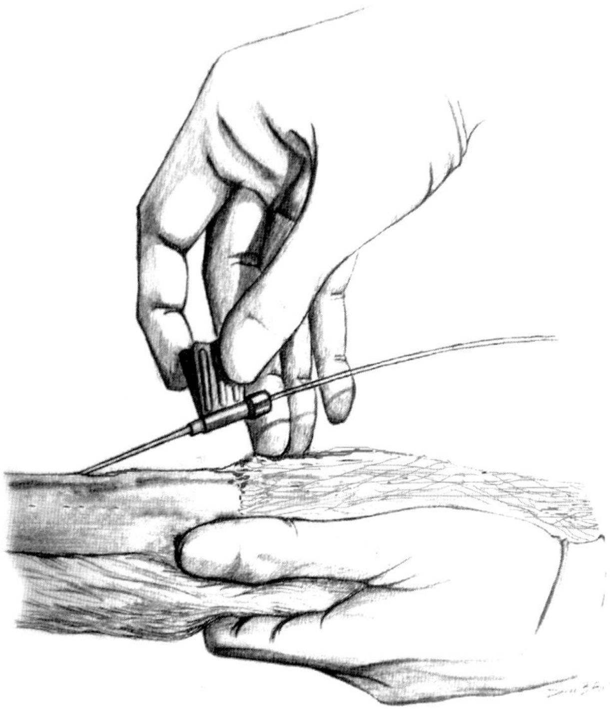

Figure 4-15 Advancing intravenous catheter with break-away needle into vein.

Technical Action	Rationale/Amplification
2. Put on gloves. Place sterile drape around catheterization site.	**2.** Strict attention to asepsis is essential to decrease the possibility of infection.
3. If catheter will be placed in jugular vein, premeasure catheter length from insertion site on animal's neck to third rib space. Then cut catheter to proper length with sterile scissors.	**3.** If the catheter is too long, its distal end will reach the right atrium where it could initiate cardiac arrhythmia.
4. Insert needle (with catheter withdrawn inside needle) into vein with needle bevel up.	**4.** A through-the-needle catheter is inserted downward into the jugular vein toward the thoracic inlet (Fig. 4-8).
5. Advance needle into vein until at least 1.5 cm is within vein lumen (Fig. 4-15).	**5.** Venipuncture is confirmed when a flash of blood is seen in the catheter. Entry of the catheter into the lumen of the vein is ensured by placing a sufficient portion of the needle within the vein before the catheter is threaded.
6. Hold needle firmly with one hand and thread flexible catheter into vein until proximal end reaches needle hub.	

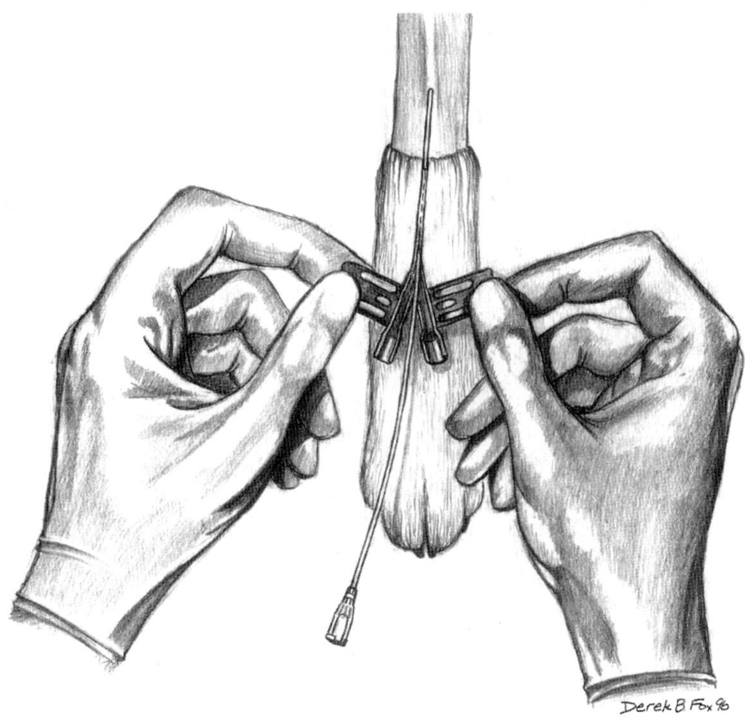

Figure 4-16 Peeling away halves of break-away needle.

Technical Action	Rationale/Amplification
7. Withdraw metal needle from vein and skin.	**7.** The metal needle must be completely out of the skin before it is taken apart.
8. Squeeze plastic wings together to break seal on metal needle.	
9. Peel needle halves apart and discard (Fig. 4.16).	
10. Remove wire stylet.	
	11. The function of the wire stylet is to add rigidity to the catheter while it is being advanced into the vein.
12. Place injection cap or T-port on catheter.	**12.** An injection cap provides a sterile seal to the catheter. A T-port should be placed on the catheter for continuous fluid administration to allow for venous access while preventing contamination by disconnection and reconnection of fluid line.
13. Flush catheter with heparinized saline.	**13.** The heparinized saline will keep the catheter patent while the catheterization site is bandaged.
14. If desired, suture catheter flange to animal's skin.	

Technical Action	Rationale/Amplification
15. Follow complete bandaging procedures previously described for bandaging, care, and removal of catheter (Fig. 4-14). (**See Insertion of Over-The-Needle Catheter**, Nos. 11 to 17.)	

MULTIPLE LUMEN INTRAVENOUS CATHETERS

Multiple lumen intravenous catheters are useful when administering two continuous infusions at the same time, such as a balanced electrolyte solution and total parenteral nutrition (TPN) formulas. The catheter is inserted with the aid of a guide wire and a vein dilator. Completely sterile technique must be used for placement of these catheters.

Additional Equipment Needed

- 1 or 2 assistants
- Clippers
- Appropriate size sandbag, or roll gauze for very small animals
- 2% chlorhexidine scrub and alcohol
- Appropriate size jugular catheter
- 2 sterile field drapes
- Cap and mask
- Sterile gloves
- Local anesthetic (2% lidocaine)
- Scalpel blade
- Package of sterile 4″ × 4″ gauze sponges
- Sterile suturing instruments
- Sterile 6 mL syringe
- 20 g needle
- Alcohol cotton ball
- Heparinized saline
- Suture material
- 18 or 20 g peripheral catheter
- 2 inch × 2 inch sterile gauze
- Tape
- Roll gauze of appropriate size

Procedure

Preparation

1. Place a sterile drape over Mayo stand. Aseptically place all sterile items and second drape onto sterile field.

2. Place alcohol ball on top of heparinized saline bottle.
3. Don cap, mask, and sterile gloves
4. While holding 6 mL syringe, have an assistant place 20-gauge needle onto syringe and remove needle guard.
5. Draw 6 mL of heparinized saline into syringe using aseptic technique.
6. Remove intermittent infusion plug from brown distal port and leave open.
7. Flush all ports with heparinized saline.

Technical Action	Rationale/Amplification
1. Assess jugular veins for visibility, thrombosis, hematoma, dermatopathy, or anything else that might make catheterization difficult or impossible. Select a vein to catheterize.	
2. Assistant: Restrain animal in lateral recumbency with sandbag or gauze roll under neck or shoulder.	**2.** Support material under the neck will bow the neck toward the operator while providing physical comfort for the animal. Sedation may be necessary. Avoid general anesthesia because most patients requiring multiple lumen catheters are in critical condition.
3. Measure from expected insertion site to caudal edge of triceps muscles.	**3.** This measurement is the length to which the catheter should be inserted. The end of the catheter should reach the vena cava half way between the thoracic inlet and the right atrium. If the catheter is too long, its distal end will contact the right atrium where it could initiate a cardiac arrhythmia.
4. Clip and remove hair from neck over jugular vein.	**4.** Clip widely so that long hairs at the edge cannot fall into the aseptic area.
5. Prepare skin with dilute chlorhexidine scrub and alcohol (3 times each, ending with alcohol).	**5.** Strict attention to asepsis is essential to decrease the possibility of infection.
6. Cut a hole of appropriate size in middle of drape and place drape over intended puncture site.	**6.** A sterile drape helps to prevent inadvertent contamination of the catheter and guide wire.
7. Tent skin and make a small skin puncture/incision.	**7.** The incision must be large enough to allow easy passage of the intended catheter through the skin at the insertion site.
8. *Assistant*: Reach under drape and occlude jugular vein by applying digital pressure near thoracic inlet.	

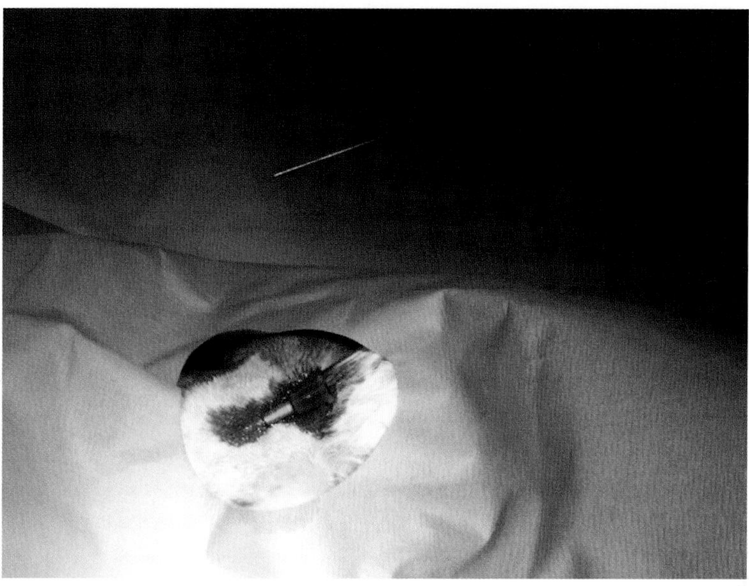

Figure 4-17 Inserting introducer catheter/needle for multilumen catheter in jugular vein.

Technical Action	Rationale/Amplification
9. Insert introducer catheter/needle into vein (Fig. 4-17) with point directed toward thorax; then remove needle, leaving catheter in vein.	
10. Feed guide wire into catheter and down jugular vein 5–8 cm (Fig. 4-18).	**10.** The length of guide wire remaining visible should be longer than the length of the multilumen catheter and the central port. Control the end of the wire so that it does not make contact with a nonsterile area.
11. Remove catheter, leaving guide wire in vein.	**11.** Do not let go of the guide wire. It can be drawn into the vessel and cause an emergency situation.
12. Feed vessel wall dilator over guide wire and advance it into vein as far as it will go (Fig. 4-19).	**12.** This step requires an aggressive, forceful insertion. A twisting/turning technique may facilitate dilator insertion.
13. Remove dilator from vein and guide wire and quickly apply digital pressure at skin entry site to control hemorrhage.	**13.** Use sterile gauze to apply pressure to the dilated vessel to avoid excessive blood loss.
14. Feed tip of multilumen catheter over guide wire until about 2.5 cm of wire protrudes from brown/distal port (Fig. 4-20).	

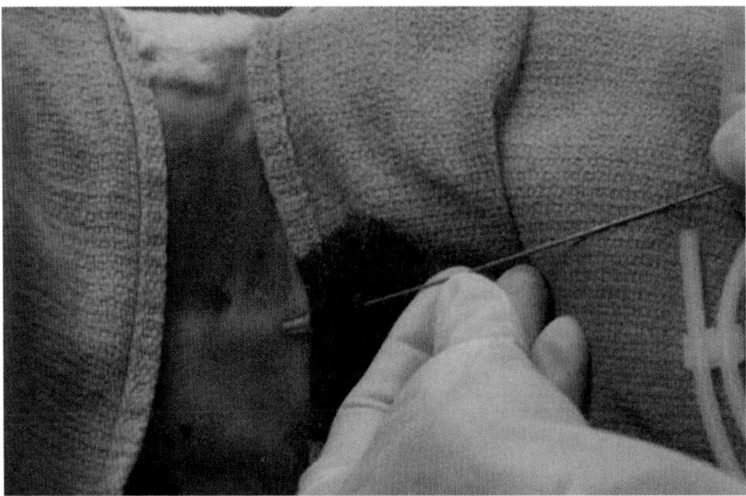

Figure 4-18 Guide wire fed into jugular vein through introducer catheter. With permission from: Advanced Monitoring and Procedures for Small Animal Emergency and Critical Care, Burkitt Creedon J and Davis H. Catheterization of Venous Compartment. p. 58, Copyright Wiley-Blackwell (2012).

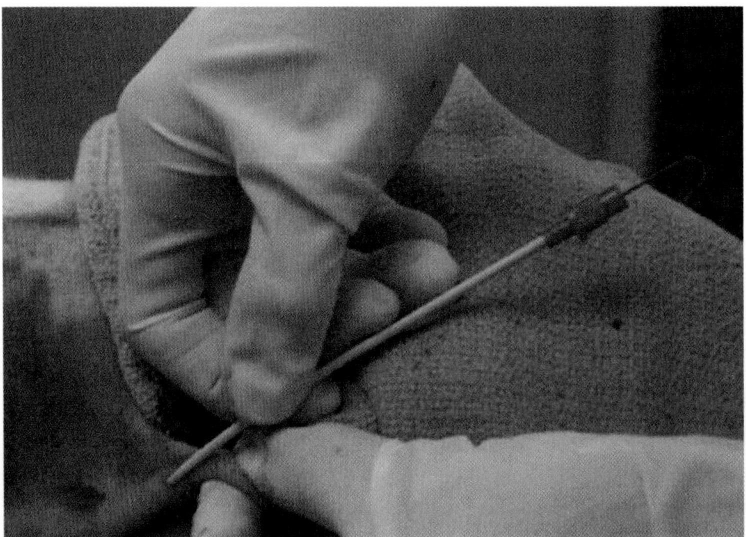

Figure 4-19 Feeding vessel wall dilator over guide wire into the jugular vein. With permission from: Advanced Monitoring and Procedures for Small Animal Emergency and Critical Care, Burkitt Creedon J and Davis H. Catheterization of Venous Compartment. p. 58, Copyright Wiley-Blackwell (2012).

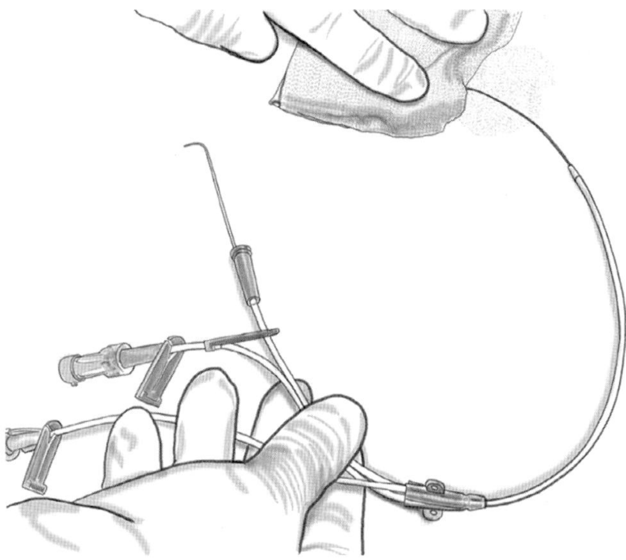

Figure 4-20 Passing multilumen catheter over guide wire until ~2.5 cm of the wire extends out end of middle (brown) port.

Technical Action	Rationale/Amplification
15. Hold end of guide wire firmly so that it is not inserted with catheter and slide catheter into vein to predetermined length (Fig. 4-21).	**15.** Never let go of the guide wire. If lost in the catheter, the catheter and guide wire will need to be removed and the procedure started over.
16. Remove guide wire and place an infusion plug on brown extension tube port; aspirate any air and flush line with heparinized saline.	**16.** An infusion plug provides a sterile seal to the catheter. The heparinized saline will keep the catheter patent while the skin incision is sutured and the catheterization site is bandaged.

NOTE: *Secure catheter in following manner if it has been partially inserted (less than full length):*

Technical Action	Rationale/Amplification
17. *Assistant:* Hold catheter and animal so that catheter does not accidentally back out of vein.	**17.** Do not allow the catheter to back out and become contaminated.
18. Place rubber butterfly sheath around catheter at prescribed level, as close to skin puncture site as possible.	**18.** This step allows a portion of the catheter to be secured outside of the vessel. Insure that the catheter is not pinched or occluded.
19. Suture rubber butterfly sheath to catheter by placing ligatures around indented portion at either end of rubber sheath.	
20. Place fastener clamp over rubber butterfly.	

NOTE: *Secure catheter in the following manner if it has been inserted to full length:*

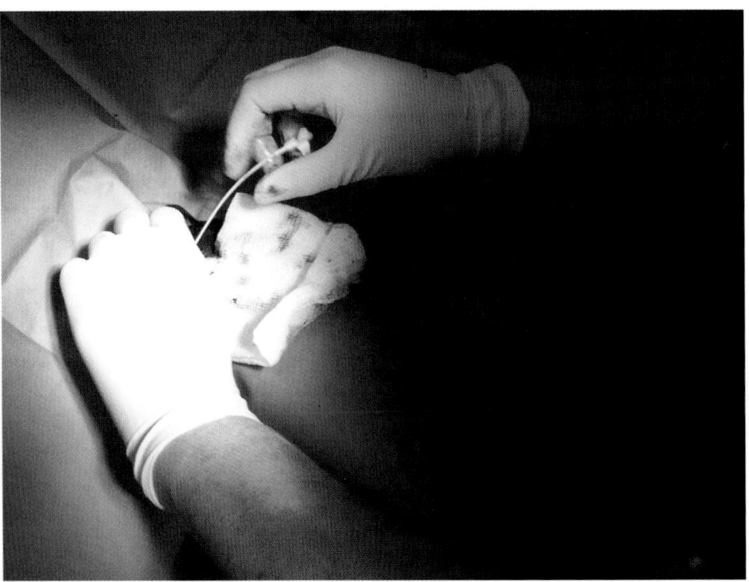

Figure 4-21 Slide catheter over guide wire into jugular vein.

Technical Action	Rationale/Amplification
21. *Assistant:* Hold catheter and patient so that catheter does not accidentally become dislodged.	
22. Place catheter on neck, behind ear, making sure that there are no kinks in catheter.	
23. Place a stay suture in skin next to side holes in fastener clamp.	**23.** These sutures will facilitate catheter exchange if/when it is necessary to do so.
24. Suture wings of clamp to these stay sutures. Suture hub of catheter to neck skin also (Fig. 4-22).	
25. Check each port to make sure that they can be aspirated and flushed.	**25.** If the catheter ports cannot be aspirated, the catheter may need to be repositioned or backed out.
26. Clean area of blood and antiseptic solution.	**26.** Blood is a good culture medium for bacterial growth. Removal of any blood extravasated during the procedure will help to decrease the possibility of infection.
27. Place a sterile 2 inch × 2 inch gauze over insertion site and wrap catheter and neck with roll gauze (Fig. 4-23).	**27.** CDC guidelines advise placing a sterile gauze square over the insertion site to help avoid catheter related infections.
28. Secure gauze and ports with tape.	

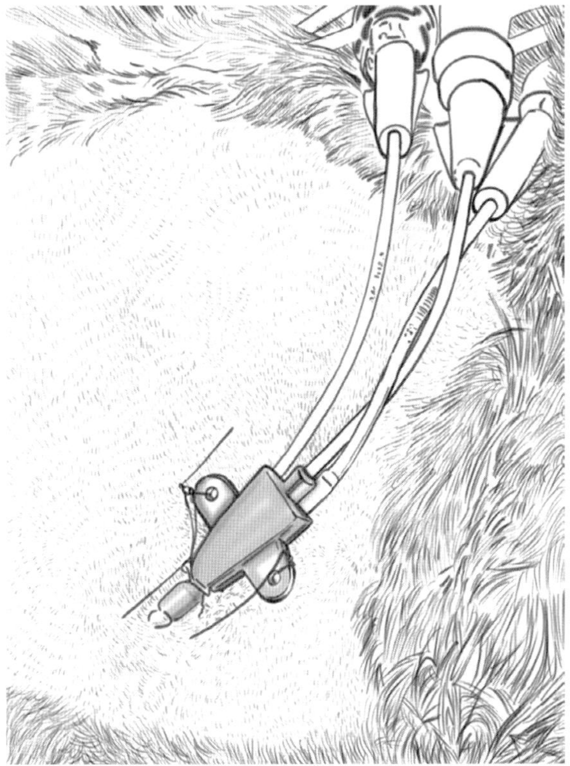

Figure 4-22 Multilumen catheter secured to neck by sutures.

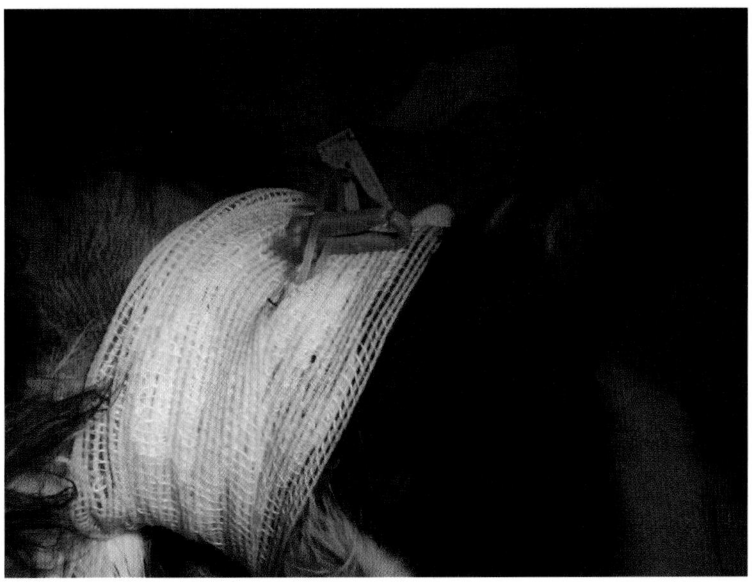

Figure 4-23 Multilumen jugular catheter wrap. Photo courtesy of C Knightly.

INSERTION OF CUT-DOWN CATHETER

*** The following procedure is considered invasive and is typically performed exclusively by veterinarians.**

Additional Equipment Needed

- Sterile drapes
- Surgeon's gloves
- Cap and mask
- Scalpel blade
- Curved hemostat
- Suture material
- Local anesthetic (2% lidocaine)

Procedure

Technical Action	Rationale/Amplification
1. Prepare for catheterization of jugular vein.	**1.** A through-the-needle catheter is suitable for use in the cut-down procedure. In hypotensive, debilitated, or very young animals, the veins may not be visible or palpable, rendering a cut-down procedure necessary for intravenous catheterization.
2. Don cap, mask, and sterile gloves. Place sterile drapes around catheterization site.	**2.** Strict attention to asepsis is essential to decrease the possibility of infection.
3. Infiltrate region of incision with local anesthetic (2% lidocaine).	**3.** General anesthesia should be avoided because of the critical condition of the patient.
4. Make a longitudinal skin incision over jugular vein.	
5. Using blunt dissection, isolate vein and use curved hemostat to preplace two 12–15-cm lengths of absorbable suture material under vein on each side of proposed insertion site (Fig. 4-24).	**5.** These ligatures will be needed above and below the venipuncture site to prevent hemorrhage. The normal compressing effect of the surrounding tissues will be disrupted by the surgical dissection.
6. Tie distal ligature (ligature closer to animal's head), but do not cut ends of ligature yet.	
7. Insert through-the-needle catheter into vein routinely, but do not remove wire stylet at this time.	**7.** See **Insertion of Through-The-Needle Catheter** (Nos. 3 to 6).
8. Ligate vein around catheter proximal to insertion site (Fig. 4-25).	**8.** The wire stylet prevents the ligature from crushing the catheter.
9. Tie loose ends of distal ligature around catheter to hold it to outside wall of vein distal to insertion site (Fig. 4-26).	**9.** Tying the distal ligature stabilizes the catheter further and prevents kinking at the insertion site.

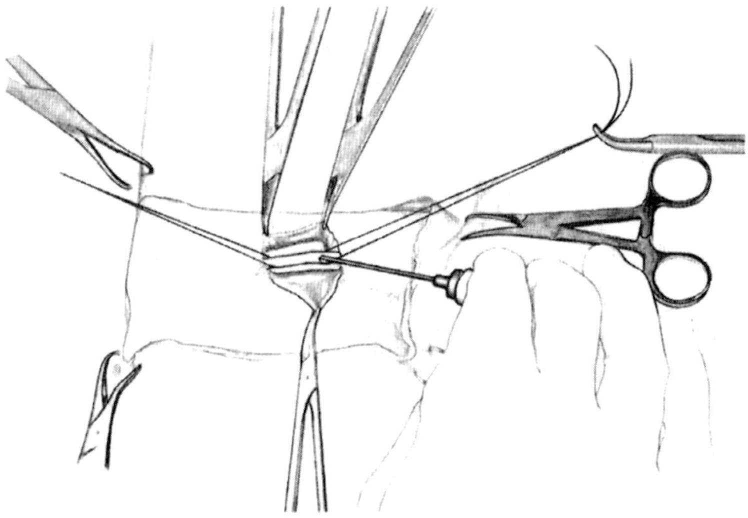

Figure 4-24 Preplacing suture material during cut-down intravenous catheterization.

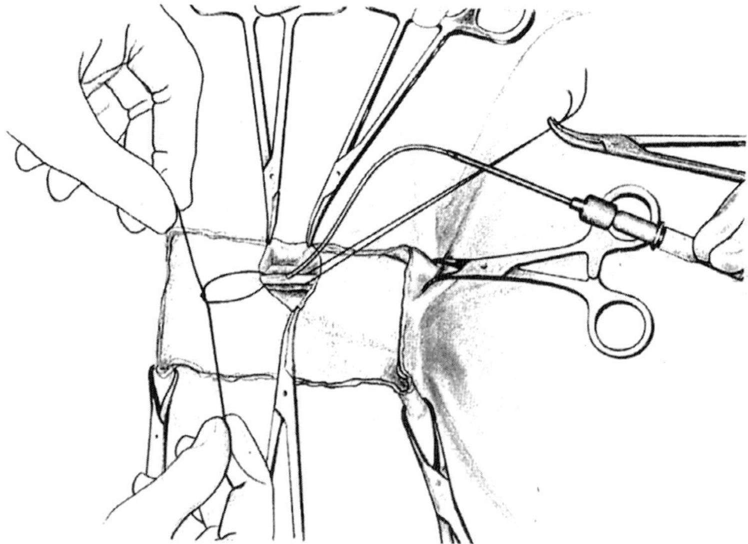

Figure 4-25 Tying proximal ligature around vein.

Technical Action	Rationale/Amplification
10. Remove wire stylet.	
11. Place injection cap or T-port on catheter.	**11.** An injection cap provides a sterile seal to the catheter. A T-port should be placed on the catheter for continuous fluid administration to allow for venous access while preventing contamination by disconnection and reconnection of fluid line.

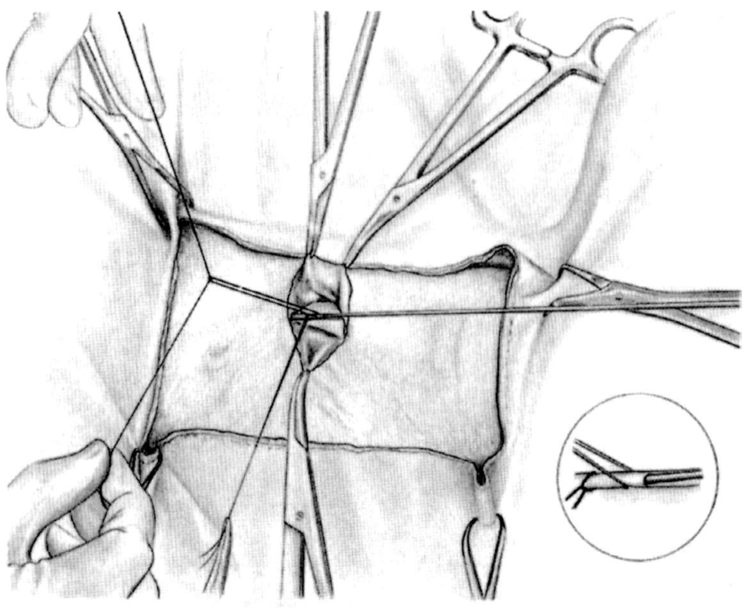

Figure 4-26 Tying distal ligature around vein and catheter.

Technical Action	Rationale/Amplification
12. Flush catheter with heparinized saline.	**12.** The heparinized saline will keep the catheter patent while the skin incision is sutured and the catheterization site is bandaged.
13. Place needle guard over point at which catheter emerges from tip of needle, and snap it shut.	**13.** The needle guard protects the catheter from being severed by the needle.
14. Suture skin incision.	**14.** The skin sutures can be removed when the incision has healed (7–10 days).
15. Double back external portion of catheter to facilitate bandaging (Fig. 4-13).	**15.** Be careful not to kink the catheter.
16. Follow complete procedure previously described for bandaging, care, and removal of catheter Fig. 4-14). (See **Insertion of Over-The-Needle Catheter**, Nos. 11 to 17.)	
17. If hypertonic fluids are to be administered, take thoracic radiograph to check catheter position within jugular vein.	**17.** It is important to make sure that the catheter is properly positioned (e.g. not folded back on itself or positioned in a small vein such as the internal thoracic vein). Hypertonic solutions should be given only in large veins, where the volume of blood will decrease the possibility of thrombophlebitis.

NOTE: *Certain complications of intravenous therapy, such as pyrogenic reaction, circulatory overload, and air embolism, are beyond the scope of this book but are discussed in depth in The Lippincott Manual of Nursing Practice, third edition.*

Bibliography

Bistner SI, Ford RB: Kirk and Bistner's Handbook of Veterinary Procedures and Emergency Treatment, 6th edition. Philadelphia, WB Saunders, 1995

Brunner LS, Suddarth DS: The Lippincott Manual of Nursing Practice, 3rd edition. Philadelphia, JB Lippincott, 1982

Burrows CF: Techniques and complications of intravenous and intraartrial catheterization in dogs and cats. JAVMA 163(12): 1357–1363, 1973

CDC: Guideline for Prevention of Surgical Site Infection. www.cdc.gov/ncidod/dhqp/gl_ surgicalsite.html, 1999

Cook L, Bellini S, Cusson RM : Heparinized saline vs normal saline for maintenance of intravenous access in neonates: an evidence-based practice change. Adv Neonatal Care 11(3): 208–15, June 2011

Haskins SC: Fluid and electrolyte therapy. Comp Contin Educ for Pract Vet 6(3): 244–257, 1984

Kirk RW, Bistner SI: Handbook of Veterinary Procedures and Emergency Treatment, 4th edition. Philadelphia, WB Saunders, 1985

Lane DR, Cooper B: Veterinary Nursing (Formerly Jones's Animal Nursing, 5th edition). Oxford, England, Pergamon Press, 1994

Managing IV Therapy, A Nursing Photobook, In Nursing '81 Photobook. Springhouse, PA, Intermed Communications, 1980

O'Grady NP *et al.*: Guidelines for the prevention of intravascular catheter-related infections. MMWR 51(RR10):1–26. www.cdc.gov/mmwr/preview/mmwrhtml/rr5110a1.htm, 2002

Schallom M, Prentice D, Sona C; Micek S, Skrupky L: Heparin or 0.9% sodium chloride to maintain central venous catheter patency: a randomized trial. Crit Care Med 40(6): 1820–6, June 2012

Chapter 5

Oral Administration of Medications

Patience is the companion of wisdom.
ANONYMOUS

Oral administration of medications is the placement of solid or liquid material in the oral cavity so that specific quantities of the material are swallowed.

Purposes

1. To administer medications, water, and nutritional supplements
2. To administer certain radiographic contrast materials

Contraindications

1. Dysphagia, regurgitation, and vomiting
2. Acute pancreatitis
3. Esophageal and gastrointestinal obstruction
4. Esophageal surgery within the past 2–7 days, depending on extent of injury
5. Gastric or intestinal surgery within the past 12–24 hours
6. Head and neck trauma

Complications

1. Aspiration of medications into respiratory tract
2. Inaccurate dosing

Crow and Walshaw's Manual of Clinical Procedures in Dogs, Cats, Rabbits, and Rodents, Fourth Edition. Edited by Jennifer E. Boyle. Published 2016 by John Wiley & Sons, Inc.
Companion Website: www.wiley.com/go/boyle/manual4e

Equipment Needed

- For capsules or tablets:
  - Lubricant or canned food
  - Syringe of water
  - Pilling device
- For liquids:
  - Syringe, small bottle, or spoon

Restraint and Positioning

The procedure may be accomplished with the animal standing, sitting, or in sternal recumbency. Minimal restraint should be used. When handling vicious animals, oral medication can be offered in small amounts of palatable food. It is imperative that the animal be fully conscious whenever medications are administered orally.

ADMINISTRATION OF CAPSULE OR TABLET

Procedure

Technical Action	Rationale/Amplification
1. Check medication to be administered with regard to "The Five Rights": right patient, right drug, right dose, right route, right time and frequency.	**1.** It is important to take measures to prevent errors of medication administration.
2. Wash hands.	**2.** Washing hands between patients is important in controlling communicable diseases in a hospital. It is advisable to wear nonsterile examination gloves when administering oral medication to an animal with a communicable disease.
3. Lubricate capsule or tablet.	**3.** Lubrication of the capsule or tablet, with lubricant or canned food, makes it easier to swallow. Also see Rationale No. 11.
4. Place capsule or tablet in pilling device (Fig. 5-1) or hold between thumb and index finger of one hand (Fig. 5-2).	**4.** A pilling device is useful for administering capsules or tablets to a cat or a dog that resists attempts to hold the mouth open during the procedure.
5. Place palm of other hand on dorsal surface of animal's snout.	
6. Insert thumb behind one upper canine tooth into mouth and stroke animal's hard palate.	**6.** Rolling the animal's lips inward over its teeth may minimize the possibility of the person being bitten. Tactile

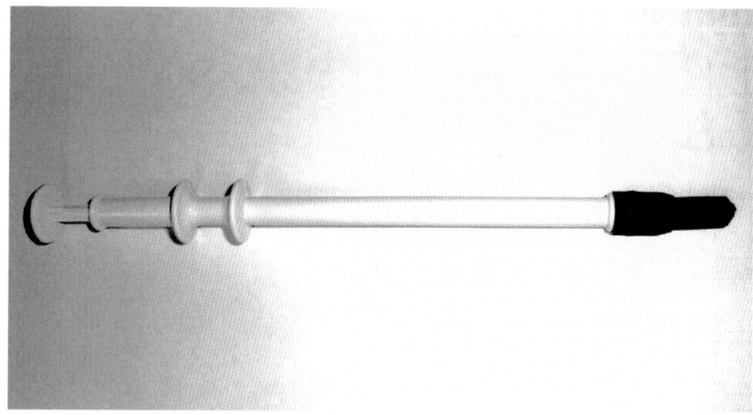

Figure 5-1 Commercial pilling device.

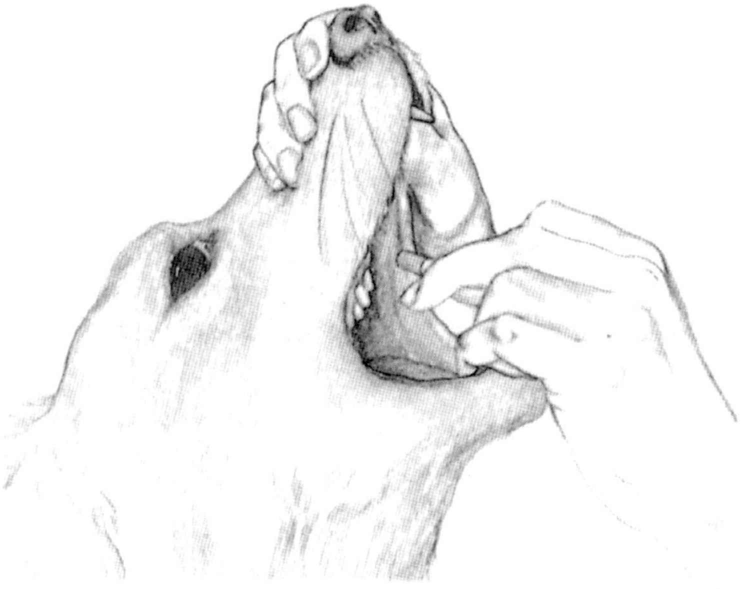

Figure 5-2 Manually placing capsule on base of dog's tongue.

Technical Action	Rationale/Amplification
	stimulation of the hard palate often leads to spontaneous opening of the mouth.
7. Tilt animal's nostrils toward ceiling.	**7.** This head position causes relaxation of the lower jaw muscles in many animals, thereby eliminating the need for forceful attempts to pry open the animal's mouth.

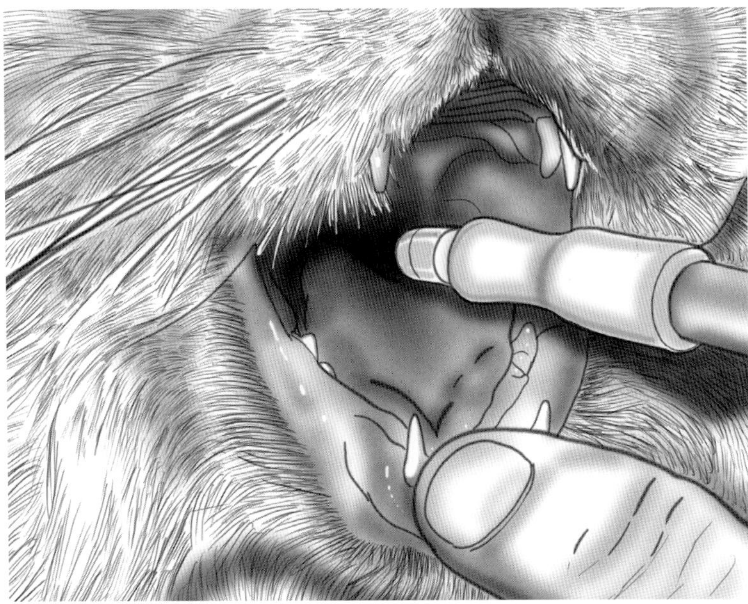

Figure 5-3 Placing capsule on base of cat's tongue with pilling device.

Technical Action	Rationale/Amplification
8. Press downward on animal's lower incisors with fourth and fifth fingers of hand holding medications.	**8.** At this point, the animal's mouth should be open wide.
9. Place capsule or tablet on base of animal's tongue (Figs. 5-2 or 5-3).	**9.** An animal can easily eject from its mouth a capsule or tablet placed on the rostral portion of the tongue.
10. Withdraw hand or pilling device from animal's mouth.	
11. Close animal's mouth quickly and hold it closed, while at same time gently rubbing laryngeal area.	**11.** Licking of the nasal planum indicates that the animal has swallowed.

Note: *Administration of tablets and capsules to cats should be chased with water to prevent risk of esophagitis and stricture.*

Technical Action	Rationale/Amplification
12. Note in animal's medical record that medication was given.	**12.** The following information should be noted in the medical record: date, time, medication, dosage, route, initials of individual administering medication, and comments.

ADMINISTRATION OF LIQUID MEDICATION

Procedure

Technical Action	Rationale/Amplification
1. Check medication to be administered, using "The Five Rights": right patient, right drug, right dose, right route, right time and frequency.	**1.** It is important to take measures to prevent errors of medication administration.
2. Wash hands.	**2.** Washing hands between patients is important in controlling communicable diseases in a hospital. It is advisable to wear nonsterile examination gloves while administering oral medication to an animal with a communicable disease.
3. Place liquid medication in syringe or small bottle.	**3.** A spoon may be used to administer palatable liquids to animals of quiet temperament.
4. With one hand, form a pouch from animal's cheek just caudal to commissures of its lips by placing finger or thumb inside cheek and pulling laterally on lip (Fig. 5-4).	**4.** The animal's jaws therefore can remain closed during the procedure.
5. Place liquid medication into cheek pouch, small amounts at a time (Fig. 5-5).	**5.** The dorsal surface of the animal's snout should be parallel to the ground or only slightly elevated while liquids

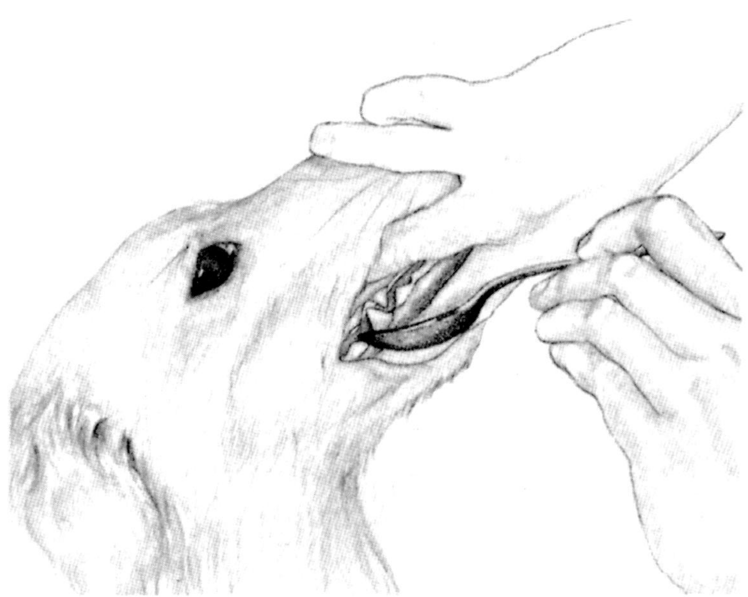

Figure 5-4 Forming a cheek pouch for administration of liquids.

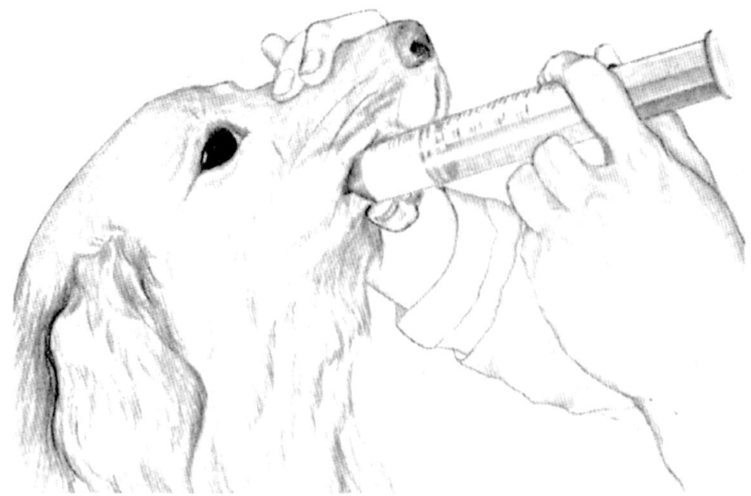

Figure 5-5 Administering liquid medication orally.

Technical Action	Rationale/Amplification
	are administered. Avoiding pointing the animal's nostrils toward the ceiling minimizes the possibility of aspiration of the liquid into the respiratory tract.
6. Give medication slowly.	**6.** To ensure adequate dosing, it is advisable to administer a small amount of liquid and wait until the animal swallows before placing any more liquid into the cheek pouch.
7. Note in animal's medical record that medication was given.	**7.** The following information should be noted in the medical record: date, time, medication, dosage, route, initials of individual administering medication, and comments.

Bibliography

Bassert J, Thomas J: McCurnin's Clinical Textbook for Veterinary Technicians, 8th edition. Philadelphia, WB Saunders, 2013

Bistner SI, Ford RB: Kirk and Bistner's Handbook of Veterinary Procedures and Emergency Treatment, 6th edition. Philadelphia, WB Saunders, 1995

Burkitt Creedon J, Davis H: Advanced Monitoring and Procedures for Small Animal Emergency and Critical Care. Oxford, England, Wiley-Blackwell, 2012

Giving Medications, A Nursing Photobook. In Nursing '80 Photobook. Springhouse, PA, Intermed Communications, 1980

Kirk RW, Bistner SI: Handbook of Veterinary Procedures and Emergency Treatment, 4th edition. Philadelphia, WB Saunders, 1985

Westfall DS, Twedt DC, Steyn PF, Oberhauser EB, VanCleave JW: Evaluation of esophageal transit of tablets and capsules in 30 cats, J Vet Intern Med 15(5): 467–70, Sept–Oct 2001

Chapter 6

Dermatologic Procedures

What we see depends mainly on what we look for.
JOHN LUBBOCK

This chapter describes several procedures that are useful for gathering diagnostic information about skin diseases.

SKIN CULTURE

Skin culture is the inoculation of suitable media with material from the skin.

Purposes

1. To identify bacterial and fungal pathogens of the skin
2. To determine the antibiotic sensitivity of bacterial skin pathogens

Equipment Needed

- Cotton
- Culture media
- Sterile 22-gauge needle or scalpel blade (for bacterial culture)
- Scalpel blade
- Hemostatic forceps (for fungal culture)
- 70% alcohol (for bacterial culture)

Crow and Walshaw's Manual of Clinical Procedures in Dogs, Cats, Rabbits, and Rodents, Fourth Edition. Edited by Jennifer E. Boyle. © 2016 John Wiley & Sons, Inc. Published 2016 by John Wiley & Sons, Inc.
Companion Website: www.wiley.com/go/boyle/manual4e

Restraint and Positioning

An assistant restrains the animal in a position that affords access to the skin lesion(s) (see Chapter 1).

BACTERIAL CULTURE OF A SKIN PUSTULE

Procedure

Technical Action	Rationale/Amplification
1. Clip hair around pustule.	**1.** Clipping must be done carefully to avoid rupturing the pustule. A 2.5-cm square area is usually adequate for culturing a skin pustule.
2. Cleanse clipped area gently with cotton moistened with 70% alcohol.	**2.** Disinfection of the pustule with 70% alcohol removes surface contaminants that might invalidate the culture results.
3. Let the skin air dry.	**3.** Do not collect material while skin is still moist because excess alcohol may be transferred to the swab.
4. Insert tip of swab into pustule after puncturing it with sterile 22-gauge needle or after incising the pustule with point of No. 11 scalpel blade.	
5. Inoculate material into suitable bacterial culture media.	**5.** The culture media can be inoculated directly, or the swab can be placed in transport medium.
6. Cleanse open pustule with 70% alcohol.	

CULTURE FOR DERMATOPHYTES

Procedure

Technical Action	Rationale/Amplification
1. Clean edge of lesion with cotton moistened with water.	**1.** Gentle cleansing with water removes superficial debris but will not interfere with fungal culture results.
2. Using scalpel blade or hemostat, scrape or pluck several hairs from edge of lesion.	**2.** Recovery of dermatophytes is most successful if visibly diseased hairs from the edge of the lesion are cultured.

Technical Action	Rationale/Amplification
3. Inoculate dermatophyte culture medium with hairs by forcing hairs below surface of medium.	**3.** Forcing of hairs below the surface of the medium ensures contact of dermatophytes on the hair with the culture medium.
4. In absence of lesions or when carrier status is suspected, use a new toothbrush to briskly brush hair on animal's body.	**4.** A new toothbrush in its package is free of fungal organisms.
5. Inoculate dermatophyte culture medium by pressing toothbrush several times to surface of medium.	**5.** The toothbrush collection procedure is especially useful for diagnosing feline dermatophytosis.
6. Place cover on culture medium but do not close tightly.	**6.** Fungal growth may be enhanced by placing the medium in the dark.
7. Incubate at room temperature and check daily for growth.	**7.** Dermatophyte organisms will cause a color change in dermatophyte test medium when minimal growth is visible.

SKIN SCRAPING

Skin scraping is a diagnostic procedure involving intentional abrasion of a skin lesion with a scalpel blade.

Purpose

To detect the presence of microscopic skin parasites.

Complications

Minor hemorrhage.

Equipment Needed

- New, dulled scalpel blade*
- Glass slides
- Mineral oil or potassium hydroxide

*Note: *Reusing scalpel blades is not recommended for skin scraping due to possible contamination of transmittable diseases. The blade can be dulled by passing it over a clean metal surface several times before using it on the patient.*

Restraint and Positioning

An assistant restrains the animal in a position that affords access to the skin lesion(s) (see Chapter 1).

Procedure

Technical Action	Rationale/Amplification
1. Place one drop of mineral oil on each of several glass slides.	
2. Insert edge of scalpel blade into mineral oil on glass slide or apply mineral oil directly to skin to be scraped.	2. Moistening the scalpel blade with mineral oil provides a sticky surface for collecting mites and ova during the scraping. Applying mineral oil to the skin helps dislodge debris on the skin in addition to making it easier to collect the scraped material.
3. Select lesion(s) to be scraped, avoiding areas of severe excoriation.	3. If sarcoptic mange is suspected, lesions on the ears, elbows, and hocks should be scraped.
4. Pinch fold of skin and scrape surface until drops of capillary blood appear (Fig. 6-1).	4. Pinching the skin helps to move the demodectic mites out of the deeper parts of the hair follicles. The normally deep location of demodectic mites within the skin necessitates scraping to the level of capillaries.

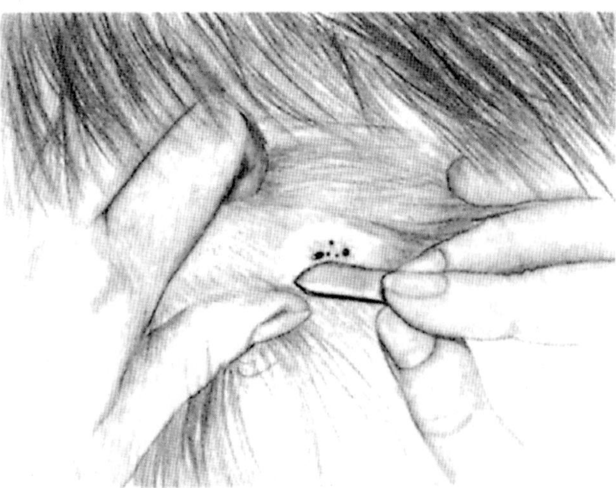

Figure 6-1 Skin scraping. Note that a fold of skin is pinched between the fingers to move mites out of hair follicles.

Technical Action	Rationale/Amplification
5. Transfer hair and epithelial debris collected from skin scraping into drop of mineral oil on glass slide by swirling or scraping material on slide edge.	5. Several scrapings should be made and the site of the scraping indicated on each glass slide. As many as 20 scrapings may be necessary to obtain sarcoptic mites.
6. Examine immediately.	6. If potassium hydroxide is used, waiting several minutes may result in some clearing of the prepared specimens.
7. Note results of skin scrapings in animal's medical record.	7. Note date, scraping sites, number of live and dead mites, larvae, and ova at each site. This is especially important in following the progress of animals being treated with parasiticides.

CELLOPHANE TAPE PREPARATION

A *cellophane tape preparation* is used to collect material from the surface of the skin and hair coat.

Purpose

To detect the presence of certain skin parasites, including flea larvae, lice, and mites.

Equipment Needed

- Clear cellophane tape
- Glass slides
- Mineral oil

Restraint and Positioning

The animal is restrained in sternal recumbency or in a sitting or standing position.

Procedure

Technical Action	Rationale/Amplification
1. Select site for sampling.	1. Choose an area in which seborrhoea or black debris is present, usually along the dorsal midline.

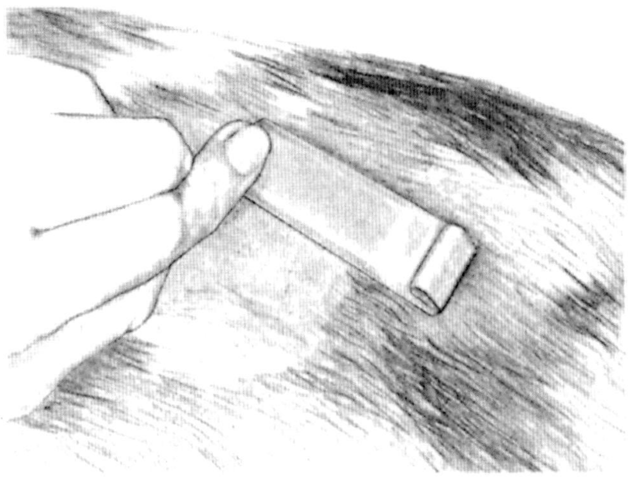

Figure 6-2 Collecting specimen from skin, using cellophane tape.

Technical Action	Rationale/Amplification
2. Tear off a 3–5-cm piece of cellophane tape, attach one end to a glass slide, and double it back onto slide so that sticky side does not contact slide.	
3. Part hair and touch sticky side of clear cellophane tape to hair and skin (Fig. 6-2).	**3.** Loose particles will adhere to the tape. The attached slide adds rigidity to the tape and may improve collection of parasites.
4. Place a drop of mineral oil on glass slide and flip tape so that sticky side with collected debris attaches to slide and covers oil.	
5. Examine under microscope and note findings in animal's medical record.	**5.** Note date, sampling site, number, and identity of parasitic organisms collected.

SKIN VACUUMING FOR ECTOPARASITES

Skin vacuuming is a diagnostic procedure for enhancing the recovery of superficial ectoparasites.

Purpose

To detect the presence of microscopic skin parasites.

Equipment Needed

- Small vacuum cleaner with wand attachment
- Blunt scalpel
- Filter paper, for example, in-line, non-gauze milk filter
- Hand lens or dissecting microscope
- 10% potassium hydroxide
- Beaker and test tube
- Hot plate
- Glass slides and cover slips
- Centrifuge
- Fecal flotation solution

Procedure

Technical Action	Rationale/Amplification
1. Assemble apparatus with filter paper between wand attachment and vacuum cleaner hose (Fig. 6-3).	**1.** The filter paper will trap hair, debris, and ectoparasites.
2. If vacuum cleaner noise frightens animal, position vacuum cleaner in adjacent room with vacuum tubing brought through a door slightly ajar.	**2.** Some animals are frightened by the sound of the vacuum, but others seem to enjoy the vacuuming procedure.
3. Vacuum animal's hair coat while scraping it with edge of vacuum	**3.** Blunt scraping of areas most likely to harbor certain ectoparasites or

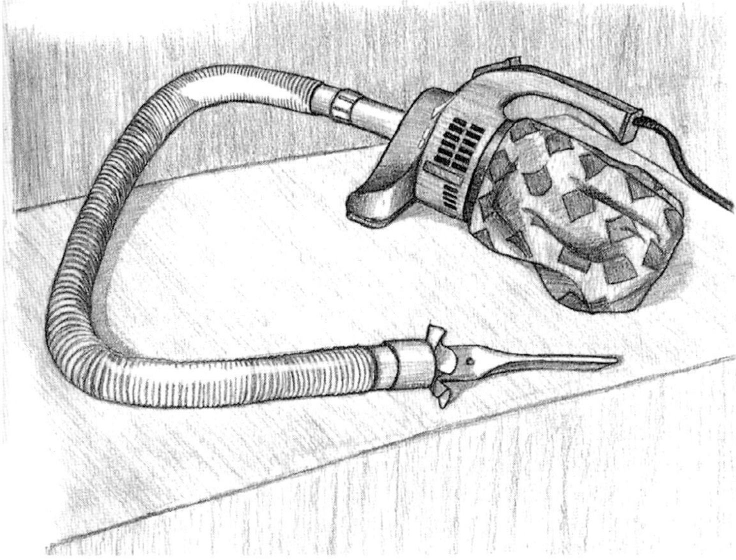

Figure 6-3 Small vacuum cleaner with wand attachment and filter paper in place.

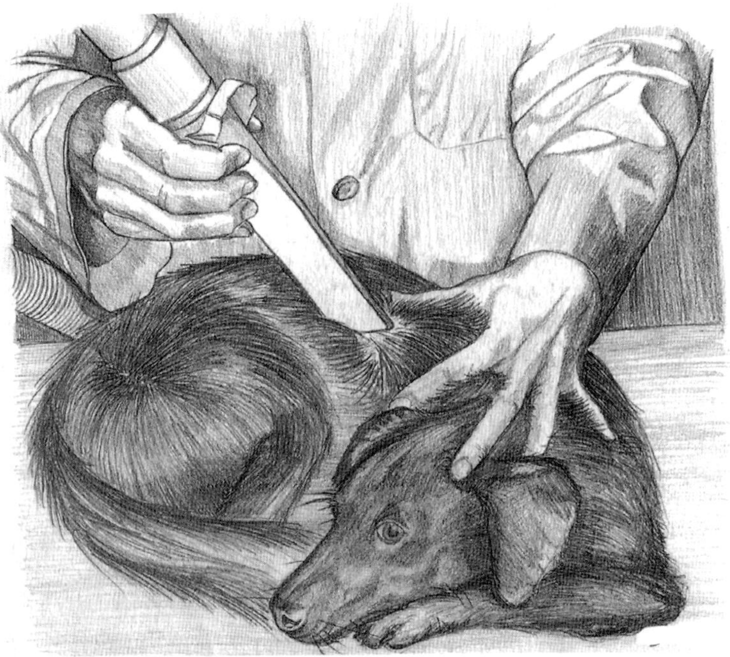

Figure 6-4 Skin vacuuming a dog.

Technical Action	Rationale/Amplification
wand or with blunt scalpel (Fig. 6-4).	suspicious lesions may increase the recovery of parasites during the vacuuming process.
4. Remove filter and examine with hand lens or dissecting microscope.	**4.** Certain parasites, such as lice and *Cheyletiella* mites, may be seen with a hand lens or dissecting microscope crawling about in the debris on the filter paper.
5. Place filter in beaker with 10% potassium hydroxide and heat until just boiling.	**5.** The hot potassium hydroxide dissolves debris in the sample.
6. Pour suspension from beaker into test tube and centrifuge at 1000 RPM for 5 minutes.	**6.** Centrifuging the suspension helps to concentrate any ectoparasites or their eggs in the sample.
7. Pour off supernatant, add fecal flotation solution and centrifuge for 5 minutes.	**7.** Any ectoparasites or their eggs will be further concentrated.
8. Fill test tube to top with fecal flotation solution, place cover slip on top of test tube, and wait for 5 minutes.	**8.** Ectoparasites and/or their eggs will float to the top of the solution.
9. Place cover slip on microscope slide and examine with regular light microscope.	**9.** This procedure is especially valuable in recovering elusive ectoparasites, such as *Sarcoptes*.

SKIN BIOPSY

*** The following procedures are considered invasive and are typically performed exclusively by veterinarians.**

Skin biopsy is the removal of a small section of skin for histopathology or for making impression smears. A very small skin lesion may be excised completely by means of the biopsy procedure.

Purposes

1. To demonstrate the presence of bacterial, fungal, or parasitic organisms responsible for a particular skin disorder
2. To diagnose immune-mediated skin diseases
3. To identify skin tumors
4. To further characterize skin lesions for which fine-needle aspiration did not provide a definitive diagnosis

Complications

1. Minor hemorrhage
2. Infection
3. Scar formation

Equipment Needed

Clipper with No. 40 blade
- Skin preparation materials:
  - Cotton
  - Mild soap (*not* povidone-iodine)
  - 70% alcohol
  - Sterile gauze sponges (2 inch × 2 inch)
- Sterile equipment for biopsy procedure:
  - Surgeon's gloves
  - Surgical drape
  - Gauze sponges (2 inch × 2 inch)
  - Fine-tooth forceps
  - 4-mm Keyes cutaneous biopsy punch* or No. 15 scalpel blade
  - Needle-holding forceps

Suture material:
- Equipment for local anesthesia:
  - 1-mL syringe
  - 25-gauge needle
  - Local anesthetic solution (e.g. 2% lidocaine)
- Materials for handling biopsy specimen:
  - 25-gauge needle
  - Paper towels

* J. Sklar Manufacturing Co., Long Island City, N.Y.

- Container with preservative: 10% formalin
- Glass slides for impression smears
- Drugs for sedation (if necessary)

Restraint and Positioning

An assistant restrains the animal in a position that affords access to the skin lesion(s). It may be necessary to tranquilize or sedate uncooperative animals.

PREPARATION FOR SKIN BIOPSY

Procedure

Technical Action	Rationale/Amplification
1. Select appropriate biopsy site.	1. Avoid traumatized, crusted, or atypical lesions. Biopsies should be obtained from different-stage lesions as well as normal tissue. If possible, try to take a sample that includes the transition from normal to abnormal tissue.
2. Clip hair carefully from site.	2. It is important to avoid traumatizing the biopsy area during clipping.
3. Prepare clipped area by washing gently with mild soap and applying 70% alcohol.	3. Vigorous scrubbing may distort the microscopic findings and therefore should be avoided. Iodine preparations should not be used because they can interfere with histology staining.
4. Instill 0.5 mL to 1 mL of local anesthetic intradermally and subcutaneously around and beneath biopsy site.	4. Avoid instilling local anesthetic directly into the lesion because this may cause artifacts in the preparation.
5. Place surgical drape around biopsy site and don sterile gloves.	

CUTANEOUS PUNCH BIOPSY

Procedure

Technical Action	Rationale/Amplification
1. Prepare for biopsy.	1. See **Preparation for Skin Biopsy**.
2. Press skin biopsy punch firmly onto chosen site while applying rotary motion, until entire skin has been penetrated (Fig. 6-5).	2. Use fingers of the other hand to stretch the skin over the biopsy site while the punch is introduced.

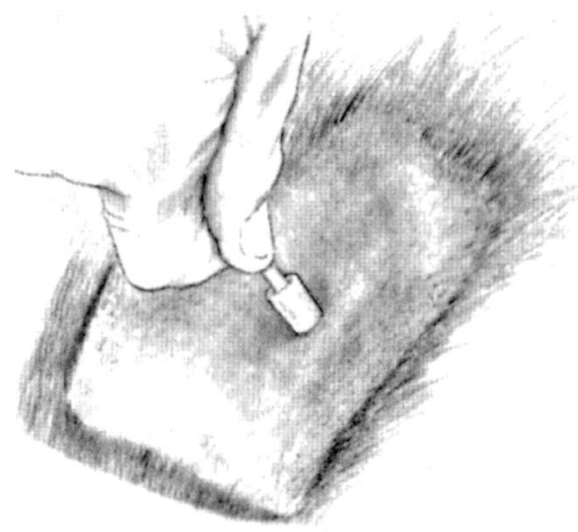

Figure 6-5 Using skin biopsy punch.

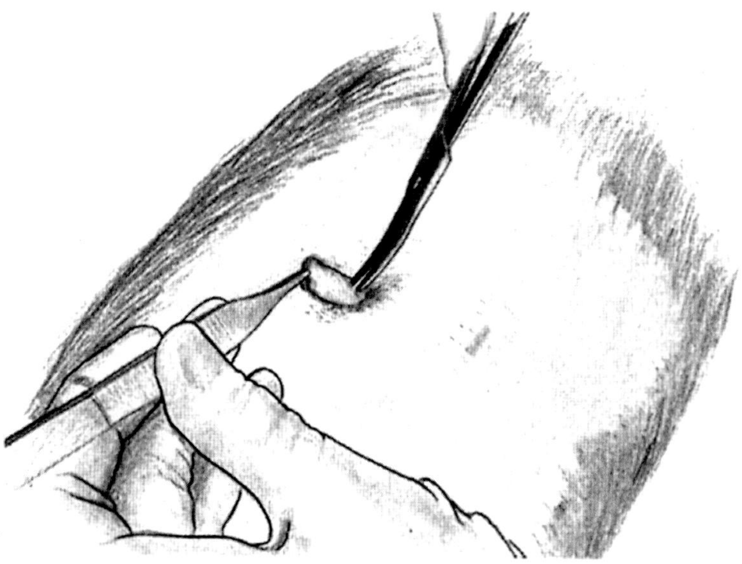

Figure 6-6 Severing base of biopsy specimen from underlying tissues.

Technical Action

3. Remove punch from site and hold firm pressure on site with sterile gauze sponges to stop bleeding.

4. If necessary, use a 25-gauge needle to skewer biopsy core and raise it above skin level. Cut base off with sharp scissors or scalpel blade (Fig. 6-6).

Rationale/Amplification

3. Hemostasis after biopsy is best achieved with firm pressure because cauterizing agents may enhance scar formation.

4. In many instances, the biopsy core will remain in situ instead of being contained in the instrument lumen.

Technical Action	Rationale/Amplification
5. Carefully remove biopsy specimen from punch instrument with 20-gauge needle.	**5.** An additional specimen may be taken for the purpose of making impression smears.
6. Blot specimen on paper to remove excess blood.	**6.** See Chapter 7.
7. Make impression smears or place in container with preservative.	**7.** See Chapter 7.
8. Suture skin incision.	**8.** One or two single interrupted sutures usually are adequate to achieve primary closure.

CUTANEOUS WEDGE BIOPSY (ELLIPTICAL INCISIONAL BIOPSY)

Procedure

Technical Action	Rationale/Amplification
1. Select appropriate biopsy site and prepare for biopsy.	**1.** Avoid traumatized, crusted, or atypical lesions. Biopsies of different stages of lesions, as well as normal tissue, should be obtained. If possible, try to take a sample that includes the transition from normal to abnormal tissue. See **Preparing for Skin Biopsy**, Nos. 1 to 5.
2. Make elliptical incision, extending from normal tissue into lesion through entire skin thickness.	**2.** A 1–2-cm long incision is usually sufficient for biopsy. A slightly longer incision may be necessary if the lesion is surrounded by fibrous tissue. To facilitate skin closure, the width of the ellipse should be no more than 50% of its length.
3. Sever any subcutaneous attachments with sharp scissors, and remove wedge of tissue created by incision (Fig. 6-7).	
4. Hold firm pressure on site with sterile gauze sponges to stop bleeding.	**4.** Hemostasis after biopsy is best achieved with firm pressure because cauterizing agents may enhance scar formation.
5. Blot biopsy specimen with paper to remove excess blood.	**5.** See Chapter 7.
6. Make impression smears and place in container with preservative.	**6.** See Chapter 7.
7. Suture skin incision.	**7.** Simple interrupted, nonabsorbable sutures are appropriate for most biopsy sites.

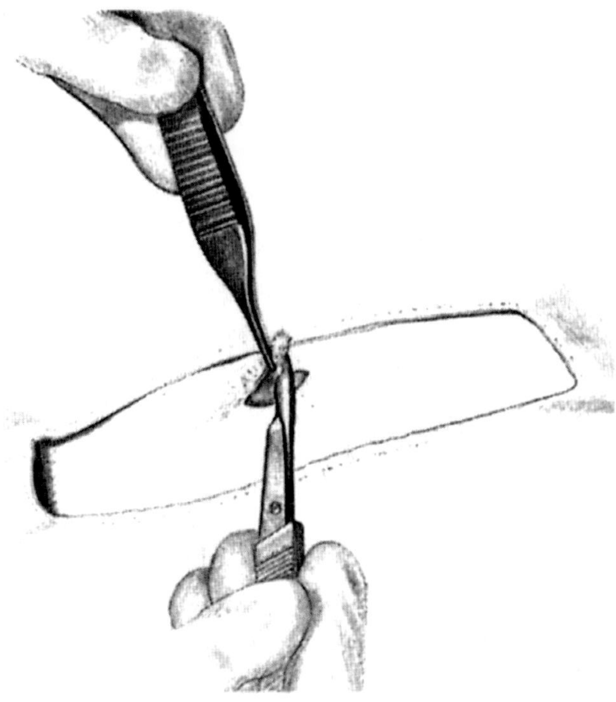

Figure 6-7 Removing cutaneous wedge by elliptical incisional biopsy.

Bibliography

Allen SK, McKeever PJ: Skin biopsy techniques. Vet Clin North Am 4(2): 269–280, 1974

Bistner SI, Ford RB: Kirk and Bistner's Handbook of Veterinary Procedures & Emergency Treatment, 6th edition. Philadelphia, WB Saunders, 1995

Clinkinbeard KD, Cowell RL, Morton RJ, Walker DB, Gowan HL, Meinkoth JH: Diagnostic cytology: Bacterial infections. Comp Con Edu for Prac Vet 17(1): 71–84, 1995

DeBoer DJ, Moriello KA: Clinical update on feline dermatophytosis—Part I. Comp Con Edu for Prac Vet 17(10): 1197–1204, 1995

Kirk RW, Bistner SI: Handbook of Veterinary Procedures and Emergency Treatment, 4th edition. Philadelphia, WB Saunders, 1985

Locke PH, Harvey RG, Mason IS, eds: BSAVA Manual of Small Animal Dermatology. Cheltenham, England, British Small Animal Veterinary Association, 1993

Medleau L, Hnilica K: Small Animal Dermatology: A Color Atlas and Therapeutic Guide, 2nd edition. Philadelphia, Saunders, 2006

Muller GH, Kirk RW: Small Animal Dermatology, 2nd edition. Philadelphia, WB Saunders, 1976

Murphy A, Schillhorn Van Veen T: Personal Communication, 1993

Stannard AA: Current concepts in small animal dermatology, 59th Annual Postgraduate Conference for Veterinarians, Michigan State University, East Lansing, MI, January 27, 1982

Chapter 7

Impression Preparations

Aim for perfection. Half right is always half wrong.
LAWRENCE LEVESON

Impression preparations (also known as touch preparations or impression smears) are samples for cytology evaluation, obtained by imprinting removed masses, biopsy specimens, or masses in situ onto microscope slides. Specimens that can be used for impression smears include ulcerated tumors, surgically excised tumors, and core biopsy specimens.

Purposes

1. To differentiate among causes of organomegaly involving lymph nodes, spleen, kidneys, liver, prostate, mammary glands, and other organs
2. To differentiate among inflammation, hyperplasia, and neoplasia as the cause of skin, subcutaneous, and other accessible tumors
3. To differentiate benign from malignant neoplasia for diagnostic and therapeutic planning purposes
4. To differentiate carcinomas from sarcomas for diagnostic and therapeutic planning purposes

Equipment Needed

- Scalpel blade
- Glass slides
- Sterile gauze
- Paper towel or blotter

Crow and Walshaw's Manual of Clinical Procedures in Dogs, Cats, Rabbits, and Rodents, Fourth Edition. Edited by Jennifer E. Boyle. © 2016 John Wiley & Sons, Inc. Published 2016 by John Wiley & Sons, Inc.
Companion Website: www.wiley.com/go/boyle/manual4e

Procedure

Technical Action	Rationale/Amplification
1. Prepare specimen in following manner: • Excised mass: Slice mass with sharp scalpel blade to expose an internal surface, and then blot until dry. • Biopsy sample: Blot specimen repeatedly until no visible fluid soils paper (Fig. 7-1). • Mass in situ: Clean surface by scraping with sterile gauze or scalpel blade. Blot mass repeatedly.	1. To ensure adequate cellular material for interpretation, a freshly cut surface free of contamination by blood and exudate is needed. Care should be taken not to crush the specimen.
2. Touch biopsy or mass lightly to a clean glass slide and withdraw immediately.	2. Firm pressure is not required. If exfoliation does not occur, the specimen may be lightly scraped. Do not rub specimen against slide. Rubbing or smearing causes distortion or rupture of cells.
3. Make several imprints on each slide (Fig. 7-2).	
4. Make several slides.	4. Having several slides allows the cytologist to use multiple stains, if necessary, for diagnosis.

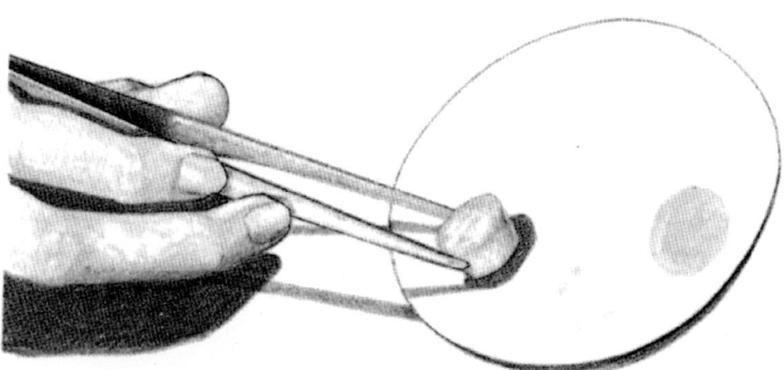

Figure 7-1 Blotting tissue specimen on filter paper until dry.

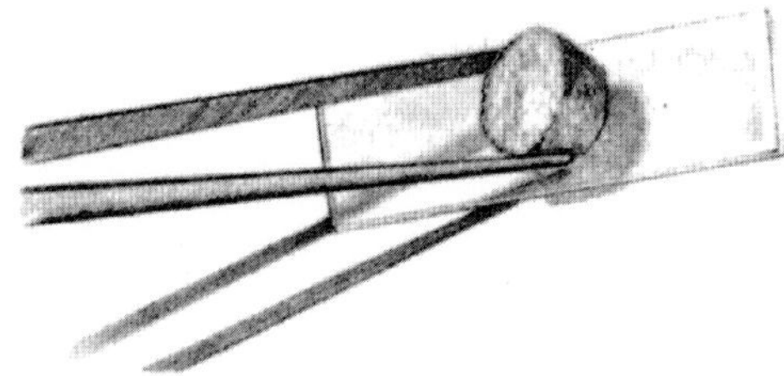

Figure 7-2 Touching tissue specimen to glass slide to make impression preparation.

Bibliography

Allen SK, McKeever PJ: Skin biopsy techniques. Vet Clin N Am 4: 269–280, 1974

Perman V, Alsaker RD, Riis RC: Cytology of the Dog and Cat, pp. 1–5. South Bend, Indiana, American Animal Hospital Association Monograph, 1979

Rebar AH: Handbook of Veterinary Cytology. St. Louis, Purina Company Monograph, 1981

Stevens JB, Perman V, Osborne CA: Biopsy sample management, staining, and examination. Vet Clin North Am 4: 233–253, 1974

Valenciano A, Cowell R: Cowell and Tyler's Diagnostic Cytology and Hematology of the Dog and Cat, 4th edition. St.Louis, Elsevier, 2014

Chapter 8

Fine-Needle Aspiration Biopsy

Not failure, but low aim, is a crime.
LOWELL

Fine-needle aspiration biopsy is a diagnostic procedure involving introduction of a narrow-gauge, rigid hypodermic needle into a tissue or organ and removal of a small amount of tissue by suction.

Purposes

1. To differentiate among causes of organomegaly involving lymph nodes, spleen, mammary glands, and other organs
2. To differentiate among inflammation, hyperplasia, and neoplasia as the cause of skin, subcutaneous, and other accessible tumors
3. To differentiate benign from malignant neoplasia for diagnostic and therapeutic planning purposes
4. To differentiate carcinomas from sarcomas for diagnostic and therapeutic planning purposes

Complications

1. Minor hemorrhage
2. Tissue damage

Equipment Needed

- 22–25-gauge, ¾-inch to 3½-inch sterile needles
- 3-mL syringe
- Glass slides

Crow and Walshaw's Manual of Clinical Procedures in Dogs, Cats, Rabbits, and Rodents, Fourth Edition. Edited by Jennifer E. Boyle. © 2016 John Wiley & Sons, Inc. Published 2016 by John Wiley & Sons, Inc.
Companion Website: www.wiley.com/go/boyle/manual4e

Procedure

Technical Action

1. With animal restrained in an appropriate position, isolate lesion in one hand.
2. Prepare skin overlying lesion.

Rationale/Amplification

1. Local or general anesthesia is not required, except in rare instances.
2. For most lesions, simple cleansing and disinfection of the skin is all that is required. Intracavitary tumors or heavily soiled areas should have the hair clipped and the skin carefully scrubbed and disinfected.

Attached syringe technique:

3. Carefully introduce needle, with syringe tightly attached, into lesion.
4. Apply negative pressure at needle bevel end by withdrawing syringe plunger (Fig. 8-1).

Attached syringe technique:

3. In large lesions, the needle is directed into the peripheral parts of the lesion to avoid the necrotic center
4. Several brisk excursions of the syringe plunger are made.

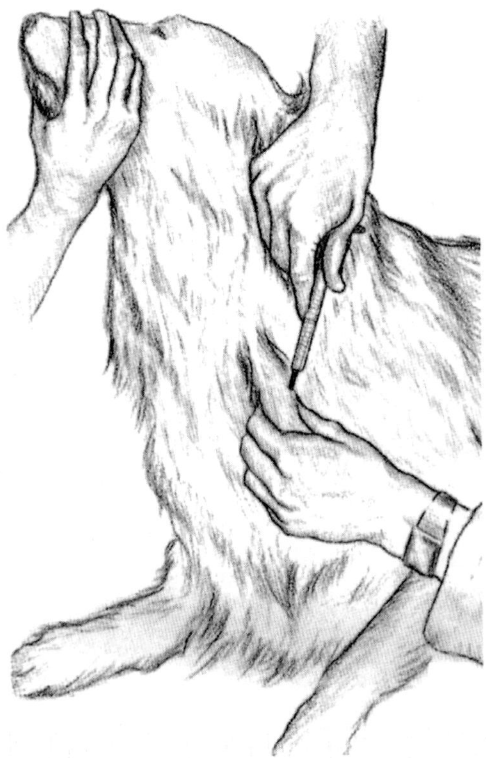

Figure 8-1 Aspiration of lymph node or other mass by brisk withdrawal of syringe plunger, creating suction at needle bevel.

Technical Action

Attached syringe technique:

5. Partially withdraw needle and redirect it into lesion (Fig. 8-2).
6. Again apply suction by several brisk movements of syringe plunger.
7. Release negative pressure by allowing syringe plunger to retract, and withdraw needle from lesion.
8. Separate needle from syringe and draw air into syringe.

Detached needle technique: (in place of steps 3–8 above).

Rationale/Amplification

Attached syringe technique:

5. This step helps to ensure adequate sampling of the lesion.

7. Release of the negative pressure retains the sample within the needle lumen.

Detached needle technique: This technique is easier and safer in animals that will not hold still and affords better control of the needle direction and depth for the operator. It also decreases the chances of accidental contamination/dilution of blood in the sample.

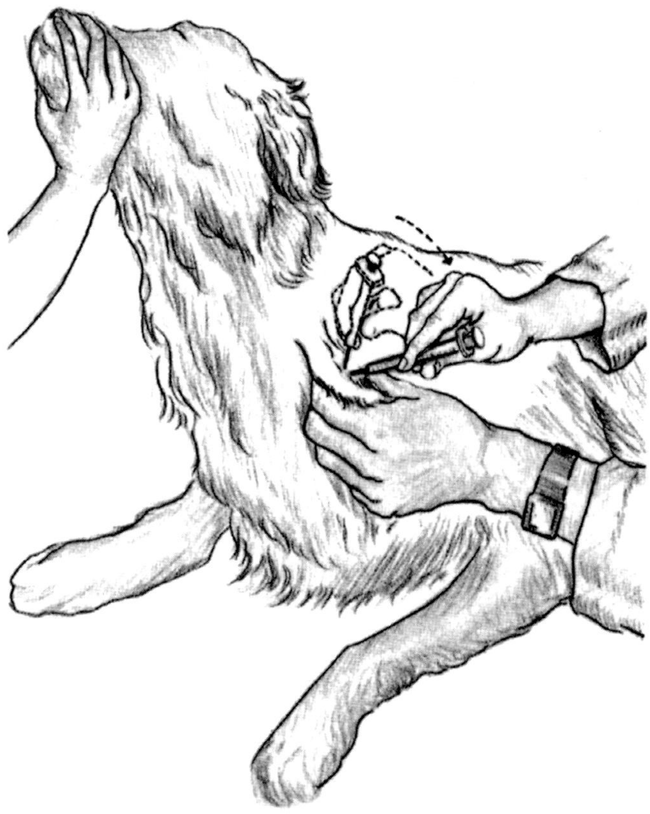

Figure 8-2 Partial withdrawal and redirection of needle/syringe assembly.

Technical Action	Rationale/Amplification
Attached syringe technique:	**Attached syringe technique:**
3. Detach needle from syringe.	
4. Carefully introduce needle into lesion.	**4.** Direct the needle into the specific portion of the nodule or cyst to be sampled. When uncertain which part to use, select the periphery rather than the center of a mass or lymph node, because the center is often necrotic and will yield a poor cytology specimen.
5. In a back and forth motion, slide needle in and out of lesion several times.	**5.** A very small amount of fluid is forced into the lumen of the needle with each pass.
6. Change direction of needle and slide needle in and out of lesion again.	**6.** Second and third passes of the needle should be in slightly different directions.
7. Repeat step 6 a third time, then withdraw needle from lesion.	
8. Draw air into syringe.	**8.** The air is used to expel the contents from the needle lumen.
9. Reattach syringe to needle and expel contents of needle lumen onto clean microscope slides (Fig. 8-3).	**9.** Expulsion should be rapid and forceful to remove all material from the needle lumen. Only a small drop of fluid is obtained in most aspirations.
10. Make smears of aspirated fluid immediately (Figs. 8-4 and 8-5).	**10.** Push smears or squash preparations are made, depending on fluid

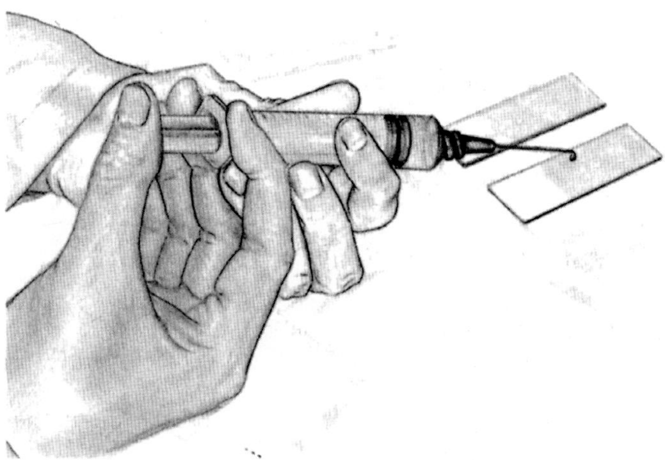

Figure 8-3 Expelling aspirated fluid from needle lumen with air-filled syringe.

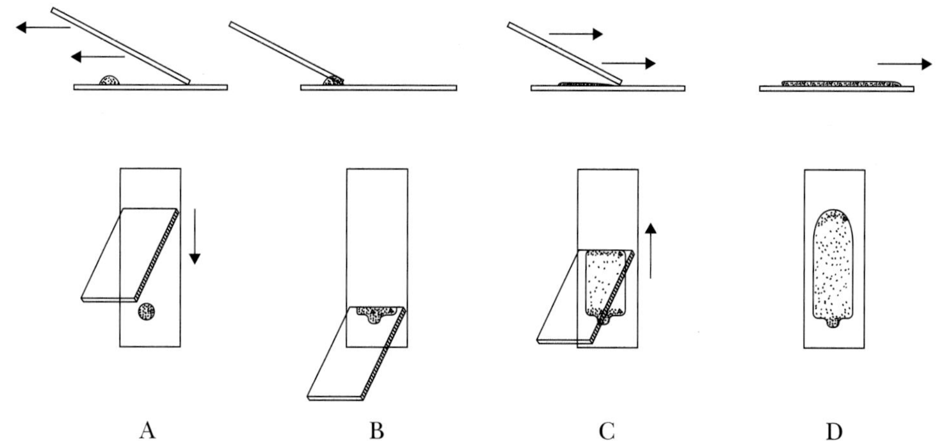

Figure 8-4 Blood smear (Push smear) technique. (A) A drop of fluid sample is placed on a glass microscope slide close to one end, then another slide is slid backward to contact the front of the drop. (B) When the drop is contacted, it rapidly spreads along the juncture between the two slides. (C) and (D) The spreader slide is then smoothly and rapidly slid forward the length of the slide, producing a smear with a feathered edge. With permission from: Diagnostic Cytology and Hematology of the Dog and Cat, Meinkoth JH, Cowell RL, Tyler RD, Morton RJ. Sample Collection and Preparation. p. 9, Copyright Elsevier (2014).

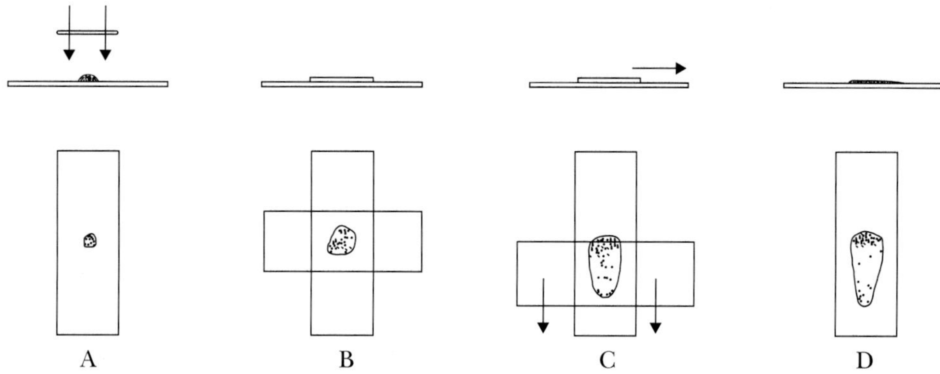

Figure 8-5 Squash smear technique (A) A portion of the aspirate is expelled onto a glass microscope slide, and another slide is placed over the sample. (B) This spreads the sample. If the sample does not spread well, gently digital pressure can be applied to the top slide. Care must be taken not to place excessive pressure on the slide, causing the cells to rupture. (C) The slides are smoothly slid apart. (D) This usually produces well- spread smears but may result in excessive cell rupture. With permission from: Diagnostic Cytology and Hematology of the Dog and Cat, Meinkoth JH, Cowell RL, Tyler RD, Morton RJ. Sample Collection and Preparation. p. 9, Copyright Elsevier (2014).

Technical Action	Rationale/Amplification
Attached syringe technique:	**Attached syringe technique:**
	viscosity. Squash preparations are more successful in producing thin smears when the fluid is highly viscous. Mix thick fluids with a small drop of physiologic saline prior to making smears to decrease shredding/shearing of nuclei. Smears may be stained with a variety of pigments. Whenever possible, three or four slides should be made.

Bibliography

Rebar AH: Handbook of Veterinary Cytology. St. Louis, Purina Company, 1981

Soderstrom N: Fine-Needle Aspiration Biopsy. New York, Grune & Stratton, 1996

Valenciano A, Cowell R: Cowell and Tyler's Diagnostic Cytology and Hematology of the Dog and Cat, 4th edition. St. Louis, Elsevier, 2014

Chapter 9

Ophthalmic Procedures

You can observe a lot just by watching.
YOGI BERRA

This chapter describes a number of diagnostic and therapeutic procedures that are commonly used in caring for the eye.

Diagnostic Procedures

Schirmer tear test
- Corneoconjunctival culture
- Staining of the cornea
- Corneoconjunctival smear and scraping
- Measuring intraocular pressure

NOTE: *These procedures are listed in an order conducive to proceeding from one procedure to the next. For proper management and use of the procedures, consideration of the animal's signs and careful planning of the appropriate sequence is recommended. Read the rationale/amplification comments in each section thoroughly.*

Therapeutic Procedures

- Topical administration of ophthalmic medication
- Subconjunctival injection
- Flushing of nasolacrimal duct

Restraint and Positioning

An assistant restrains the animal in sternal recumbency or in a sitting position for most of the procedures. Topical administration of ophthalmic medication can usually be

Crow and Walshaw's Manual of Clinical Procedures in Dogs, Cats, Rabbits, and Rodents, Fourth Edition. Edited by Jennifer E. Boyle. Published 2016 by John Wiley & Sons, Inc.
Companion Website: www.wiley.com/go/boyle/manual4e

accomplished without the aid of an assistant. If the animal is fractious, it will be necessary to apply a muzzle or to tranquilize the animal.

SCHIRMER TEAR TEST

Purpose

To assess the amount of tear production in each eye.

Complications

1. Corneal irritation
2. Corneoconjunctival infection

Equipment Needed

- Topical ophthalmic anesthetic
- Schirmer tear test strips* (Fig. 9-1)

Procedure

Technical Action	Rationale/Amplification
1. Perform Schirmer tear test I before any other procedures on eye.	1. The results of the test will be affected by other procedures involving eyelid manipulations, instillation of topical materials, and procurement of specimens.
2. While keeping test strip within sterile package, fold the strip at a right angle at the notch above the rounded tip.	2. The notched end of the strip should be kept sterile because this is the portion that will be placed in contact with the eye.
3. Remove sterile strip from package and insert folded end in the conjunctival sac with the calibrated end facing out of the eye (Fig. 9-2).	3. Avoid moving the strip across the cornea. In the Schirmer tear test I, the rate of basal and reflex tear production is measured as the animal forms tears in response to the sensation of the strip contacting the eye.

* http://www.merck-animal-health-usa.com

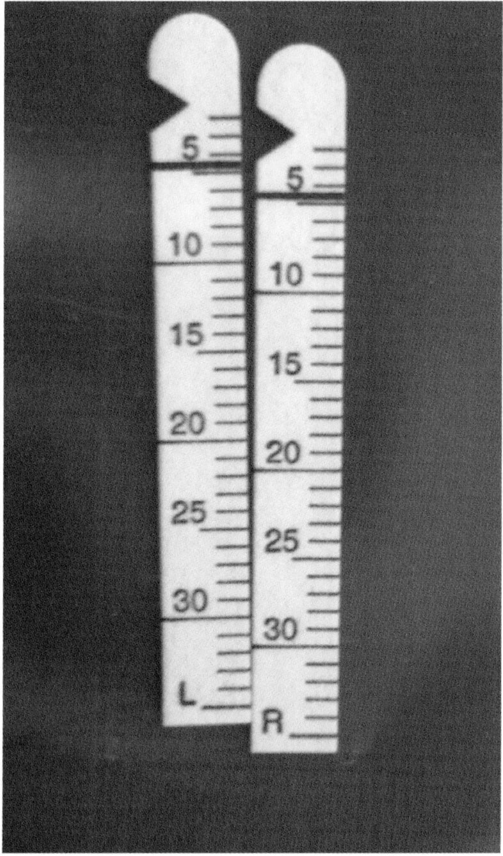

Figure 9-1 Schirmer tear test strips with millimeter scale.

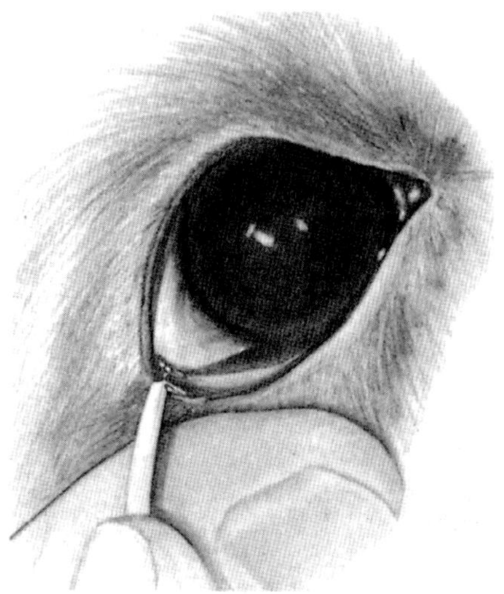

Figure 9-2 Schirmer tear test strip in place between lower eyelid and cornea.

Technical Action	Rationale/Amplification
4. Hold strip in place for 1 minute and prevent animal from rubbing eye.	
5. Remove strip and measure length of strip from notch to wet/dry interface according to package instructions.	**5.** Read quickly to avoid false migration of dye (higher than actual result) or drying of the strip (lower than actual result). The normal rate of tear production, as measured by the Schirmer tear test I, in cats is 20.2 ± 4.5 mm and in dogs is 18.64 ± 4.47 mm/min to 23.90 ± 5.73 mm/min, with greater than 15 mm/min desired.
6. To perform Schirmer tear test II **a)** Lift upper eyelid with index finger and instill 1–2 drops of topical ophthalmic anesthetic at 12 o'clock position on globe (Fig. 9-3). **b)** Wait 30 to 60 seconds. **c)** Prevent animal from rubbing its eye.	**6.** Specimens for bacteriologic cultures should be obtained before conducting Schirmer tear test II because topical solutions can interfere with culture results.
7. Repeat Nos. 2–5 as for Schirmer tear test I.	**7.** The Schirmer tear test II measures basal tear flow. The value obtained should be approximately one half that of the Schirmer tear test I.

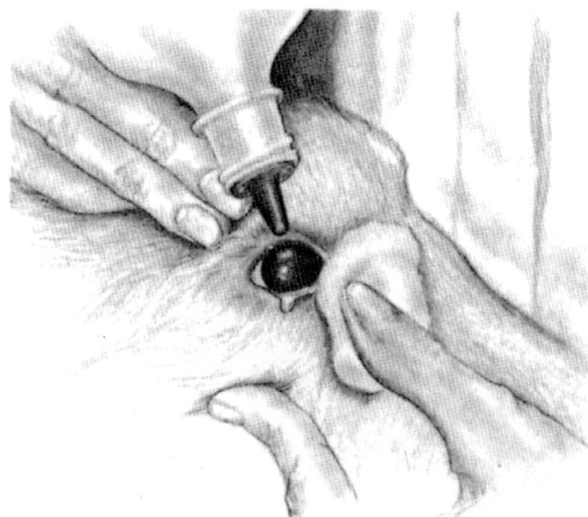

Figure 9-3 Instilling topical ophthalmic anesthetic. Note that the drops are placed at the 12 o'clock position on the globe.

CORNEOCONJUNCTIVAL CULTURE

Purposes

1. To identify bacterial, fungal, and other pathogens of the cornea and conjunctiva, especially in severe, chronic, or nonresponsive conditions
2. To determine the antibiotic sensitivity of corneoconjunctival pathogens

Complication

Corneal irritation

Equipment Needed

- Sterile swabs for bacterial and fungal cultures
- Tube with transport medium
- Specific bacterial and fungal culture media (if desired)

Procedure

Technical Action	Rationale/Amplification
1. Obtain specimens for culture before instilling any topical ophthalmic medications.	1. Topical medications, including anesthetics, can interfere with culture results.
2. Moisten end of culture swab with liquid transport medium.	2. There is better recovery of organisms and less chance of corneal irritation if a moistened swab is used to obtain the specimen.
3. Evert lower eyelid by pulling skin of lower eyelid ventrally with index finger.	3. Do not put finger in palpebral fissure.
4. Gently rub swab on cornea and/or conjunctival sac, avoiding eyelid margins (Fig. 9-4).	4. Debris and normal skin flora on eyelid margins can interfere with the accuracy of culture results.
5. Replace swab in transport tube or inoculate culture media immediately	5. Transport inoculated media to laboratory as soon as possible.

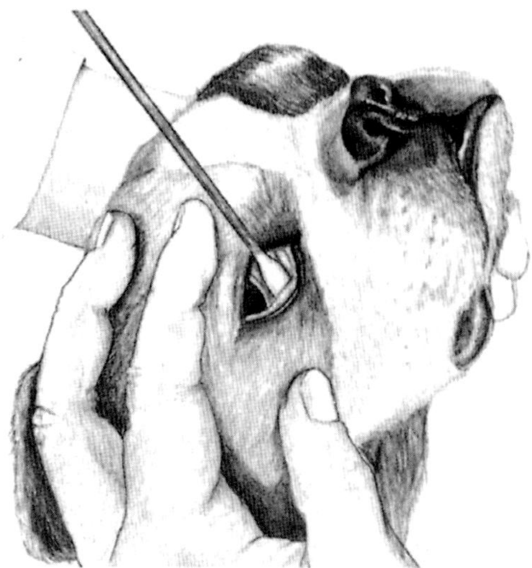

Figure 9-4 Obtaining specimen for corneoconjunctival culture.

STAINING THE CORNEA

Purposes

1. To determine presence, location, and severity of corneal ulcers
2. To demonstrate patency of nasolacrimal duct

Equipment Needed

- Ophthalmic irrigating solution
- Sterile fluorescein impregnated strips or fluorescein ophthalmic solution

Procedure

Technical Action

1. Perform corneal staining after Schirmer tear test I and after specimens have been obtained for bacteriologic culture and cytology but before instilling topical ophthalmic anesthetic.

Rationale/Amplification

1. The stain will interfere with the results of these tests. Use of a topical ophthalmic anesthetic may result in a false-positive stain reaction.

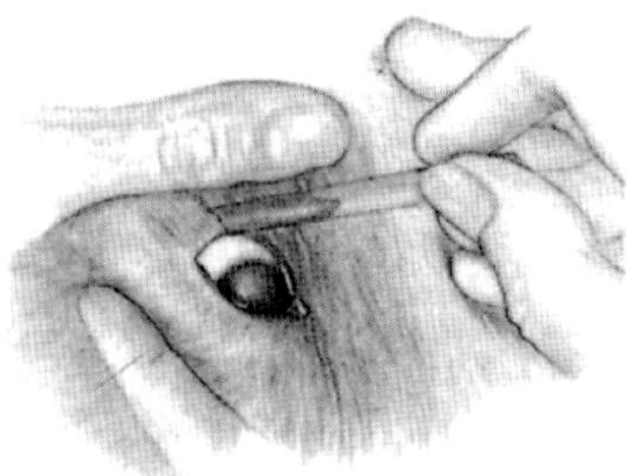

Figure 9-5 Staining of cornea with fluorescein. Note that fluorescein strip is applied to the bulbar conjunctiva rather than directly to the cornea.

Technical Action	Rationale/Amplification
2. Moisten end of sterile fluorescein strip with ophthalmic irrigating solution or artificial tear solution.	**2.** Sterile fluorescein strips are recommended rather than the fluorescein solution because the solution can easily become contaminated with microorganisms.
3. Elevate upper eyelid by pulling dorsally on skin of upper lid.	
4. Place moistened tip of fluorescein strip against bulbar conjunctiva for one or two seconds (Fig. 9-5).	**4.** It is important to avoid touching the fluorescein strip directly to the cornea because this may cause staining artifacts.
5. Remove strip and allow animal to blink.	**5.** Blinking helps to distribute the stain.
6. Liberally flush eye with ophthalmic irrigating solution.	**6.** The sodium ions in the solution will enhance the stain.
7. Examine cornea in a partially darkened room.	**7.** The exposed corneal stroma in an ulcer stains bright green with fluorescein. Use of an ultraviolet light source (i.e. Wood's lamp) may enhance the observer's perception of stromal stain retention.
8. Observe external nares for emergence of green dye.	**8.** The appearance of fluorescein dye at the nostril indicates patency of the nasolacrimal duct.

NOTE: *An alternate method of staining the cornea is to aseptically drop a fluorescein stain applicator into a 3 or 5ml syringe with the plunger removed and needle attached, then sterile saline or water (label bottle specifically and only for this purpose) can be drawn into the syringe, the needle removed and the stain dripped into the patient's eye. This will alleviate concerns about damaging the cornea. Do not reuse due to risk of contamination* (Figs. 9-6 and 9-7).

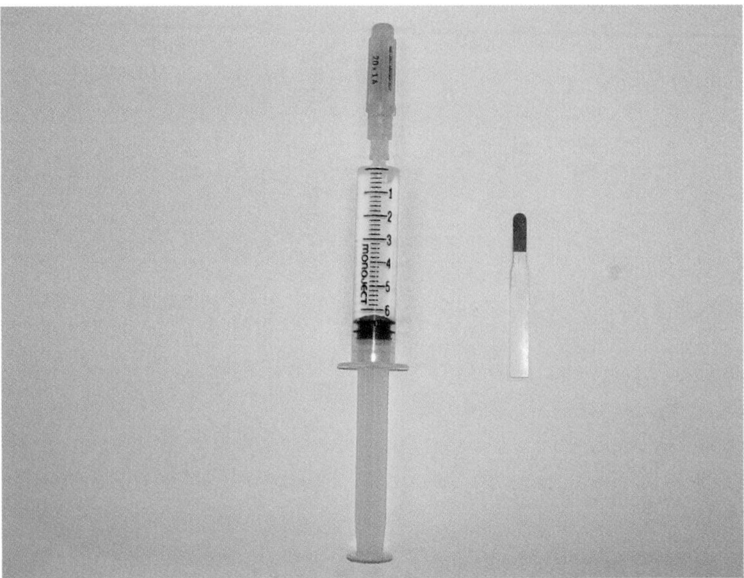

Figure 9-6 Fluorescein stain applicator added to a 5 ml syringe of sterile saline. Photo courtesy of C Knightly.

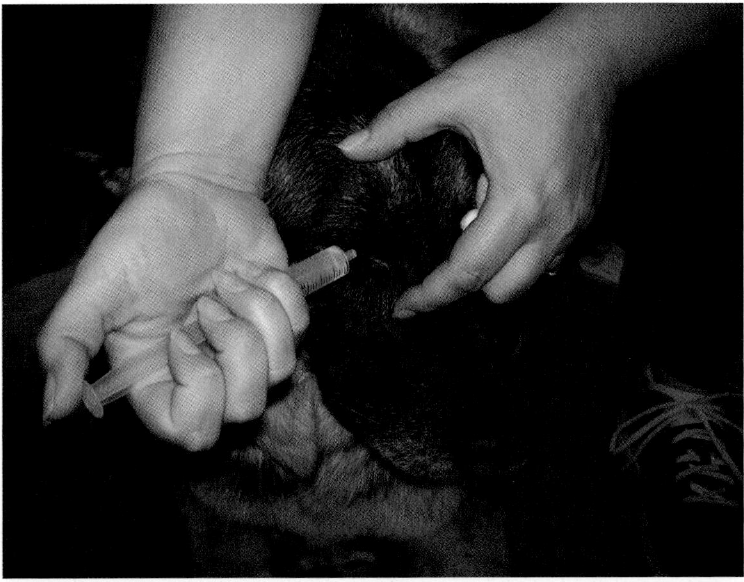

Figure 9-7 Applying fluorescein stain solution to eye. Photo courtesy of C Knightly.

CORNEOCONJUNCTIVAL SMEAR AND SCRAPING

Purpose

To obtain specimen(s) for cytology examination.

Complication

Corneal irritation.

Equipment Needed

- Topical ophthalmic anesthetic
- Glass slides
- Stains (one or more may be selected)
  - Gram's stain
  - Modified Giemsa stain
  - 2 mL of Wolbach modified Giemsa tissue stain
    - 2 mL of Wright's buffer (pH 6.8)
    - 50 mL of distilled water
  - New methylene blue stain
- Sterile cotton swabs for smear
- Sterile metal ocular spatula for scraping

Procedure

Technical Action	Rationale/Amplification
1. Remove mucus or exudate from eyelids (Fig. 9-8).	1. Clean eyelids gently with water moistened cotton balls so that excess debris is not collected inadvertently with the specimen.
2. Lift upper eyelid with index finger to expose sclera and instill one or two drops of topical ophthalmic anesthetic at 12 o'clock position on globe.	2. It is important that the anesthetic flows down over the entire cornea for adequate desensitization to occur.
3. Wait 30 to 60 seconds.	
4. Evert lower eyelid by pulling downward on skin just below lower eyelid margin.	
5. For smear preparation, swab cornea and conjunctiva with cotton-tipped applicator, avoiding eyelid margins (Fig. 9-4). For scraping, gently rub	5. Debris and normal skin flora on eyelid margins can interfere with the accuracy of cytology examination.

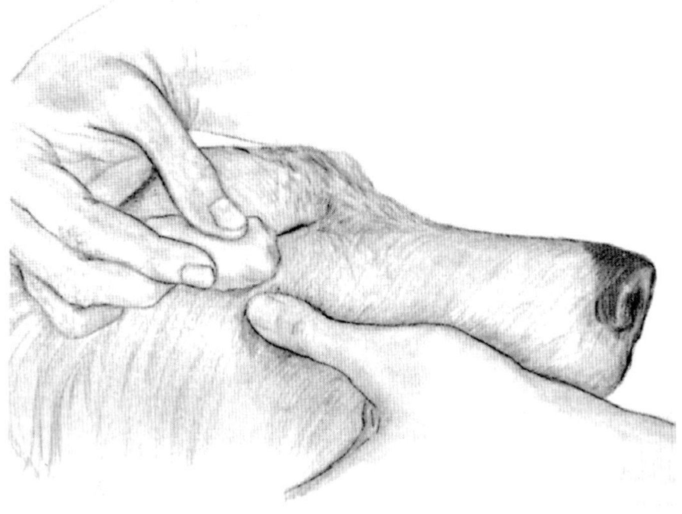

Figure 9-8 Removing mucus or exudate from eyelids.

Technical Action

area of cornea or conjunctiva with metal ocular spatula until a small droplet of material is collected (Fig. 9-9).

6. Roll material from swab onto clean glass slides (Fig. 9-10). Spread material from scraping over glass slides.

Rationale/Amplification

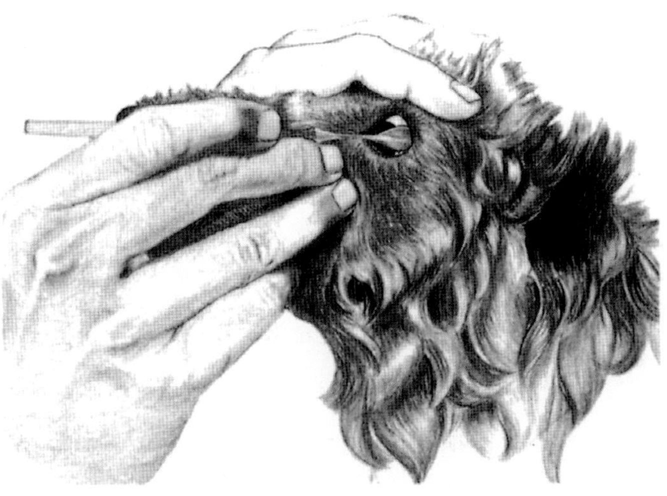

Figure 9-9 Obtaining corneoconjunctival scraping.

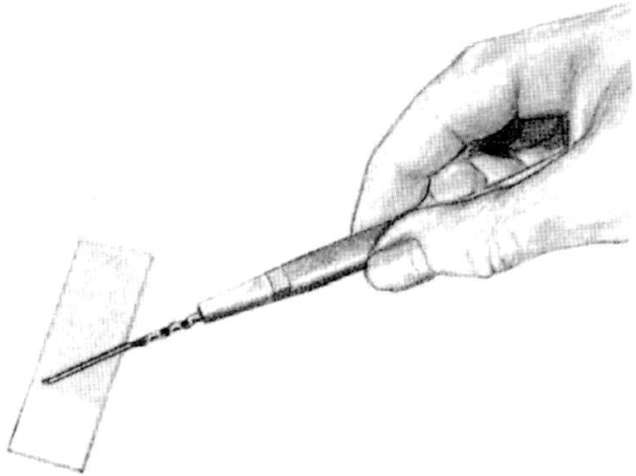

Figure 9-10 Placing corneoconjunctival specimen on glass slide.

Technical Action	Rationale/Amplification
7. Allow slides to air dry and then stain.	**7.** A Gram-stained slide can be examined for bacteria. The modified Giemsa stain is useful for cytology examination.
8. For Giemsa staining: Fix slide for 5 minutes in absolute methanol; stain with modified Giemsa stain for 20 minutes; rinse with running tap water and allow to air dry.	**8.** For Giemsa staining: Fix slide for 5 minutes in absolute methanol; stain with modified Giemsa stain for 20 minutes; rinse with running tap water and allow to air dry.
9. Prevent animal from rubbing its eye.	**9.** Instillation of topical medication often causes an animal to rub its eye.

MEASURING INTRAOCULAR PRESSURE

Purpose

To measure intraocular pressure.

Complication

Corneal irritation or erosion.

Equipment Needed

- Topical ophthalmic anesthetic
- Tonometer (Applanation or Rebound)

Procedure—Applanation Technique (TonoPen®)

Technical Action	Rationale/Amplification
1. Gently apply a sterile protective tip cover so that the edge rests in the groove at the base of the sensor tip.	**1.** The cover should sit smoothly over the applanation tip, but not be so tight as to restrict the movement of the sensor tip.
2. Lift upper eyelid with index finger to expose sclera and instill one or two drops of topical ophthalmic anesthetic at 12 o'clock position on globe.	**2.** It is important that the anesthetic flows down over the entire cornea for adequate desensitization to occur.
3. Wait 30 to 60 seconds.	
4. Tilt animal's snout upward toward ceiling and retract lower eyelid with finger of one hand.	**4.** Avoid applying pressure to the globe.
5. With other hand, grasp tonometer with thumb and index finger, while resting other fingers on animal's skull just above upper eyelid.	**5.** Resting the hand holding the tonometer on the animal's head helps to steady the instrument during the procedure.
6. Place sheathed tip of tonometer gently on central part of cornea such that tonometer is perpendicular to cornea and to floor (Fig. 9-11).	**6.** An applanation tonometer works with only a light touch to the cornea. It is not necessary or desirable to press it firmly against the eye. Pressure on the jugular vein or excessive pressure on the eye will falsely elevate the tonometry results.

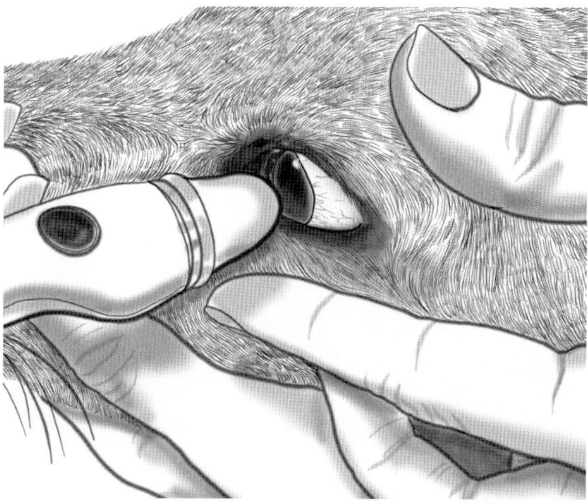

Figure 9-11 Touching applanation tonometer to cornea.

Technical Action	Rationale/Amplification
7. When instrument beeps, note reading.	**7.** In general, the tonometer will beep right away if the instrument is held exactly perpendicular to the cornea so that the flat tip is parallel to the cornea.
8. Lift instrument off cornea slightly.	
9. Repeat procedure two more times.	**9.** The average of three readings is used. Normal IOP values in dogs and cats are 15–25 mm Hg.
10. Remove rubber sheath and wipe tonometer clean after each use. Enclose in container.	**10.** The rubber sheath prevents cross-contamination between animals.
11. Prevent animal from rubbing its eye.	**11.** Instillation of topical medication often is followed by the animal attempting to rub its eye.

Procedure- Rebound Technique (TonoVet®)

Technical Action	Rationale/Amplification
1. Insert a new (arrow) rebound tip in the hand piece, and activate the hand piece according to manufacturer instructions.	**1.** Because of the limited corneal contact, topical anesthetic is not required for the rebound tonometer.
2. The animal should be positioned so that the probe can be aimed perpendicular and central to the ocular surface.	**2.** The probe shoots and rebounds on a flat plane.
3. Hold the rebound probe slightly in front of the cornea and parallel to the floor with thumb on the lower button.	**3.** The rebound probe launched from the tonometer contacts the cornea and rebounds back into the instrument.
4. 4. Press the lower button. Repeat until the tonometer's audible tone changes, indicating that 3 readings have been accepted and averaged.	**4.** Normal IOP values in dogs and cats are 15–25 mm Hg.

TOPICAL ADMINISTRATION OF OPHTHALMIC MEDICATION

Purpose

To medicate cornea, conjunctiva, and anterior uveal tract.

Complication

Self-trauma to the eye by the animal.

Equipment Needed

- Ophthalmic irrigating solution
- Cotton
- Ophthalmic solution or ointment
- Bandaging materials for paws (if necessary):
- Gauze
- Adhesive tape, 1 or 2 inches in width
- Elizabethan collar (if necessary)

Procedure

Technical Action	Rationale/Amplification
1. Clean eyelids and adjacent facial skin with cotton moistened with warm water.	**1.** Keep animal's lids closed during cleansing to prevent trauma to cornea
2. Remove debris on cornea and conjunctival sac by everting eyelids and flushing thoroughly with ophthalmic irrigating solution.	**2.** The eye and eyelids should be cleaned before instilling medication to ensure effectiveness of treatment.
3. Hold solution or ointment container between thumb and index finger of one hand while using third finger or heel of hand to lift upper eyelid.	
4. Instill one or two drops of solution or small ribbon of ointment on sclera at 12 o'clock position (Fig. 9-12). Then release eyelid.	**4.** It is important to avoid contaminating the medicine bottle or tube by letting it touch the eye or eyelid.
5. If instilling several medications, wait at least 1 minute between applications, and always instill solutions before ointments.	**5.** Solutions cannot readily penetrate a film of ointment. Topical medications will enter the nasolacrimal duct and therefore may be licked from the nose. Atropine has a bitter taste and may induce salivation.
6. Apply petroleum-based ointment to facial skin adjacent to eye if ocular discharge is present.	**6.** The petroleum-based ointment will prevent scalding of the skin by the ocular discharges.
7. Note in animal's medical record that medication was given.	**7.** Note date, time, medication, eye(s) medicated, comments, and initials.

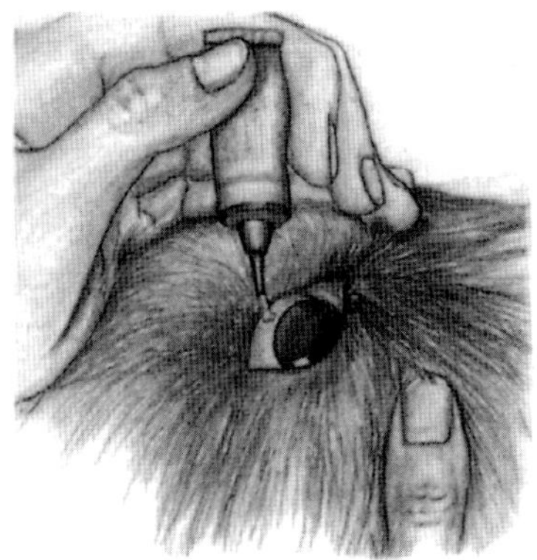

Figure 9-12 Instilling ophthalmic ointment.

Technical Action

8. Prevent self-trauma to eye by bandaging dewclaws or entire feet, or by placing Elizabethan collar on animal.

Rationale/Amplification

8. Animals commonly try to rub the eyes after topical medications, particularly solutions, are instilled.

SUBCONJUNCTIVAL INJECTION

Purpose

To medicate the anterior uveal tract.

Complications

1. Systemic over dosage
2. Penetration of the globe by needle

Equipment Needed

- Cotton
- Ophthalmic irrigating solution
- Topical ophthalmic anesthetic
- 25-gauge needle
- Tuberculin syringe
- Ocular fixation forceps
- Magnifying loupe (if desired)

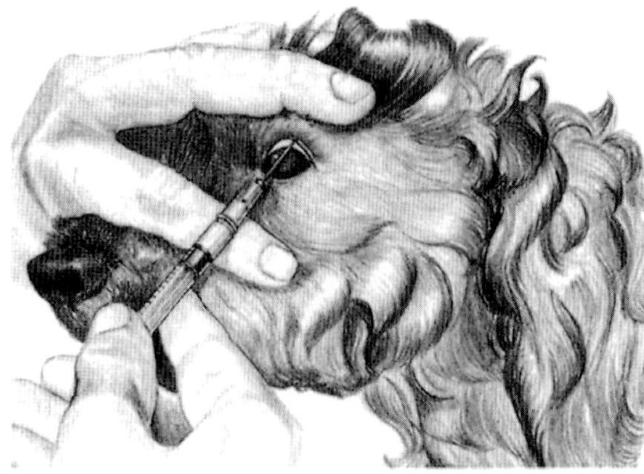

Figure 9-13 Performing subconjunctival injection.

Procedure

Technical Action	Rationale/Amplification
1. Clean eyelids and cornea as previously described.	
2. Lift upper eyelid to expose sclera and instill one or two drops of topical ophthalmic anesthetic at 12 o'clock position on globe.	2. It is important that the anesthetic flows down over the entire eye for adequate desensitization to occur.
3. Wait 30 to 60 seconds.	
4. Ask assistant to lift animal's upper eyelid.	
5. Grasp bulbar conjunctiva with ocular fixation forceps and insert needle under bulbar conjunctiva (Fig. 9-13).	
6. Withdraw syringe plunger slightly. If no blood appears in syringe, inject medication. If blood appears in syringe, remove needle and select different site for injection.	6. No more than 0.25 mL should be injected at any one site.
7. Note in animal's medical record that medication was given.	7. Note date, time, medication, eye(s) medicated, comments, and initials.

FLUSHING NASOLACRIMAL DUCTS

Purposes

1. To determine patency of nasolacrimal duct
2. To relieve minor obstruction of nasolacrimal duct

Complication

Corneal irritation.

Equipment Needed

- Cotton
- Ophthalmic irrigating solution
- Topical ophthalmic anesthetic
- Sterile blunt metal probe (lacrimal duct dilator), 18–22-gauge
- Sterile cannula
- Syringe containing 5 mL sterile saline

Procedure

Technical Action	Rationale/Amplification
1. Clean eyelids and cornea as previously described.	
2. Lift upper eyelid to expose sclera and instill one or two drops of topical ophthalmic anesthetic at 12 o'clock position on globe.	
3. Wait 30 to 60 seconds.	
4. Dilate upper and lower openings (puncta) of nasolacrimal duct with blunt metal probe of appropriate diameter (Fig. 9-14).	**4.** The puncta are located close to the medial canthus. Entering the opening is facilitated by slowly moving the metal probe along the inner lid margin toward the medial canthus while tensing the lid. The upper punctum is entered more easily than the lower.
5. Cannulate upper or lower punctum with commercial lacrimal cannula or with 20-gauge (or 22-gauge) Teflon or polyethylene intravenous catheter (with needle removed).	**5.** Flushing of the duct can be accomplished by cannulating only one of the puncta.
6. Flush 3–5 mL sterile saline through cannulated punctum (Fig. 9-15).	**6.** If all of the flushing solution exits through the other punctum rather than at the nostril, occlude the other punctum with finger tip or cotton swab.
7. See Staining the Cornea for use of fluorescein stain as an alternative method for determining patency of nasolacrimal duct.	**7.** The emergence of fluorescein at the external naris indicates the patency of the nasolacrimal duct.

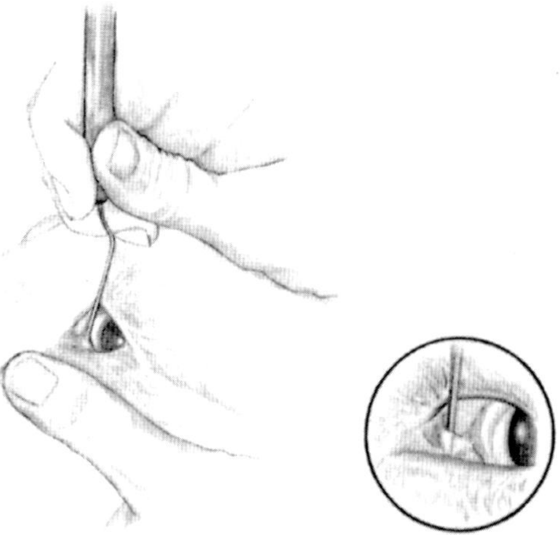

Figure 9-14 Dilating puncta of nasolacrimal duct with blunt metal probe.

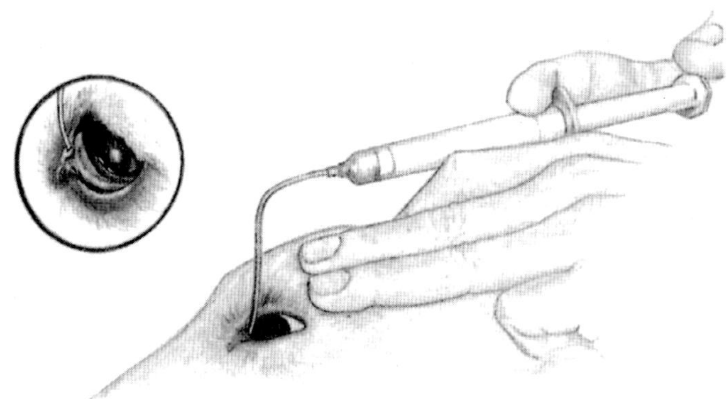

Figure 9-15 Flushing nasolacrimal duct.

Bibliography

Brightman AH: Current concepts in ocular pharmacology. Vet Clin North Am 10(2): 261–280, 1980

Brunner LS, Suddarth DS: The Lippincott Manual of Nursing Practice, 3rd edition. Philadelphia, JB Lippincott, 1982

Glaze MB: Care of the ophthalmic patient. Compend Contin Educ for AHT 1(4): 173–178, 1980

Helper LC: Magrane's Canine Ophthalmology, 4th edition. Philadelphia, Lea and Febiger, 1989

Kural E, Lindley D, Krohne S: Canine glaucoma Part I. Comp Contin Educ for Prac Vet 17(8): 1017–1026, 1995

Leiva M, Naranjo C, Peña MT: Comparison of the rebound tonometer (ICare) to the applanation tonometer (Tonopen XL) in normotensive dogs. Vet Ophthalmol 9: 17–21, 2006

Magrane WC: Canine Ophthalmology, 3rd edition. Philadelphia, Lea & Febiger, 1977

Plumb D, Veterinary drug handbook, 8th edition. Oxford, Wiley-Blackwell, 2015

Pratt PW (ed): Medical Nursing for Animal Health Technicians. Santa Barbara, CA, American Veterinary Publications, 1985

Severin GA: Veterinary Ophthalmology Notes, 2nd edition. Fort Collins, Colorado State University Press, 1979
Slatter DH: Fundamentals of Veterinary Ophthalmology. Philadelphia, WB Saunders, 1981
Whitley RD: Diagnostic and treatment techniques of corneal diseases in small animals. Compend Contin Educ for AHT 1(2): 64–69, 1980
Wilkie, D: Determining Intraocular Pressure, NAVC Clinician's Brief 11(2): 77–80, Feb 2013
Williams, D and Kraetz de Oliveira J: Potential Variation in Tonometry Values Using the Tonovet Rebound Tonometer in the Canine Eye, British Small Animal Veterinary Congress, 2014

Chapter 10

Ear Care

Use what talents you possess: the woods would be very silent if no birds sang there except those that sang best.

HENRY VAN DYKE

Ear care includes obtaining samples for cytology and/or culture as well as cleaning and medicating the external ear canal.

Purposes

1. To obtain specimens for diagnosis of external ear canal diseases
2. To remove cerumen (waxy material), foreign objects, matted hair, and other debris
3. To treat otitis externa
4. To prepare site for surgical procedures on the external ear canal

Complications

1. Rupture of tympanic membrane
2. Injury to external ear canal

Equipment Needed

- Cotton
- Bulb syringe or 10-mL hypodermic syringe
- Solution and waste bowls
- Cotton-tipped swabs
- Hemostat for hair removal (if necessary)
- Mild soap or ceruminolytic agents
- Otoscope—fiber optic, if possible
- Prescribed medication

Crow and Walshaw's Manual of Clinical Procedures in Dogs, Cats, Rabbits, and Rodents, Fourth Edition. Edited by Jennifer E. Boyle. Published 2016 by John Wiley & Sons, Inc.
Companion Website: www.wiley.com/go/boyle/manual4e

NOTE: *When using a standard otoscope, the edges of the eardrum are partially obscured by the ear canal walls, even in animals with healthy ears. In general, only the central 40–60% of the tympanic membrane is visualized through an otoscope cone. Consequently, perimeter tears or avulsions of the tympanum may not be seen. Most fiber optic otoscopes, when used properly, provide visualization of the tympanic membrane perimeter.*

Restraint and Positioning

Most tractable animals will tolerate ear cleaning and medicating with minimal restraint. An assistant holds the animal in sitting position or sternal recumbency, using one hand around the animal's snout to stabilize the animal's head. Fractious animals or those with painful ear infections may require general anesthesia or chemical tranquilization.

Procedure

Technical Action	Rationale/Amplification
1. Examine each ear carefully. Check for odor, ulceration, reddening, proliferation of tissue, discharge, or debris. If signs of inflammation or exudate are noted, aseptically inoculate sterile cotton-tipped swabs with ear canal contents by inserting swab tip 1–2 cm into vertical canal.	**1.** The external ear canal is composed of a lateral vertical segment, which leads to a horizontal portion that terminates medially at the tympanic membrane. It may be difficult to see the eardrum in inflamed ears or in older dogs due to narrowing and hardening of the ear canal. When collecting ear swabs, obtain a sample for microbiologic culture first, and then make a second swab for cytology. In severe cases, it is wise to sample from each ear and submit separate cultures for each ear. Cytology examination may reveal a preponderance of yeast organisms, Gram positive bacteria, or Gram negative bacteria. Such information is useful when initiating treatment.
2. Examine each ear with otoscope starting with more normal ear (Fig. 10-1).	**2.** Apply lateral tension to ear pinna (flap) to straighten ear canal as otoscope is advanced. A fiber optic otoscope, with or without video attachment, affords significantly better visualization of the ear canal and tympanic membrane. It is important to avoid contaminating a normal ear with debris from an infected one.

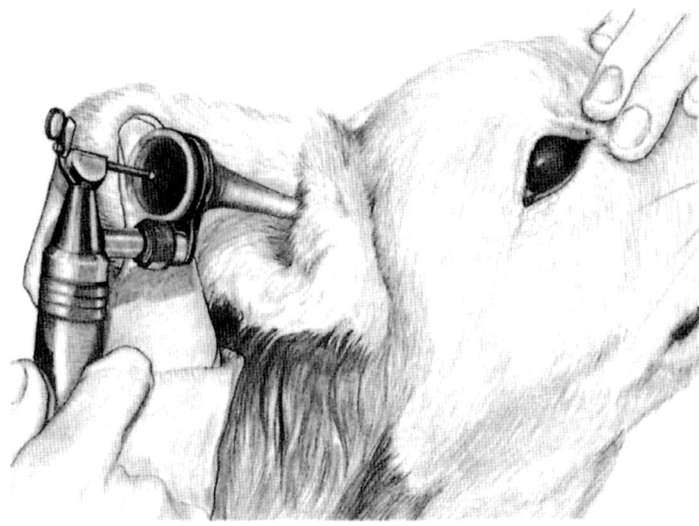

Figure 10-1 Examining ear with otoscope.

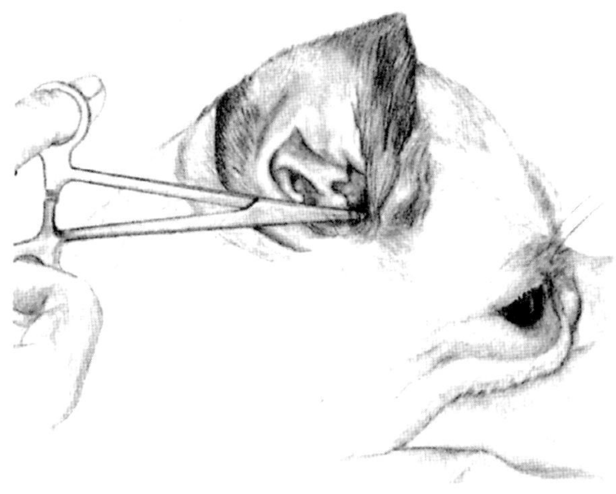

Figure 10-2 Removing hairs from external ear canal.

Technical Action

3. Remove hair, if present, by grasping groups of hairs with hemostat and twisting handle of hemostat until hairs are gently removed (Fig. 10-2).

Rationale/Amplification

3. Poodles and some terriers normally have hair growing in their external ear canals. An alternative method of hair removal is simply to pluck the hairs out using fingers.

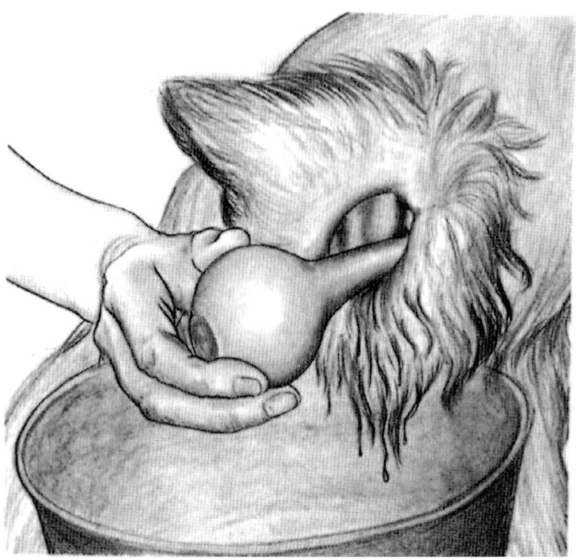

Figure 10-3 Instilling liquid agents into ear with bulb syringe.

Technical Action	Rationale/Amplification
4. If eardrum appears intact, instill ceruminolytic agent by dropper or mild soapy water by bulb syringe (Fig. 10-3) and gently massage skin over external ear canal. If tympanic membrane cannot be seen, use only sterile water or saline for flushing.	**4.** Excess irrigating solution can be caught in a waste bowl held beneath the ear. Massaging the skin over the external ear canal helps to loosen accumulated debris. Using a new bulb syringe for each animal will prevent contamination.
5. Use pieces of cotton to remove loosened debris and discharge from ear canal (Fig. 10-4).	**5.** Cleansing of the ear canal with cotton wrapped around an index finger is a method that involves virtually no danger of rupturing the tympanic membrane.
6. Repeat procedure as needed to remove all visible debris.	**6.** Allowing the animal to shake its head from time to time will help dislodge debris in the deeper portions of the ear canal.
7. Rinse ear canal with warm water or normal saline.	**7.** Residual soap or other cleansing agent may be irritating and can interfere with otic medication.
8. Cleanse folds of skin on interior part of pinna with cotton-tipped swabs (Fig. 10-5.	**8.** Cotton-tipped swabs may be safely used on the ear flap, but their use in the deeper portions of the ear canal is not recommended unless the animal is anesthetized.
9. Dry ear canal as thoroughly as possible.	**9.** Use pieces of cotton and allow the animal to shake its head.

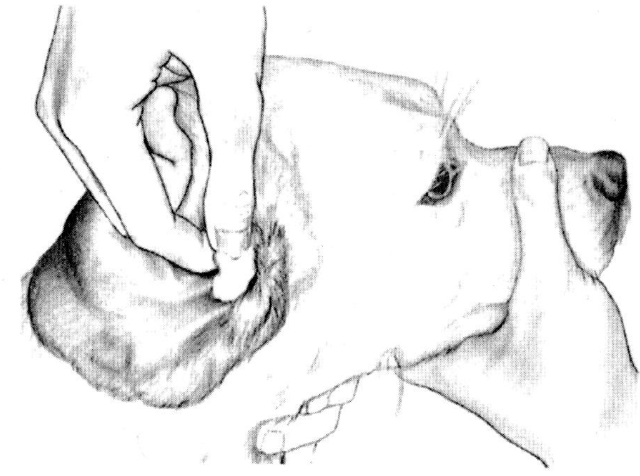

Figure 10-4 Removing loosened debris from ear canal with cotton.

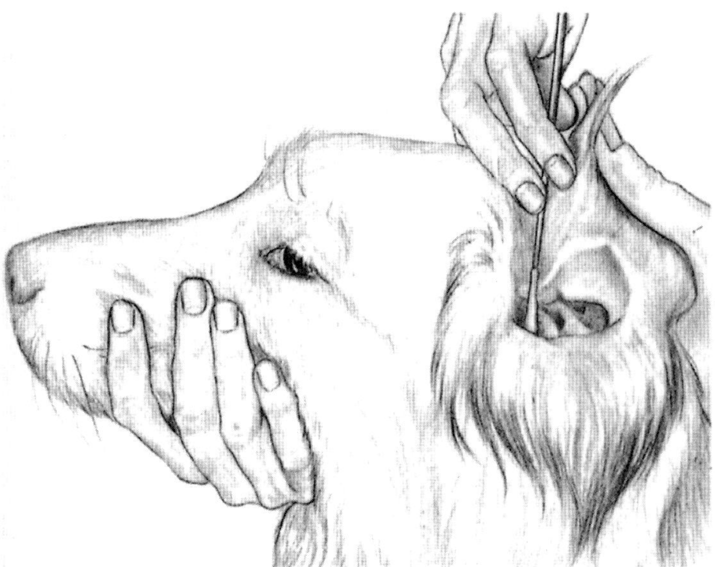

Figure 10-5 Cleaning interior folds of pinna with cotton-tipped swab.

Technical Action	Rationale/Amplification
10. Inspect ear canal with otoscope.	**10.** Thoroughness of cleaning can be evaluated, and any lesions previously obscured by debris may be visible now.

Technical Action	Rationale/Amplification
11. Instill prescribed medication (drops or ointment) and massage external ear canal gently.	**11.** As a rule, do *not* instill any potentially irritating solution or medication into the ear canal if the eardrum may be damaged. Massaging the ear aids in dispersal of the medication throughout the external ear canal. Note in animal's medical record: date, time, medication, dosage, ear(s) medicated, initials, and comments.

Bibliography

Bistner SI, Ford RB: Kirk and Bistner's Handbook of Veterinary Procedures & Emergency Treatment, 6th edition. Philadelphia, WB Saunders, 1995

Brunner LS, Suddarth DS: The Lippincott Manual of Nursing Practice, 3rd edition. Philadelphia, JB Lippincott, 1982

Kirk RW, Bistner SI: Handbook of Veterinary Procedures and Emergency Treatment, 4th edition. Philadelphia WB Saunders, 1985

McCurnin DM: Clinical Textbook for Veterinary Technicians. Philadelphia, WB Saunders, 1985

Chapter 11

Pedicure

You may not have to declaw him, think of all the animals that have horrific nail bed injury and end up with no or strange growing nails.

Small deeds done are better than great deeds planned.

PETER MARSHALL

Pedicure in cats and dogs consists of prophylactic or therapeutic trimming of the toenails.

Purposes

1. To prevent traumatic nail fracture
2. To trim or amputate damaged or ingrown toenails
3. To allow normal ambulation on footpads
4. To minimize physical damage to property, human beings, and other animals

Complications

1. Minor hemorrhage
2. Loss of toenail
3. Permanent deformity of toenails
4. Thermal injury

Equipment Needed

- Commercial pet toenail clippers (guillotine type or scissors type) for dogs, or human toenail clippers for cats
- Dremel drill with appropriate bits
- Cauterizing agent (e.g. silver nitrate or ferric subsulfate applicators)

Crow and Walshaw's Manual of Clinical Procedures in Dogs, Cats, Rabbits, and Rodents, Fourth Edition. Edited by Jennifer E. Boyle. Published 2016 by John Wiley & Sons, Inc.
Companion Website: www.wiley.com/go/boyle/manual4e

Restraint and Positioning

Nail trimming can be accomplished with the animal standing or in lateral recumbency. An assistant may be needed to restrain the animal. A muzzle or Elizabethan collar, and sometimes even chemical tranquilization, may be necessary if the animal objects to the procedure (see Chapter 1).

Procedure

Technical Action

1. If animal has light-colored toenails, note location of vascular matrix.
2. When using a guillotine-type nail clippers
   a) Slide ring over nail and position clippers so that screws on clipper face base of toenail.
   b) Place ring 2 mm from end of vascular matrix.
   c) Clip nail by forcefully squeezing clipper handles together, thereby advancing cutting blade (Fig. 11-1).

Rationale/Amplification

1. It is easy to see and avoid the pink matrix containing blood vessels and nerve supply if the animal has light-colored toenails.
2. This type of clipper is recommended for general use because it is inexpensive and can be used safely by pet owners for regular nail trimming.
   a) Holding the clippers in this way helps to prevent inadvertent clipping of the nail too short.
   b) If animal has dark-colored toenails, clip small amount of nail at a time and look at clipped cross-section. When the matrix is near the clipped edge, the cross-section will begin to appear "meaty" and lighter in color.
   c) The nail is severed by the bevelled cutting blade as the latter slides across the rigid metal ring encircling the nail.

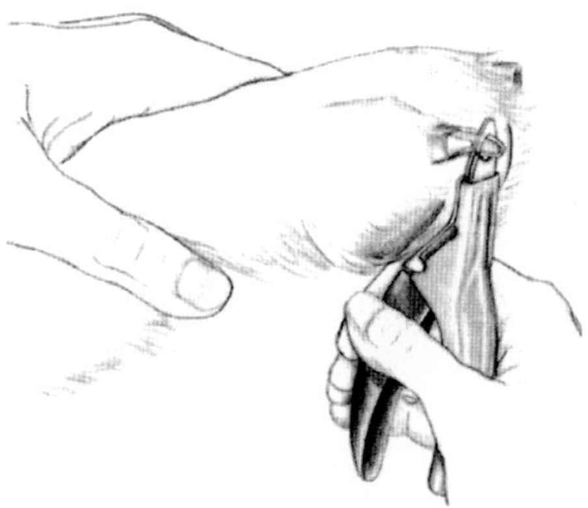

Figure 11-1 Clipping toenail using guillotine-type clippers.

Technical Action	Rationale/Amplification
3. If bleeding from toenail occurs, apply cauterizing agent (Fig. 11-2).	**3.** Silver nitrate–impregnated applicators or cotton swabs moistened with ferric subsulfate solution are effective cauterizing agents. Electrocautery can cause nail deformity and should not be used to stop hemorrhage from toenails, even if the animal is under general anesthesia.
4. Use scissors-type nail clippers for clipping toenails that have grown into foot pads (Fig. 11-3).	**4.** Ingrown toenails can result in painful inflammation or infection of the footpad. Aftercare may include soaking the foot several times daily in warm Epsom salt solutions.

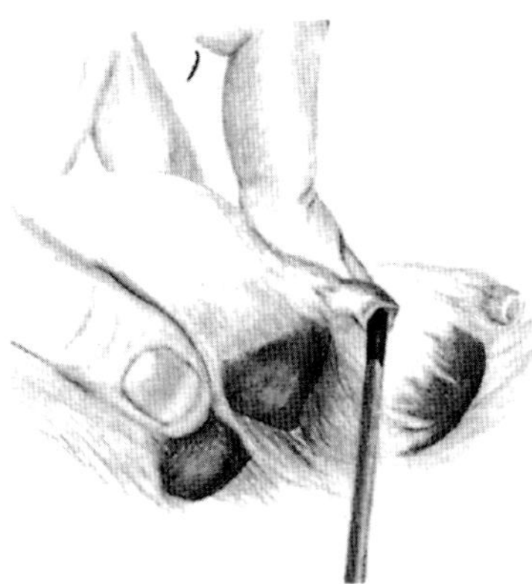

Figure 11-2 Cauterizing bleeding toenail matrix.

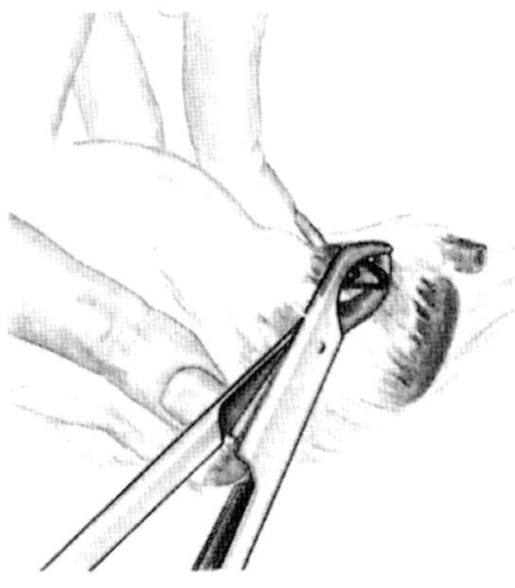

Figure 11-3 Clipping toenail using scissors-type clippers.

Technical Action	Rationale/Amplification
5. Use human toenail trimmer to clip claws of most cats (Fig. 11-4).	**5.** Cat claws are much thinner and delicate; the matrix of the nail is usually readily visible. Also good for young puppies.
6. A dremel drill can be used for large dogs or pets with thick nails (Fig. 11-5) This method produces a smooth, rounded nail (Fig. 11-6).	**6.** Use on low speed as drill bit can cause thermal burns from friction. Long hair can also get caught up in rotating mechanism. Masks/googles may be needed due to nail dust.

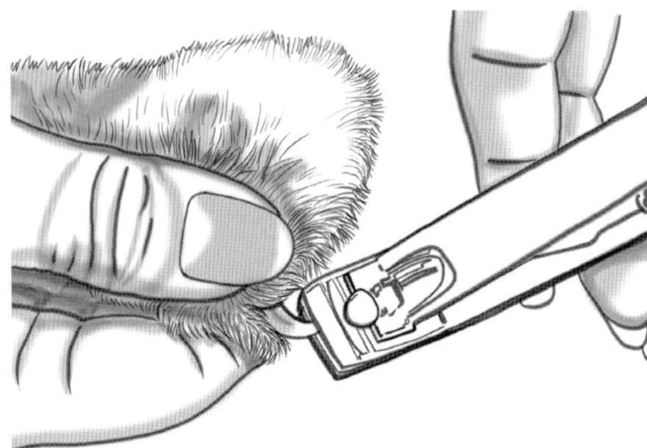

Figure 11-4 Clipping toenails of cat using human toenail clippers.

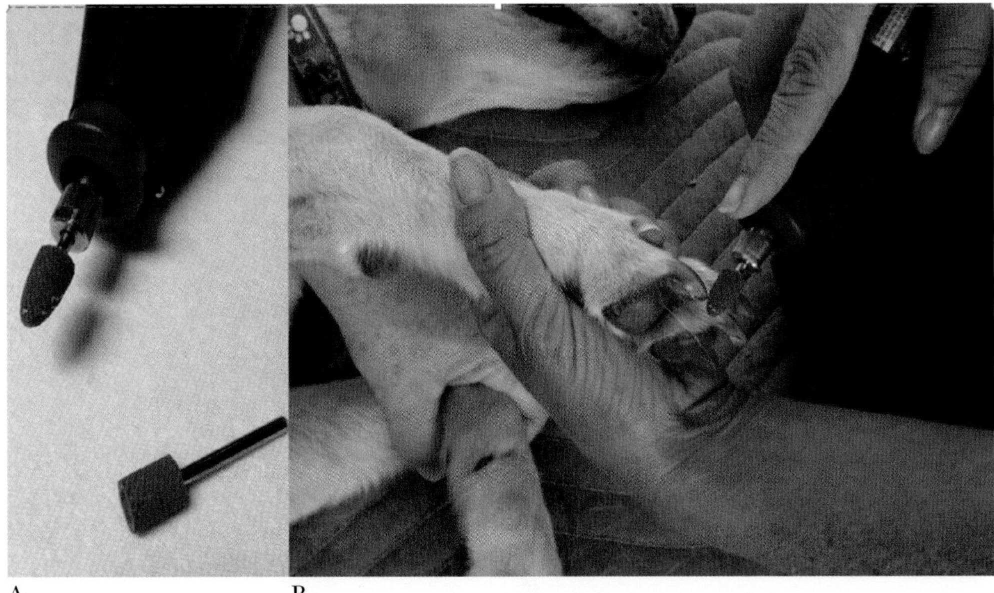

A B

Figure 11-5 (A) Dremel drill and drill bits and (B) Trimming toenails of dog using dremel drill.

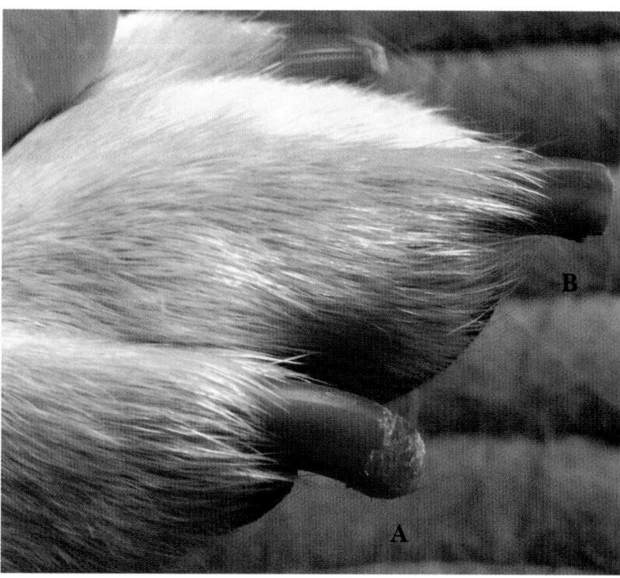

Figure 11-6 (A) Nail trimmed with dremel (B) Nail trimmed with scissors-type clippers.

Technical Action

7. Examine feet to make certain all toenails, including dewclaws, have been trimmed.

Rationale/Amplification

7. Regular monthly trimming or grinding of toenails will help prevent trauma and discomfort and may cause the matrix to retract so that the nail length can gradually be shortened.

Bibliography

Jack C and Watson P: Veterinary Technician's Daily Reference Guide. 3rd edition. Oxford, Wiley-Blackwell, 2014

McCurnin DM: Clinical Textbook for Veterinary Technicians. Philadelphia, WB Saunders, 1985

Novy, JE: Canine nail trimming, Mod Vet Pract 63(5): 381, May 1982

Chapter 12

Urethral Catheterization

If at first you don't succeed, try, try, again. Then give up. There's no use being a damn fool about it.

WC FIELDS

Urethral catheterization is the placement of a hollow tube, that is, a catheter, into the urethra.

Purposes

1. To collect urine for analysis or bacteriologic culture if the specimen cannot be obtained by percutaneous cystocentesis
2. To administer medication or radiographic contrast media directly into the urinary bladder
3. To provide closed continuous drainage of urine (e.g. when careful monitoring of urine output is necessary)
4. To relieve urethral obstruction

Complications

1. Trauma to urethra or urinary bladder
2. Urinary tract infection

Equipment Needed

- For urethral catheterization of male dog:
- Cotton

Crow and Walshaw's Manual of Clinical Procedures in Dogs, Cats, Rabbits, and Rodents, Fourth Edition. Edited by Jennifer E. Boyle. Published 2016 by John Wiley & Sons, Inc.
Companion Website: www.wiley.com/go/boyle/manual4e

- Chlorhexidine scrub
- Mild soap
- Dilute chlorhexidine or sterile saline flush
- Sterile surgeon's gloves
- Sterile urinary catheter
- Sterile lubricating jelly
- Container for urine
- Tubing and antimicrobial ointment (if continuous urine drainage is to be established)

For urethral catheterization of female dog:

- Cotton
- Chlorhexidine scrub
- Dilute chlorhexidine or sterile saline flush
- Sterile surgeon's gloves
- Sterile urinary catheter
- Sterile lubricating jelly or antimicrobial ointment
- 0.3 mL topical ophthalmic anesthetic or 0.5% lidocaine in tuberculin syringe with needle removed
- Container for urine
- Tubing and antimicrobial ointment (if continuous urine drainage is to be established)
- Light source and sterile vaginal speculum for visual technique

For urethral catheterization of cat:

- Cotton
- Chlorhexidine scrub
- Sterile surgeon's gloves
- Sterile urinary catheter
- Sterile lubricating jelly
- Container for urine
- Adhesive tape, monofilament nonabsorbable suture material, tubing, antimicrobial ointment (if continuous urine drainage is to be established)
- Drugs for tranquilization or anesthesia (if necessary)
- 0.2 mL topical ophthalmic anesthetic or 0.5% lidocaine in tuberculin syringe with needle removed (for female cat)
- Elizabethan collar

Restraint and Positioning

An assistant is needed to restrain the animal so that aseptic technique can be maintained throughout the procedure. The position preferred for urethral catheterization is lateral recumbency for the male dog. The male cat and the female cat can be positioned in lateral or sternal recumbency. Ideally, the female dog should be restrained in a standing position for urethral catheterization, but other acceptable positions are sternal or lateral recumbency.

PREPARATION FOR URETHRAL CATHETERIZATION

Procedure

Technical Action	Rationale/Amplification
1. Clip and clean area around prepuce or vulva using chlorhexidine scrub. For male and female dogs, flush prepuce or vestibule with dilute chlorhexidine or sterile saline. Repeat cleaning around prepuce or vulva. Rinse thoroughly and dry.	1. It is advisable to clip long hairs from the area immediately surrounding the prepuce or vulva if continuous urine drainage is to be established. Flushing the prepuce or vestibule assists in maintaining asepsis.
2. Select catheter of appropriate size and type (see Table 12-1).	2. To minimize trauma to the urinary tract, use the most flexible and the smallest diameter catheter that can be inserted easily. The Foley self-retaining catheter with an inflatable tip is available in sizes 6 F and larger for continuous urine drainage.
3. Wash hands thoroughly and don sterile surgeon's gloves.	3. Every precaution must be taken to reduce the chance of iatrogenic infection. Persons experienced in urinary catheterization may be able to advance the catheter slowly out of its sterile package and thus maintain asepsis without wearing surgeon's gloves. Urethral catheterization requires two or more persons. It should not be attempted without assistance.
4. Examine catheter for flaws.	4. Discard any catheter that has a rough surface, eyes (holes) that are occluded, or a weakened area.

TABLE 12-1 Recommended urethral catheter sizes for routine use in dogs and cats.

Animal	Urethral Catheter Type	Size
Cat	Flexible vinyl, red rubber, or Tomcat catheter (polyethylene)	3½ F
Male dog (<25 lb.)	Flexible vinyl, red rubber, or polyethylene	3½ or 5 F
Male dog (>25 lb.)	Flexible vinyl, red rubber, or polyethylene	8 F
Male dog (>75 lb.)	Flexible vinyl, red rubber, or polyethylene	10 or 12 F
Female dog (<10 lb.)	Flexible vinyl, red rubber, metal, or polyethylene	5 F
Female dog (10–50 lb.)	Flexible vinyl, red rubber, metal, or polyethylene	8 F
Female dog (>50 lb.)	Flexible vinyl, red rubber, metal, or polyethylene	10, 12, or 14 F

URETHRAL CATHETERIZATION OF MALE DOG

Procedure

Technical Action	Rationale/Amplification
1. Prepare for catheterization. Tranquilize or anesthetize, if necessary.	**1.** See **Preparing for Urethral Catheterization**.
2. Estimate length of catheter needed to enter urinary bladder by holding catheter above dog in approximate position for catheterization (Fig. 12-1).	**2.** If a flexible catheter is advanced too far into the urinary bladder, the catheter can become knotted or folded back on itself within the bladder.
3. *Assistant*: Place dog in lateral recumbency and abduct dog's upper rear leg. Then retract dog's prepuce such that distal 3–4 cm of glans penis is exposed (Fig. 12-2).	**3.** To retract the prepuce, the assistant should grip the prepuce caudal to the os penis with one hand and slide the prepuce caudally with the other hand.
4. *Assistant*: Clean distal glans penis with mild soap.	**4.** Any preputial glandular secretions are thereby removed.
5. *Operator*: Lubricate end of catheter liberally with sterile lubricating jelly and insert catheter tip into urethral orifice at distal end of glans penis (Fig. 12-3).	**5.** In addition to facilitating passage, thorough lubrication of catheters reduces the chance of forcing bacteria from the distal urethra into the bladder. To prevent contamination of the catheter as it is being advanced, retain rest of catheter within sterile package or coiled within gloved hand.

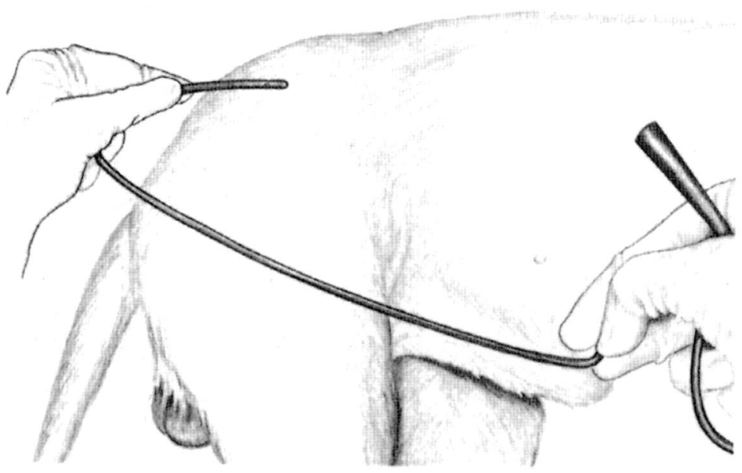

Figure 12-1 Estimating length of urethral catheter for male dog.

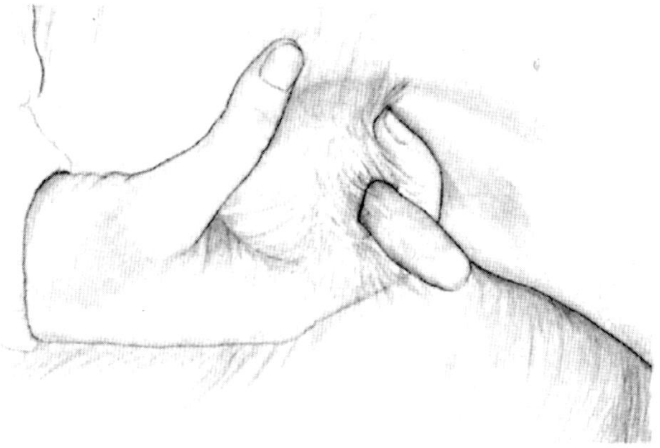

Figure 12-2 Retracting dog's prepuce.

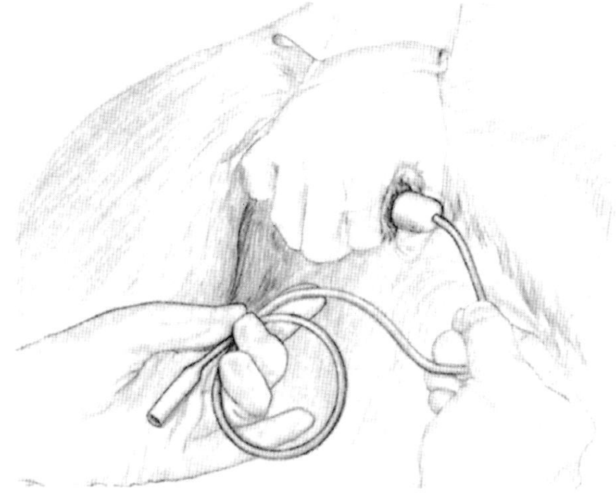

Figure 12-3 Inserting urethral catheter into penile urethra.

Technical Action	Rationale/Amplification
6. Advance catheter into urinary bladder.	**6.** Slight resistance may be encountered as the catheter passes over the ischial arch.
7. If no urine appears when catheter has been advanced sufficiently to enter bladder, try to aspirate urine from catheter by a syringe.	**7.** Advance catheter 2–4 cm farther, if necessary. Manual compression of the urinary bladder to start urine flow is not recommended because this increases the risk of iatrogenic infection.

Technical Action / **Rationale/Amplification**

8. Collect urine specimen.

   Rationale: We do not advise instilling dilute antiseptic solutions into the bladder after routine catheterization. Stock solutions of antiseptics may be contaminated with resistant bacteria.

9. Withdraw catheter, using gentle traction, and note in animal's medical record that catheterization was performed.

   Rationale: Note date, time, catheter type and size, amount of urine collected, any medication instilled, comments, and initials.

10. If catheter will be indwelling, a closed collection system must be connected to catheter.

    Rationale: See **Management of Indwelling Urethral Catheter and Closed Drainage System**.

URETHRAL CATHETERIZATION OF FEMALE DOG (VISUAL TECHNIQUE)

Procedure

Technical Action / **Rationale/Amplification**

1. Prepare for catheterization. Tranquilize or anesthetize, if necessary.

   Rationale: See **Preparing for Urethral Catheterization**.

2. *Assistant*: Restrain dog in standing position or sternal recumbency and hold dog's tail to side (Fig. 12-4).

   Rationale: If dog's tail is held straight up, some dogs will strain or defecate during the procedure.

3. *Operator*: Insert lubricated sterile tuberculin syringe (with needle removed) containing 0.3 mL topical ophthalmic anesthetic or 0.5%

   Rationale: Instillation of topical anesthetic will decrease the dog's discomfort and thus lessen struggling during the procedure.

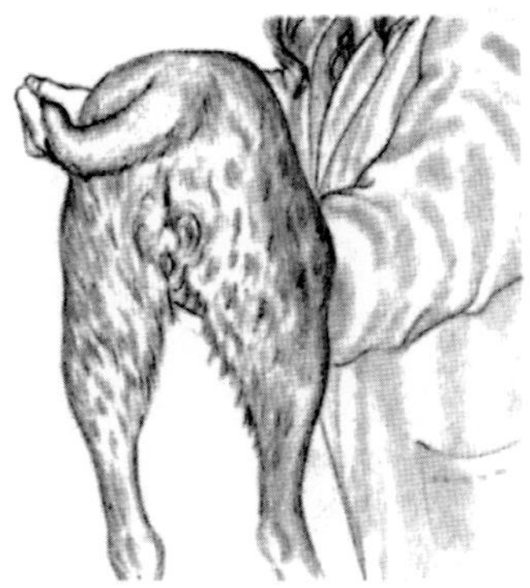

Figure 12-4 Restraint of female dog for urethral catheterization.

Technical Action

lidocaine approximately 3–5 cm into vagina and instill anesthetic.

4. Lubricate vaginal speculum and end of catheter liberally with sterile lubricating jelly.

Rationale/Amplification

4. For the visual technique, the catheter most easily introduced is either the rigid metal type or a Foley catheter equipped with a metal stylet.

Technical Action

5. Insert speculum into vagina with tip of speculum directed first dorsally, then cranially, to avoid clitoral fossa.

Rationale/Amplification

5. The clitoral fossa is a blind sac just inside the ventral opening of the vulva. In addition to the usual vaginal speculum, a variety of instruments can be used to locate the urethral opening: laryngoscope, otoscope, modified empty syringe case, modified test tube.

Technical Action

6. *Assistant*: Hold and adjust light source as necessary.

Rationale/Amplification

6. The urethral orifice is located on the ventral surface of the vagina, approximately 2–4 cm cranial to the opening of the vulva.

Technical Action

7. *Operator*: Introduce catheter through speculum into urethral orifice and advance into urinary bladder (Fig. 12-5).

Rationale/Amplification

7. The urethra of the female dog is approximately 5–10 cm in length.

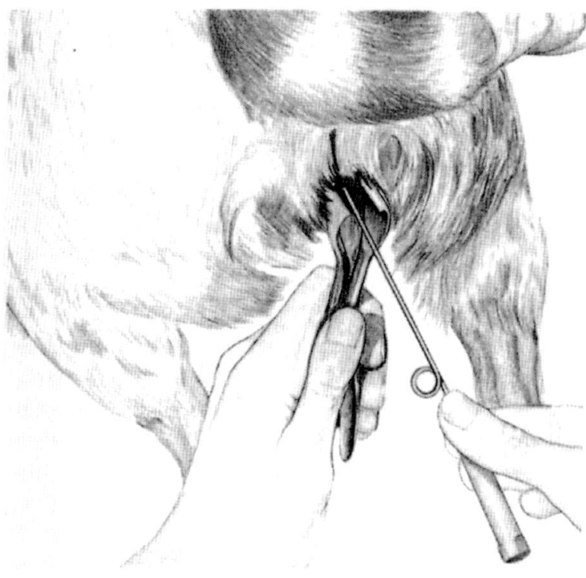

Figure 12-5 Introducing metal urethral catheter into female dog by visual technique.

Technical Action	Rationale/Amplification
8. If no urine appears when catheter has been advanced sufficiently to enter bladder, attach a syringe to distal end of catheter and try to aspirate urine.	8. Advance catheter 2–4 cm farther if necessary. Care must be taken if the dog struggles while a rigid metal catheter is in place because it could perforate the bladder wall. Manual compression of the urinary bladder to start urine flow is not recommended because this increases the risk of iatrogenic infection.
9. Collect urine specimen.	9. We do not advise instilling dilute antiseptic solutions into the bladder after routine catheterization. Stock solutions of antiseptics may be contaminated with resistant bacteria.
10. Remove catheter and note in animal's medical record that catheterization was performed.	10. Note date, time, catheter type and size, amount of urine collected, any medication instilled, comments, and initials.
11. If catheter will be indwelling, a closed collection system must be connected to catheter.	11. See **Management of Indwelling Urethral Catheter and Closed Drainage System**.

URETHRAL CATHETERIZATION OF FEMALE DOG (TACTILE TECHNIQUE)

Procedure

Technical Action	Rationale/Amplification
1. Prepare for catheterization.	1. See **Preparing for Urethral Catheterization**.
2. *Assistant*: Restrain dog in standing position or sternal recumbency and hold dog's tail to side.	2. If dog's tail is held straight up, some dogs will strain or defecate during the procedure.
3. *Operator*: Insert lubricated sterile tuberculin syringe (with needle removed) containing 0.3 mL topical ophthalmic anesthetic or 0.5% lidocaine approximately 3–5 cm into vagina and instill anesthetic.	3. Instillation of topical anesthetic will decrease the dog's discomfort and thus lessen struggling during the procedure.
4. Lubricate gloved index finger of one hand and tip of flexible urethral catheter with sterile lubricating jelly or antimicrobial ointment.	4. Theoretically, the use of an antimicrobial ointment as a lubricant could interfere with bacteriologic cultures. Right-handed persons should hold the catheter coiled in the right hand and use the left hand to palpate the urethral orifice.

Technical Action	Rationale/Amplification
5. Palpate urethral papilla (tissue surrounding urethral orifice) with gloved index finger of one hand.	**5.** The urethral papilla is a 0.5–1.5-cm round, firm or soft mass in the ventral midline of the vagina approximately 3–5 cm from the vulvar opening. The papilla is usually beneath the tip of the index finger when the finger has been inserted into the vagina to the level of the second knuckle.
6. Pass urethral catheter ventral to gloved finger in vagina and use finger to guide catheter down into urethral orifice while protecting rest of catheter from contamination with palm of hand (Fig. 12-6).	**6.** With practice, this procedure can be done as quickly as the visual method on any dog larger than 8 kg. The advantages are that it usually is tolerated better than the speculum technique and that it permits easy placement of flexible catheters. Flexible catheters must be used for continuous urine drainage.
7. If end of catheter can be palpated advancing past tip of index finger, withdraw catheter slightly and redirect it ventrally into urethral orifice.	**7.** In such an instance, the catheter is probably being inserted into the proximal vagina toward the cervix.
8. Advance catheter into urinary bladder.	**8.** The urethra of the female dog is approximately 5–10 cm long; it is relatively short as compared with that of the male dog.

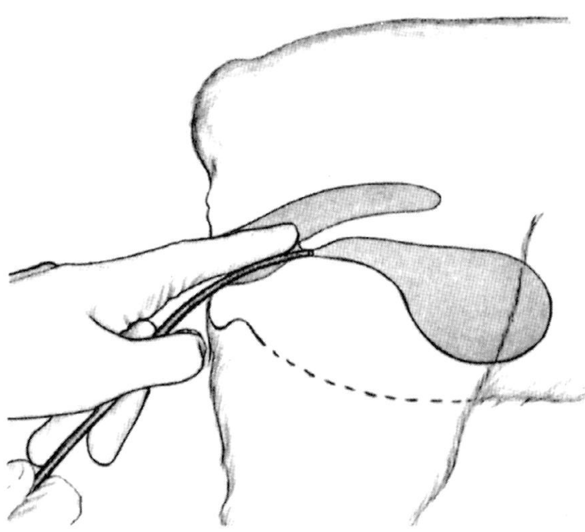

Figure 12-6 Introducing flexible urethral catheter into female dog by tactile technique.

Technical Action

9. If no urine appears when catheter has been advanced sufficiently to enter bladder, try to aspirate urine from catheter by a syringe.
10. Collect urine specimen.
11. Withdraw catheter by gentle traction and note in animal's medical record that catheterization was performed.
12. If catheter will be indwelling, a closed collection system must be connected to catheter.

Rationale/Amplification

9. Advance catheter 2–4 cm farther, if necessary. Manual compression of the urinary bladder to start urine flow is not recommended because this increases the risk of iatrogenic infection.
10. We do not advise instilling dilute antiseptic solutions into the bladder after routine catheterization. Stock solutions of antiseptics may be contaminated with resistant bacteria.
11. Note date, time, catheter type and size, amount of urine collected, any medication instilled, comments, and initials.
12. See **Management of Indwelling Urethral Catheter and Closed Drainage System**.

URETHRAL CATHETERIZATION OF MALE CAT

Procedure

Technical Action

1. Prepare for catheterization.
2. Tranquilize or anesthetize cat, if necessary.
3. *Assistant*: Restrain cat in lateral or dorsal recumbency; grasp tail base and gently deflect tail dorsally or laterally (Fig. 12-7).
4. Lubricate end of catheter with sterile jelly.
5. Place thumb and index finger of one hand on either side of prepuce so that palm of hand rests on cat's lower spine. Exert pressure with thumb and index finger in cranial direction to extrude penis from prepuce (Fig. 12-8).

Rationale/Amplification

1. See **Preparing for Urethral Catheterization**.
2. A person experienced in this procedure can perform it rapidly on a fully conscious, even-tempered cat.
3. An Elizabethan collar is a useful adjunct to restraint during this procedure. Many cats object to having their tails held, so use a light grip.
4. A polyethylene tomcat catheter is most commonly used. A catheter with side holes and closed end is less traumatic to the urethra and bladder than is the open-ended type.
5. A right-handed person should use the left hand to extrude the penis from the prepuce. Unless the penis is extruded from the prepuce at least 1 cm, catheterization will be very difficult.

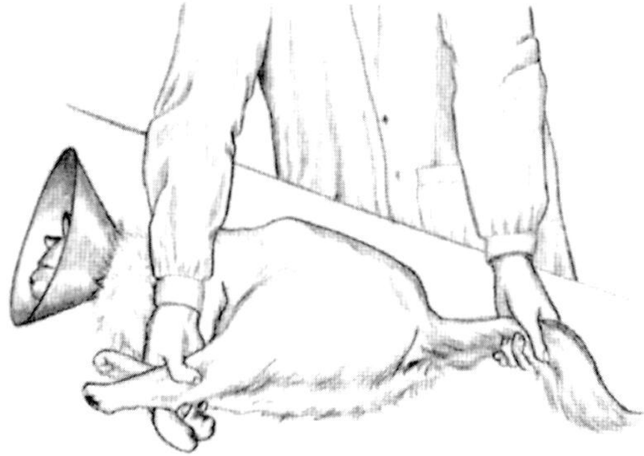

Figure 12-7 Restraint of male cat for urethral catheterization.

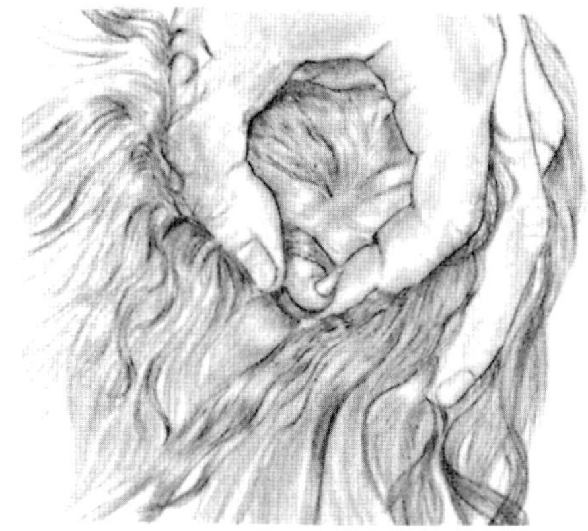

Figure 12-8 Extending cat's penis from prepuce.

Technical Action

6. Introduce catheter approximately 1.5–2.0 cm into urethra such that holes in catheter tip are no longer visible (Fig. 12-9A).
7. Allow penis to retract within prepuce, leaving catheter in place.
8. Pinch preputial skin gently between thumb and forefinger and pull prepuce caudally and ventrally while advancing catheter into urinary bladder (Fig. 12-9B).

Rationale/Amplification

8. Applying traction to the prepuce at this step straightens the flexure in the cat's penis and permits the catheter to pass over the ischial arch.

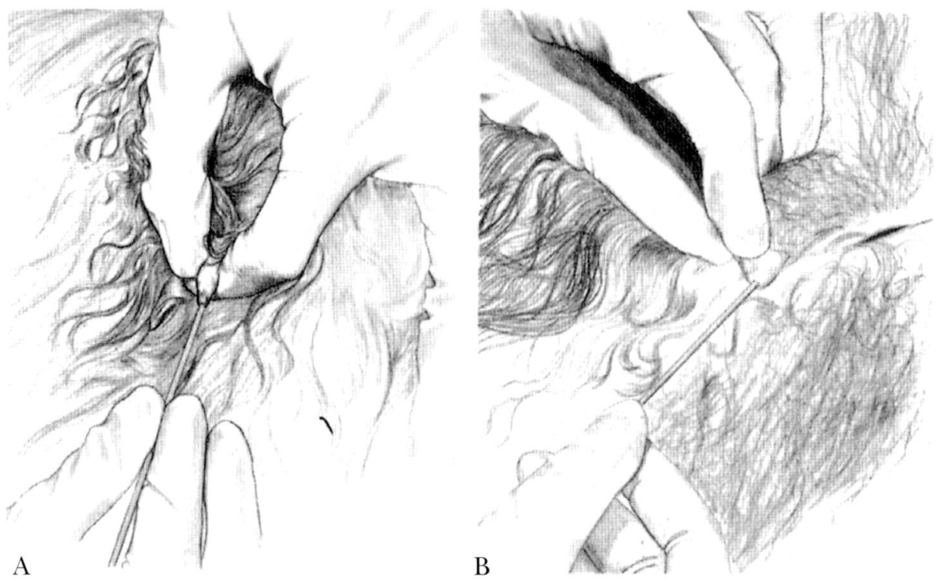

Figure 12-9 (A) and (B) Advancing urethral catheter into penile urethra.

Technical Action	Rationale/Amplification
9. If catheter cannot be advanced because of urethral blockage, repeat procedure using 22-gauge intravenous catheter (with needle removed) in place of urethral catheter. Flush catheter with sterile saline until urethral debris is dislodged.	**9.** When the urethral blockage has been relieved, insert a tomcat catheter and empty bladder by aspirating urine by a syringe attached to the catheter. Manual compression should not be attempted if a bladder has been distended by an obstruction because perforation can result.
10. Collect urine specimen.	**10.** Foley catheters are not available in sizes small enough for cats. If the catheter is to be left in place, adhesive tape is folded over the distal end of the catheter in a butterfly configuration. The "wings" of the tape are sutured once to the preputial skin on each side with nonabsorbable suture material.
11. Put Elizabethan collar on cat.	**11.** Use of an Elizabethan collar will minimize the possibility of the cat deliberately removing the catheter.
12. Remove catheter and note in animal's medical record that catheterization was performed.	**12.** Note date, time, catheter type and size, amount of urine collected, any medication instilled, comments, and initials.
13. If catheter will be indwelling, a closed collection system must be connected to catheter.	**13.** See **Management of Indwelling Urethral Catheter and Closed Drainage System**.

URETHRAL CATHETERIZATION OF FEMALE CAT

Procedure

Technical Action	Rationale/Amplification
1. Prepare for catheterization.	**1.** See Preparing for Urethral Catheterization.
2. *Assistant*: Restrain cat in lateral recumbency, grasp tail base, and deflect dorsally or laterally (Fig. 12-7).	**2.** An Elizabethan collar is a useful adjunct to restraint during this procedure.
3. Tranquilize or sedate cat, if necessary.	**3.** Many cats will fight this procedure unless they are obtunded from disease.
4. Insert lubricated sterile tuberculin syringe (with needle removed) containing 0.2 mL topical ophthalmic anesthetic or 0.5% lidocaine approximately 2 cm into vagina.	**4.** Topical anesthesia requires only a few minutes to take effect.
5. Instill anesthetic and wait 2–3 minutes.	**5.** Instillation of topical anesthetic will decrease the animal's discomfort and therefore lessen struggling during the procedure.
6. Lubricate end of catheter liberally with sterile lubricating jelly.	**6.** A 3½ F to 5 F catheter is suitable for a female cat.
7. Pull vulvar lips caudally while sliding catheter along ventral wall of vagina, until catheter slips into urethral orifice (Fig. 12-10).	**7.** In many cases, the vagina of the female cat is too small to be opened with a speculum or for the tactile technique to be utilized. The "blind" technique can be successful if the operator is gentle and patient.

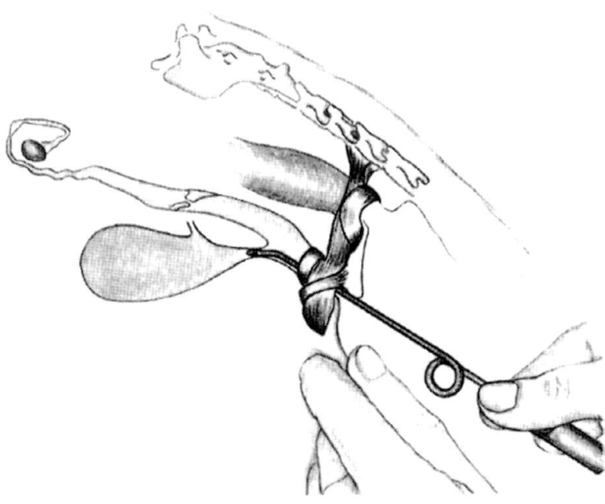

Figure 12-10 Introducing urethral catheter into female cat.

Technical Action	Rationale/Amplification
8. Collect urine specimen.	**8.** Foley catheters are not available in sizes small enough for cats. If the catheter is to be left in place, adhesive tape is folded over the distal end of the catheter in a butterfly configuration. The "wings" of the tape are sutured once to the perineal skin on each side with nonabsorbable suture material.
9. Put Elizabethan collar on cat.	**9.** Use of an Elizabethan collar will minimize the possibility of the cat deliberately removing the catheter.
10. Remove catheter and note in animal's medical record that catheterization was performed.	**10.** Note date, time, catheter type and size, amount of urine collected, any medication instilled, comments, and initials.
11. If catheter will be indwelling, a closed collection system must be connected to catheter.	**11.** See **Management of Indwelling Urethral Catheter and Closed Drainage System**.

MANAGEMENT OF INDWELLING URETHRAL CATHETER AND CLOSED URINE DRAINAGE SYSTEM

Procedure

Technical Action	Rationale/Amplification
1. For continuous urine drainage, connect urethral catheter, preferably a flexible vinyl or red rubber catheter, to collection container by means of sterile tubing (e.g. intravenous fluid administration set and empty fluid bag) or commercial urinary collection bag (Fig. 12-11).	**1.** Closed urine drainage carries less risk of urinary tract infection and prevents urine scalding of skin that can occur with an open indwelling urethral catheter. Flexible vinyl or red rubber catheters are softer and cause less damage to the urothelium than polypropylene catheters.
2. Place collection container below level of animal's urinary bladder.	**2.** Urine flow must be downhill to prevent backflow of contaminated urine into animal's bladder.
3. If Foley catheter is used: When catheter is draining well, inflate end of catheter according to manufacturer's directions.	**3.** Urethral trauma will occur if the inflatable portion has not been advanced into the urinary bladder when inflation is attempted.
4. Place Elizabethan collar on animal unless it is unconscious or can be observed constantly.	**4.** Animals can contaminate and remove urethral catheters, even if sutured to the skin.

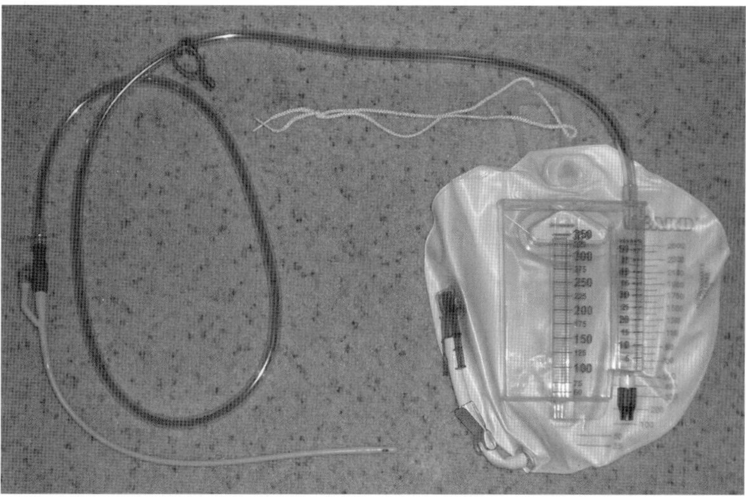

Figure 12-11 Collection apparatus for continuous urine drainage.

Technical Action	Rationale/Amplification
5. Cleanse urethral orifice–catheter junction with soap and water twice daily and apply antimicrobial ointment to junction after cleansing.	**5.** Some drainage will occur at the exit point of the catheter. Catheter care helps prevent this exudate from entering the proximal urethra and bladder. The value of daily external urethral orifice care may be greater for high-risk patients. Care of the urethral orifice–catheter junction must include the application of antimicrobial ointment because cleaning with soap alone actually increases bacteriuria in some patients.
6. If urine flow stops, check position of animal and catheter. Try flushing catheter with 5–10 mL of sterile saline.	**6.** The animal may kink or compress the catheter when changing position. Flushing the catheter may be necessary to dislodge small clots or other debris in the catheter openings or lumen.
7. If continuous urine flow cannot be reestablished, replace catheter or reevaluate necessity for continuous urine drainage.	**7.** A free flow of urine is essential in preventing catheter-associated infection.

Bibliography

Biertuempfel PH, Ling GV, Ling GA: Urinary tract infection resulting from catheterization in healthy adult dogs. JAVMA 178(9): 989–991, 1981

Brunner LS, Suddarth DS: The Lippincott Manual of Nursing Practice, 3rd edition. Philadelphia, JB Lippincott, 1982

Burke JB, Jacobson JA, Garibaldi RA *et al.*: Evaluation of daily meatal care with polyantibiotic ointment in prevention of urinary catheter-associated bacteriuria. J Urol 129: 331–334, Feb. 1983

Center for Disease Control: Engineering Out the Risk of Infection with Urinary Catheters, 2001

Comer KM, Ling GV: Results of urinalysis and bacterial culture of canine urine obtained by antepubic cystocentesis, catheterization, and the midstream voided methods. JAVMA 179: 891–895, 1981

Crow SE: Hematuria: An algorithm for differential diagnosis. Compend Contin Educ Prac Vet II (12): 941–948, 1980

Kirk RW, Bistner SI: Handbook of Veterinary Procedures and Emergency Treatment, 4th edition. Philadelphia, WB Saunders, 1985

Koskeroglu N. (2006) The role of meatal disinfection in preventing catheter-related bacteriuria in an intensive care unit: A pilot study in Turkey. Journal of Hospital Infection 56: 236–238

Lees GE: Use and misuse of indwelling urethral catheters. Vet Clin North Am 26(3): 499–505, 1996

Lees GE, Osborne CA: Urinary tract infections associated with the use and misuse of urinary catheters. Vet Clin North Am 9(4): 713–727, 1979

Lees GE, Osborne CA, Stevens JB *et al.*: Adverse effects caused by polypropylene and polyvinyl feline urinary catheters. Am J Vet Res 41(11): 1836–1840, 1980

Lees GE, Osborne CA, Stevens JB *et al.*: Adverse effects of open indwelling urethral catheterization in clinically normal male cats. Am J Vet Res 42(5): 825–833, 1981

Lees GE, Simpson RB, Green RA: Results of analyses and bacterial cultures of urine specimens obtained from clinically normal cats by three methods. JAVMA 184(4): 449–454, 1984

Lulich J: The Uses and Misuses of Urinary Catheters. Lecture notes. University of Minnesota, College of Veterinary Medicine, 2001

McCurnin DM, Poffenbarger EM: Small Animal Physical Diagnosis and Clinical Procedures. Philadelphia, WB Saunders, 1991

Osborne CA, Klausner JS, Lees GE: Urinary tract infections: Normal and abnormal host defense mechanisms. Vet Clin North Am 9(4): 587–609, 1979

Osborne CA, Klausner JS, Krawiec DR *et al.*: Canine struvite urolithiasis: Problems and their dissolution. JAVMA 179(3): 239–244, 1981

Osborne CA, Kruger JM, Lulich JP, Bartges JW, Polzin DJ: Medical management of feline urethral obstruction. Vet Clin North Am 26(3): 483–498, 1996

Osborne CA, Stevens JB: Handbook of Canine and Feline Urinalysis. St. Louis, MO, Ralston Purina, 1981

Osborne CA, Polzin DJ: Nonsurgical management of canine obstructive urolithopathy. Vet Clin North Am: Sm An Prac 16(2): 333–349, 1986

Smarick S, Haskins S, Aldrich J, Foley J, Kass P, Ling GV: Incidence of catheter-associated urinary tract infection among dogs in a small animal intensive care unit. JAVMA (2004) 224: 1936–1940

Smith CW, Schiller AG, Smith AR, *et al.*: Effects on indwelling urinary catheters in male cats. JAAHA 17: 427–433, May/June 1981

Stogdale L, Roos CJ: The use of the laryngoscope for bladder catheterization in the female dog. JAAHA 14: 616–617, Sept/Oct 1978

Wolz GC: Urinary catheterization of the small animal patient, pp 207–215. Proceedings of 12th Annual Seminar for Veterinary Technicians, Western States Veterinary Conference, Las Vegas, NV, Feb 21–23, 1983

Chapter 13

Digital Rectal Examination

If you don't know where you're going, you will probably end up somewhere else.
LAURENCE J PETER

Digital rectal examination is the palpation of perineal and pelvic structures with one finger placed into the rectal lumen through the anus.

Purpose

To identify diseases involving the rectum, anus, anal sacs, perineum, pelvic urethra, prostate, vagina, and pelvic bones.

Specific Indications

1. Standard part of complete physical examination
2. Pelvic trauma
3. Stranguria
4. Hematuria
5. Pyuria
6. Tenesmus
7. Swellings or masses in perineal region
8. Hematochezia
9. Anal pruritus
10. Preputial or anal discharge

Contraindications

1. Severe hematochezia
2. Painful tail base

Crow and Walshaw's Manual of Clinical Procedures in Dogs, Cats, Rabbits, and Rodents, Fourth Edition. Edited by Jennifer E. Boyle. Published 2016 by John Wiley & Sons, Inc.
Companion Website: www.wiley.com/go/boyle/manual4e

Equipment

- Examination gloves
- Lubricating jelly

Restraint and Positioning

Rectal palpation may be performed with the animal in a standing or recumbent position. The examiner should support the animal by gently cupping one hand under the animal's caudal abdomen while the other gloved hand examines the rectal area. An assistant should restrain the animal by cradling the head and thorax in both arms.

Procedure

Technical Action

1. Place lubricant on index or middle finger of gloved hand.
2. Slowly and gently advance lubricated finger as far as possible into rectum (Fig. 13-1).
3. Systematically palpate pelvic canal and perineum, proceeding from cranial to caudal. A recommended procedure is as follows:

   Slide finger lightly over rectal mucosa for its entire circumference.

   Palpate following structures for location, size, consistency, and shape:

   - Ventral aspect of sacrum
   - Right ilium
   - Right acetabulum
   - Pubis
   - Prostate or dorsal vaginal wall
   - Left acetabulum
   - Left ilium

   Withdraw finger 1–3 cm and repeat circumferential palpation of:

   - Rectal mucosa
   - Ventral aspect of coccygeal vertebrae
   - Right perineal fascia
   - Prostate or dorsal vaginal wall
   - Dorsal aspect of ischium

Rationale/Amplification

1. The index finger should be used for small dogs and cats.
2. If there is a large amount of fecal material present, it should be removed before proceeding.
3. Proceeding from cranial to caudal in a uniform sequence helps to avoid errors of omission. Particular attention should be paid to structures that protrude into or occlude the pelvic canal or the lumen of the rectum. In addition, note the animal's response when pressure is applied to each structure. The anal sacs are identified by squeezing them between the lubricated finger and the thumb, which is placed against the perineal skin.

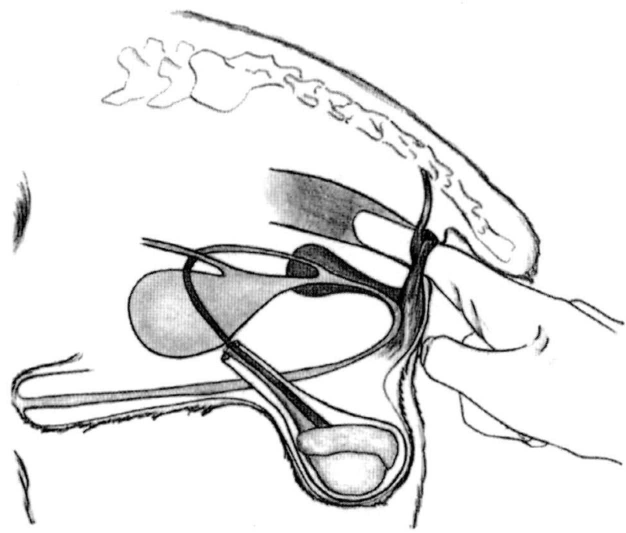

Figure 13-1 Placement of a gloved, lubricated finger in rectum for tactile inspection of the pelvic and perineal organs.

Technical Action	Rationale/Amplification
• Urethra • Left perineal fascia Continue caudally to anus and palpate: • Anal sphincter muscles (note tone and reflex contraction). • Anal sacs at 4 o'clock and 8 o'clock positions.	
4. Express contents of distended anal sacs (see also Chapter 14).	**4.** Collect secretions on cotton.
5. As finger is removed from rectum, examine mucosa visually.	**5.** One to two centimeters of the rectal mucosa can be readily everted by gentle traction at the time of withdrawal.
6. Examine soiled glove for blood, mucus, foreign materials, or parasites.	**6.** This examination should consist of both inspection and palpation.

Suggested Reading

Tilley LP, Smith F: Blackwell's Five-Minute Veterinary Consult: Canine and Feline, 6th edition, Wiley-Blackwell, 2015

Rijnberk A, van Sluijs FJ: Medical History and Physical Examination in Companion Animals, 2nd edition, Elvisier, 2009

McCurnin DM, Poffenbarger EM: Small Animal Physical Diagnosis and Clinical Procedures. Philadelphia, WB Saunders, 1991

Shell L: Rectal Deviation. Canine Associate, October 2011

Ross JT, Scavelli TD, Matthiesen, DT, Patnaik AK: Adenocarcinoma of the apocrine glands of the anal sac in dogs: A review of 32 cases. J Am Anim Hosp Assoc. 27(3): 349–355, May–June 1991

Boothe H: Colonic and Rectal Neoplasms. Western Veterinary Conference, 2003

Chapter 14

Anal Sac Expression and Cannulation

Kindness is the oil that takes the friction out of life.
MA HAMMARLUND

Anal sac expression is the manual removal of secretions that have accumulated in the animal's anal sacs. Many dogs need their anal sacs emptied frequently, but this procedure is rarely performed on cats.

Anal sac cannulation is the insertion of a tube into the anal sac orifice.

Purposes

1. To remove malodorous secretions before bathing and grooming of dogs
2. To decrease irritation (pruritus) caused by distention or inflammation of the anal sacs
3. To instill medication into diseased anal sacs

Specific Indication

Anal pruritus, usually manifest as scooting, licking, or whining.

Complications

1. Rupture of abscessed anal sac
2. Perforation of rectum

Equipment Needed

- Cotton (or paper towels)
- Examination glove(s)
- Lubricating jelly

Crow and Walshaw's Manual of Clinical Procedures in Dogs, Cats, Rabbits, and Rodents, Fourth Edition. Edited by Jennifer E. Boyle. © 2016 John Wiley & Sons, Inc. Published 2016 by John Wiley & Sons, Inc.
Companion Website: www.wiley.com/go/boyle/manual4e

- Skin disinfectant, for example, 2% chlorhexidine solution
- 6 mL syringe
- Lacrimal duct cannula or 20-gauge polyethylene intravenous catheter
- Prescribed medication

Restraint and Positioning

The dog should be restrained in the standing position by an assistant. A muzzle or Elizabethan collar may be needed (see Chapter 1).

Procedure

Technical Action	Rationale/Amplification
1. Put on examination glove.	1. Normal anal sac contents are malodorous. Use of an examination glove prevents soiling of the hands.
2. Express each anal sac externally by placing cotton over anus and pressing sac forward against perineum, while gently squeezing sac with thumb and one or two fingers (Fig. 14-1).	2. The anal sacs are located within the anal sphincter muscles ventrolateral to the anus (4 o'clock and 8 o'clock positions). The duct of each sac opens just inside the anal orifice.

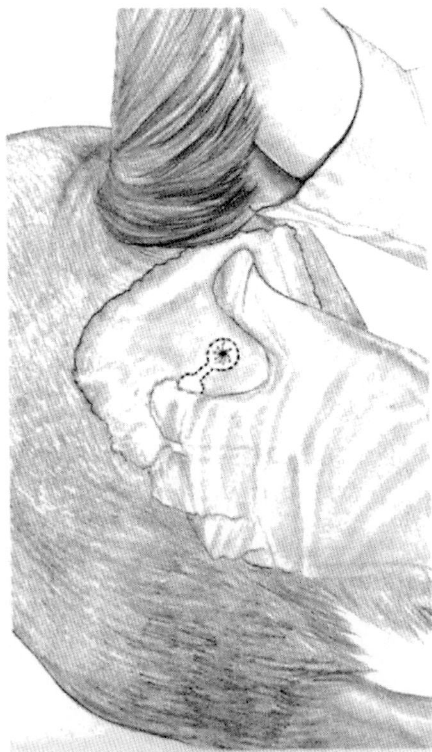

Figure 14-1 External expression of anal sac.

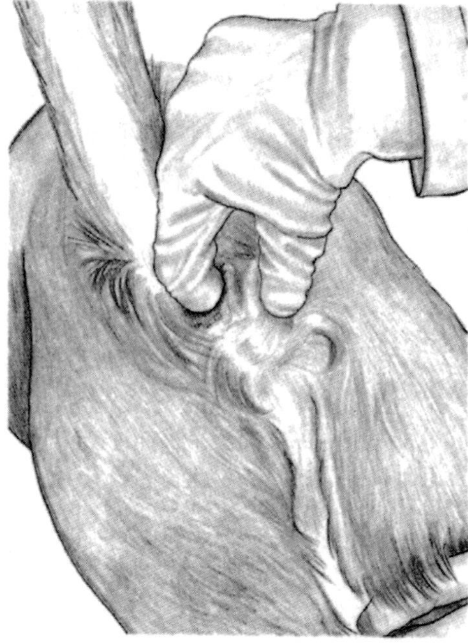

Figure 14-2 Internal expression of anal sac.

Technical Action	Rationale/Amplification
3. Apply generous amount of sterile lubricant to gloved index finger.	**3.** Liquid soaps may also be used in place of lubricants.
4. Express anal sacs more completely by inserting lubricated gloved index finger into rectum and gently milking contents of sac between finger and thumb dorsomedially into anal opening (Fig. 14-2).	**4.** This is the preferred method of anal sac expression because it ensures emptying of the sacs. Rectal perforation, a very rare complication, can be prevented by gentle technique and adequate lubrication. If sacs cannot be expressed with light to moderate pressure, consider cannulation rather than applying more pressure.
5. Examine material expressed from anal sacs.	**5.** Normal anal sacs contain a granular brown, malodorous material.
6. Invert glove and tie it in knot.	**6.** Enclosing anal sac material in this manner minimizes dispersion of odor in the examination room.
7. If material expressed from anal sacs is purulent in appearance, identify duct openings and cannulate anal sac duct. Flush sacs several times with 2% chlorhexidine solution (Fig. 14-3).	**7.** Flushing with dilute chlorhexidine solution cleanses the interior aspect of the anal sacs. A lacrimal duct cannula dedicated to this procedure attached to a 6 mL syringe is ideal. A 20-gauge polyethylene intravenous catheter is also suitable in diameter and rigidity

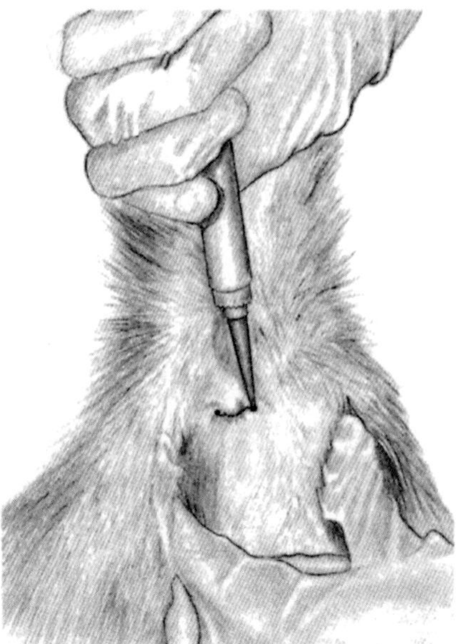

Figure 14-3 Flushing of anal sac by means of cannula inserted into anal sac duct.

Technical Action	Rationale/Amplification
	for cannulating anal sac ducts. Cannulation is facilitated by ejecting flushing solution through the cannula as it is introduced into the duct opening.
	NOTE: *A curved-tip syringe can be used in place of a syringe and cannula for anal sac flushing/infusion.*
8. Instill prescribed medication into anal sacs.	**8.** Topical ointments suitable for use in the ear have been used to treat inflammation of the anal sac.
9. Note in patient's medical record any abnormalities observed or medication instilled.	**9.** Note date, time, medication, anal sac(s) affected, dosage, initials, and comments.
10. Clean anus and surrounding skin with disinfectant.	**10.** Cleaning the area helps to dissipate odors lingering from the procedure.

Bibliography

Anal Sacs. Client education series. Indianapolis, Eli Lilly and Company

McCurnin DM, Poffenbarger EM: Small Animal Physical Diagnosis and Clinical Procedures. Philadelphia, WB Saunders, 1991

Muller GH, Kirk RW: Small Animal Dermatology, Philadelphia, WB Saunders, 1969

Pratt PW (ed): Medical Nursing for Animal Health Technicians. Santa Barbara, CA, American Veterinary Publications, 1985

Chapter 15

Enema

When a man has pity on all living creatures,
then only is he noble.

BUDDHA

Enema is the infusion of fluid in the lower intestinal tract through the anus.

Purposes

1. To remove fecal material from the colon
2. To prepare for survey and contrast radiographic studies of abdomen and pelvis
3. To administer radiographic contrast media
4. To irrigate the colon in certain types of poisoning

Specific Indications

1. Constipation or obstipation
2. Some poisonings

Complications

1. Rupture of colon
2. Leakage of enema fluid into peritoneal cavity through already-ruptured, gastrointestinal tract
3. Hemorrhage, in cases of ulcerative colitis

Crow and Walshaw's Manual of Clinical Procedures in Dogs, Cats, Rabbits, and Rodents, Fourth Edition. Edited by Jennifer E. Boyle. Published 2016 by John Wiley & Sons, Inc.
Companion Website: www.wiley.com/go/boyle/manual4e

Equipment Needed

- Examination glove
- Lubricating jelly
- Enema container with attached tubing and nozzle
- Enema solution (one or more of the following items):
  - Warm water
  - Glycerine and water (1:1)
  - Mild soap and water
  - Saline for irrigation
  - Commercial enema preparation

NOTE: *Phosphate enema solutions should not be used in cats and small dogs because these preparations may cause acute collapse associated with hypocalcemia.*

Restraint and Positioning

The animal is restrained in a standing position, usually in a wash basin or bathtub.

Procedure

Technical Action	Rationale/Amplification
1. Evaluate animal for evidence of abdominal pain or ulcerative colitis. If abdominal pain is present, eliminate possibility of intestinal perforation or obstruction before proceeding.	**1.** Enemas are contraindicated in cases of intestinal obstruction or perforation because of the risk of forcing fecal material throughout the peritoneal cavity. Enemas may increase colonic bleeding in cases of ulcerative colitis.
2. Place prescribed warm enema solution in enema container.	**2.** Approximately 150–200 mL of an enema solution can be administered safely to an adult cat; a medium-sized or large dog can be given up to 1 liter. Warm solutions are preferred to cool solutions because the former are more readily retained and more comfortable for the animal.
3. Put on examination glove.	**3.** The glove will prevent soiling of the hand with feces and potential transmission of zoonotic diseases.
4. Lubricate nozzle on end of enema tubing with lubricating jelly.	**4.** Lubrication of the nozzle facilitates atraumatic introduction of the tube into the rectum.
5. Insert nozzle into animal's rectum (Fig. 15-1).	**5.** The nozzle must be passed at least 5 cm cranial to the animal's anal sphincter.

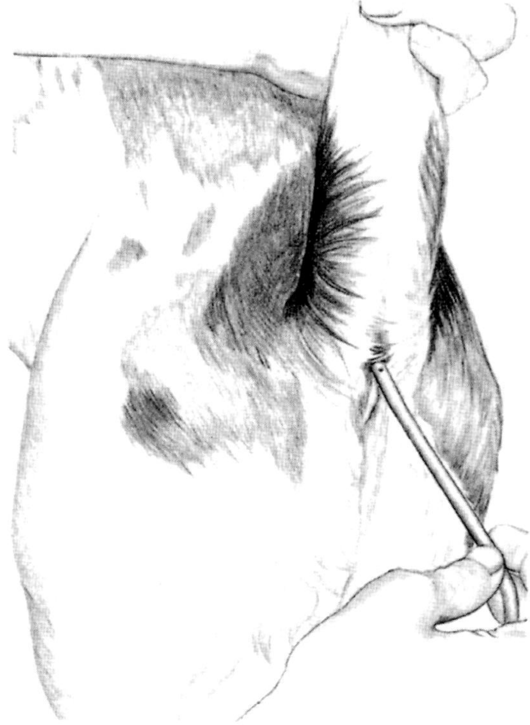

Figure 15-1 Inserting enema tube into animal's rectum.

Technical Action	Rationale/Amplification
6. Place enema container higher than animal's anus and permit solution to flow by gravity into rectum.	**6.** Elevating the animal's hindquarters and gently gripping the sphincter around the nozzle will help to prevent enema fluid from escaping. If the enema flow rate is too fast, it may cause reverse peristalsis and vomiting.
7. After administrating enema fluid, move animal immediately to suitable area for defecation.	**7.** It may be necessary to administer two or three warm-water or saline enemas to clean the bowel adequately before a barium enema procedure.
8. Note in patient's medical record that enema was given.	**8.** Note date, time, type of enema, amount, initials, and comments.
9. For a barium enema: Anesthetize animal, position in right lateral recumbency, and place barium contrast material (20–30 mL/kg) into colon.	**9.** A cuffed rectal catheter is preferred to a routine enema nozzle for this procedure because anesthesia relaxes the anal sphincter and leakage of barium can occur readily. Contamination of the animal's hair or

Technical Action	Rationale/Amplification
	skin with contrast materials may result in radiographic artifacts that interfere with diagnosis.
10. Bathe animal's hindquarters or entire body.	**10.** The hair coat becomes soiled with feces during this procedure.

Bibliography

Bistner SI, Ford RB: Kirk and Bistner's Handbook of Veterinary Procedures & Emergency Treatment, 6th edition. Philadelphia, WB Saunders, 1995

Brunner LS, Suddarth DS: The Lippincott Manual of Nursing Practice, 3rd edition. Philadelphia JB Lippincott, 1982

Jones BV: Animal Nursing, Part 2. Oxford, Pergamon Press, 1966

Kirk RW, Bistner SI: Handbook of Veterinary Procedures and Emergency Treatment, 4th edition. Philadelphia, WB Saunders, 1985

Lane DR, Cooper, B: Veterinary Nursing (Formerly Jones's Animal Nursing, 5th edition). Oxford, England, Pergamon Press, 1994

Pratt PW (ed): Medical Nursing for Animal Health Technicians. Santa Barbara, CA, American Veterinary Publications, 1985

Part II

Specialized Clinical Procedures

The procedures described in this section are described as specialized because they require considerable preparation or have very specific indications. The reader should pay particular attention to the indications and contraindications sections in applying these techniques.

As opposed to the "routine" procedures described in Part I, the specialized techniques frequently have significant inherent risk and may require specialized equipment. For the most part, however, the needed instruments are readily available and are not expensive.

Many of the procedures that were included in the first two editions of the *Manual* are still widely used today. Many of the previously described needle biopsy techniques have been replaced by procedures that use modern, often disposable equipment. In addition, sonography and endoscopy have become standards of practice in the last two decades. The safety and success of many semi-invasive techniques, such as abdominocentesis, thoracocentesis, pericardiocentesis, cystocentesis, and percutaneous needle biopsies, are greatly enhanced by concurrent use of imaging or direct visualization with an endoscope or laparoscope.

In the interest of patient comfort and safety, we routinely use endoscopic and sonographic guidance to perform many of these diagnostic procedures. Endoscopes and ultrasound machines are now commonly available in progressive small animal practices in the United States; however, not every practice may be able to incur the cost of the expensive instruments. Consequently, we continue to describe some procedures which can be performed without the benefit of these excellent clinical aids.

Because these procedures are less commonly used in everyday practice, proficiency can take much longer than for routine techniques. Appropriate care and selection of these clinical tools will help the practicing veterinarian and technician to provide clients and patients with a more complete range and greater quality of diagnostic and therapeutic services.

Things are only impossible until they're not.
JEAN-LUC PICARD

When all else fails, read the instructions.
ANONYMOUS

Chapter 16

Skin Preparation

We are held responsible not only for what we do, but for what we don't do.
CARL OSBORNE

Many of the procedures described in Part II are semi-invasive. Consequently, adequate disinfection of the skin is necessary to prevent sepsis. Methods of cleansing the skin of dogs and cats are described in almost every veterinary surgery text. For a thorough discussion of theory and principles of skin preparation, we refer our readers to those references.

Our preferred technique for skin preparation is described below. It is more than adequate for minimizing the probability of postoperative infection in all of the procedures included in this manual. Occasionally, some modifications are needed—such changes are described in the preparation section of each chapter for cases in which standard skin preparation technique is not appropriate.

Equipment Needed

- Animal hair clipper, with No. 10 or No. 40 blade
- 2 inch × 2 inch gauze sponges soaked in 2% chlorhexidine scrub
- 2 inch× 2 inch gauze sponges soaked in 70% alcohol
- Sponge forceps (optional)
- Surgical towels
- Fenestrated surgical drape
- Towel clamps (2–4)

Procedure

Technical Action	Rationale/Amplification
1. If animal's skin is heavily soiled, consider bathing whole animal before proceeding.	1. Bathing will help to minimize the chance of gross contamination of the operative site.

Crow and Walshaw's Manual of Clinical Procedures in Dogs, Cats, Rabbits, and Rodents, Fourth Edition. Edited by Jennifer E. Boyle. Published 2016 by John Wiley & Sons, Inc.
Companion Website: www.wiley.com/go/boyle/manual4e

Technical Action	Rationale/Amplification
2. Immobilize operative site.	2. Refer to recommended restraint measures for each procedure. General anesthesia is the only method that insures adequate immobilization for lengthy procedures.
3. Clip hair close to skin from a large area around operative site.	3. Do not skimp on area clipped. A wide margin is required to prevent contamination of the operative field. Clipped hairs should be less than 2 mm long.
4. Vacuum hair clippings and epithelial debris from entire area.	4. Do not touch the vacuum hose to the skin, as excessive suction may cause bruising.
5. Gently scrub skin with sponges soaked in 2% chlorhexidine scrub.	5. Start at the operative site and move the sponge outward toward the haired edges of the field, using a centrifugal spiral motion. Chlorhexidine and alcohol are recommended by the Centers for Disease Control (CDC) for skin preparation.
6. Remove soap by wiping operative site with alcohol-soaked gauze sponges.	6. Several sponges may be required.
7. Repeat Nos. 5 and 6 at least two times.	7. The alternating surgical scrub and alcohol scrubs should be continued until no soil is visible on the used sponges. Avoid applying excessive amounts of solutions.
8. After last scrub, allow operative field to air dry.	8. This delay allows the surgical scrub to kill more microorganisms.
9. Place towels and drapes around operative site and secure to skin with towel clamps.	9. Towels and drapes help to prevent inadvertent contamination of instruments.

Bibliography

CDC: Guideline for Prevention of Surgical Site Infection. www.cdc.gov/ncidod/dhqp/gl_surgicalsite.html, 1999

Knecht CD, Allen AR, Williams DJ, Johnson JH: Fundamental Techniques in Veterinary Surgery, 3rd edition. Philadelphia, WB Saunders, 1987

O'Grady NP *et al.*: Guidelines for the prevention of intravascular catheter-related infections. MMWR 51(RR10): 1–26. www.cdc.gov/mmwr/preview/mmwrhtml/rr5110a1.htm, 2002

Osuna DJ, DeYoung DJ, Walker RL: Comparison of three skin preparation techniques; Part 1: Experimental trial. Veterinary Surgery 19(1): 14–19, 1990

Osuna DJ, DeYoung DG, Walker RL: Comparison of three skin preparation techniques; Part 2: Clinical trial in 100 dogs. Veterinary Surgery 19(1): 20–23, 1990

Pratt PW (ed): Medical Nursing for Animal Health Technicians. Santa Barbara, CA, American Veterinary Publications, 1985

Riser WH: Preparation of the patient's skin. In Archibald J (ed): Canine Surgery, 1st edition. Santa Barbara, American Veterinary Publications, 1965

Slatter D: Textbook of Small Animal Surgery, 2nd edition. Philadelphia, WB Saunders, 1993

Tracy DL, Warren RG: Small Animal Surgical Nursing. St. Louis, CV Mosby, 1983

Chapter 17

Intubation

It's what you learn after you know it all that counts.
JOHN WOODEN

Intubation is the insertion of a tube into an organ or body cavity. * **With the exception of endotracheal and orogastric intubation, the following procedures are considered invasive and are typically performed exclusively by veterinarians.**

ENDOTRACHEAL INTUBATION

Endotracheal intubation is the placement of a tube that extends from the oral cavity into the trachea.

Purposes

1. To administer inhalation anesthetic drugs
2. To ensure a patent airway in unconscious animals
3. To administer oxygen
4. To provide ventilatory assistance

Complications

1. Trauma to teeth or mucous membranes of mouth, soft palate, pharynx, or larynx
2. Tracheal inflammation or necrosis
3. Subcutaneous emphysema secondary to tracheal trauma
4. Laryngospasm
5. Obstruction of the airway with secretions
6. Inadequate ventilation due to introduction of endotracheal tube into a bronchus
7. Aspiration of endotracheal tube

Crow and Walshaw's Manual of Clinical Procedures in Dogs, Cats, Rabbits, and Rodents, Fourth Edition. Edited by Jennifer E. Boyle. Published 2016 by John Wiley & Sons, Inc.
Companion Website: www.wiley.com/go/boyle/manual4e

Equipment Needed

- Endotracheal tube of appropriate size and type (Table 17-1)
- Gauze strip, 30–50 cm long
- Sterile lubricating jelly
- 6-mL syringe
- Hemostat
- Laryngoscope or other light source
- Topical anesthetic (2% lidocaine) (for cats)
- Additional equipment depending on circumstances:
  - Injectable anesthetic agents
  - Inhalation anesthesia machine
  - Ambu bag
  - Emergency drugs

Restraint and Positioning

Endotracheal intubation is performed on dogs and cats that have been rendered unconscious by sedatives or anesthetic agents, trauma, or disease. Endotracheal intubation can be accomplished most easily when an assistant holds the animal in sterna recumbency. An animal can also be intubated while in lateral or dorsal recumbency. Large dogs may be intubated more easily while in lateral recumbency.

TABLE 17-1 Recommended endotracheal tube sizes for routine use in dogs and cats.*

Animal	Body Weight (lb)	Internal Diameter of Tube (mm)
Cat	2	3
	4	3.5–4
	8	4–4.5
Dog	5	5
	10	6
	15	6–7
	20	6–7
	25	6–8
	30	7–8
	35	7–8
	40	8–10
	45	8–10
	60	11–12
	80	12–14

*Individual variations exist, and obesity must be taken into consideration. Some breeds (e.g. Bulldogs) have relatively small tracheas for their body size, and some breeds (e.g. Dachshunds) have large tracheas.

Procedure

Technical Action

1. Select endotracheal tube of appropriate diameter (see Table 17-1).
2. Premeasure length of tube against animal's neck (Fig. 17-1).
3. Check function of inflatable cuff, if present. Check that tube is clean and in good condition.
4. Lubricate tracheal end of tube with small amount of sterile lubricating jelly or water.
5. *Assistant*: (Fig. 17-2)
   a) Place animal in sterna recumbency.
   b) Extend animal's neck and open animal's mouth widely, with one hand (or gauze strip) holding upper jaw.

Rationale/Amplification

1. Attempting to use a tube that is too large can cause trauma to the larynx or trachea. A tube that is too small will not provide an adequate airway.
2. Once in place, the tip of the tube should be located midway between the larynx and the thoracic inlet. A longer tube is required for some surgical procedures (e.g. cervical decompression).
3. Inflate the cuff with air, using a 6-mL syringe. Observe and listen for leaks; submerge the cuff in water and observe for bubbles if in doubt about cuff seal.
4. Lubrication reduces irritation to the tracheal mucosa during intubation.
5. *Assistant*:
   a) Hold the animal so that the head and neck are not twisted to either side.
   b) Strips of gauze are particularly useful for holding the upper jaw of brachycephalic dogs.

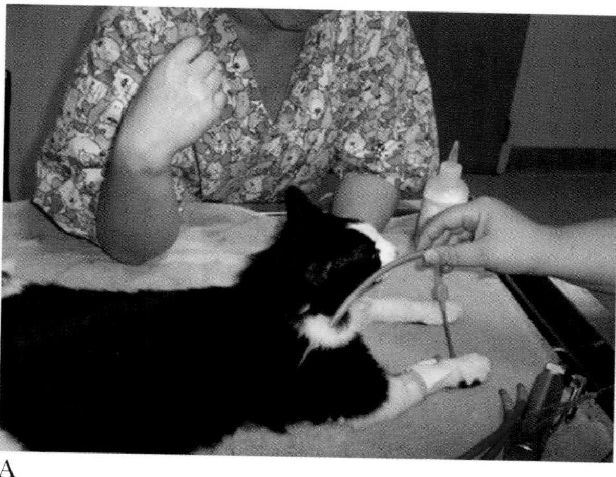
A

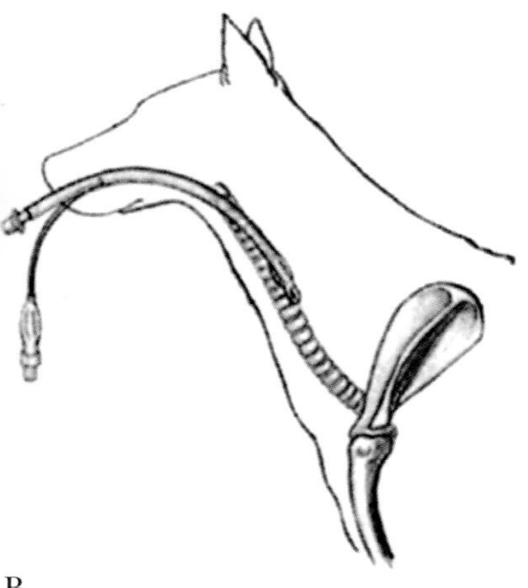
B

Figure 17-1 **(A)** Pre-measuring length of endotracheal tube required for animal. **(B)** Appropriate tube length.

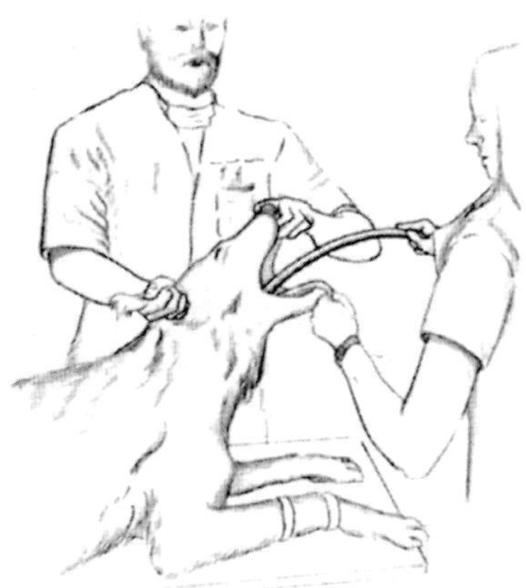

Figure 17-2 Restraint of animal for endotracheal intubation.

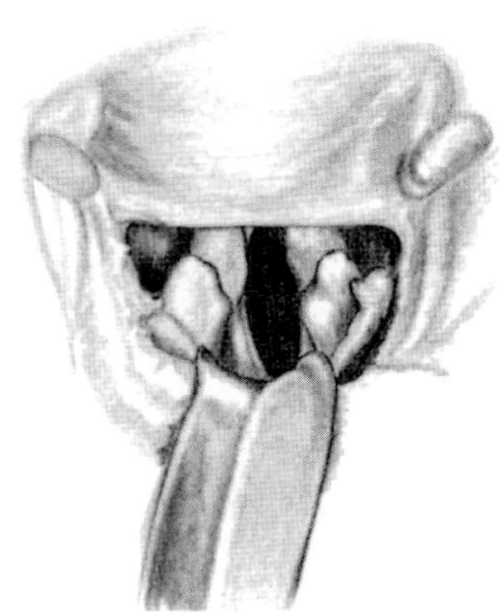

Figure 17-3 Laryngoscopic view of glottis.

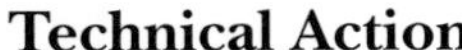

Technical Action

c) Pull animal's tongue out of mouth with other hand.

6. *Operator*: Use laryngoscope to locate larynx (Fig. 17-3). If necessary, apply topical anesthetic to larynx of cat (one drop 2% lidocaine on each arytenoid).
7. Depress epiglottis with tip of laryngoscope blade or endotracheal tube to examine arytenoid cartilages and vocal folds (Fig. 17-4).
8. Pass lubricated end of endotracheal tube through glottis and into trachea until tip of tube is midway between larynx and thoracic inlet (Fig. 17-1).
9. Check for correct placement of tube.
   a) Auscult both sides of animal's chest for breath sounds.
   b) Palpate neck for presence of two tubes.
   c) Directly palpate larynx and endotracheal tube if animal is well anesthetized.

Rationale/Amplification

c) Alternatively, the operator may grasp the tongue with one hand (see Fig. 17-2). A gauze sponge is useful for grasping a slippery tongue.

6. *Operator*: The use of a topical anesthetic is helpful in preventing laryngospasm during endotracheal intubation of the cat.
7. It is advisable to place the tip of a curved laryngoscope blade just anterior to the epiglottis in the cat so as to avoid laryngospasm, which can occur when the epiglottis is stimulated.
8. If the endotracheal tube is advanced too far down the trachea, it can enter the right or left mainstem bronchus, thus preventing ventilation of the other lung field.
9. Palpation of two firm tubes in the neck indicates that the esophagus (rather than the trachea) has been intubated.

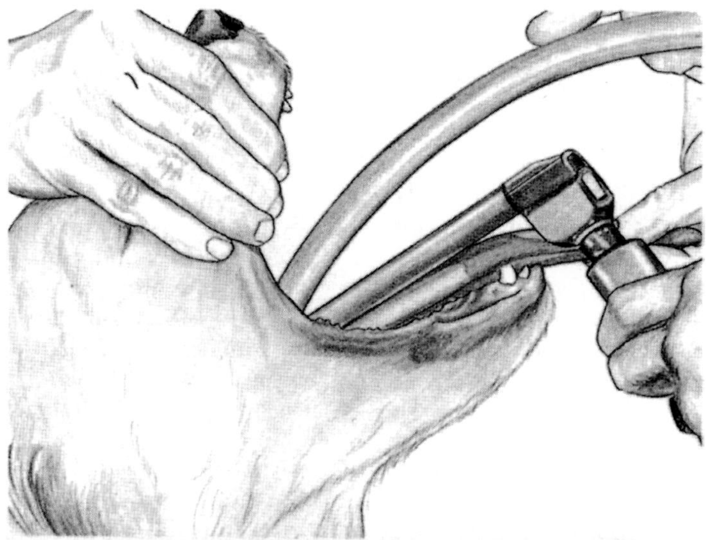

Figure 17-4 Use of laryngoscope to inspect glottis.

Technical Action

10. Tie a single half-hitch knot around tube with gauze strip and then tie tube with quick release knot to upper jaw, lower jaw, or head behind ears (Fig. 17-5).

Rationale/Amplification

10. The tie should be placed posterior to the animal's canine teeth. The position of the gauze tie will depend on whether a procedure is to be performed in the head or neck region.

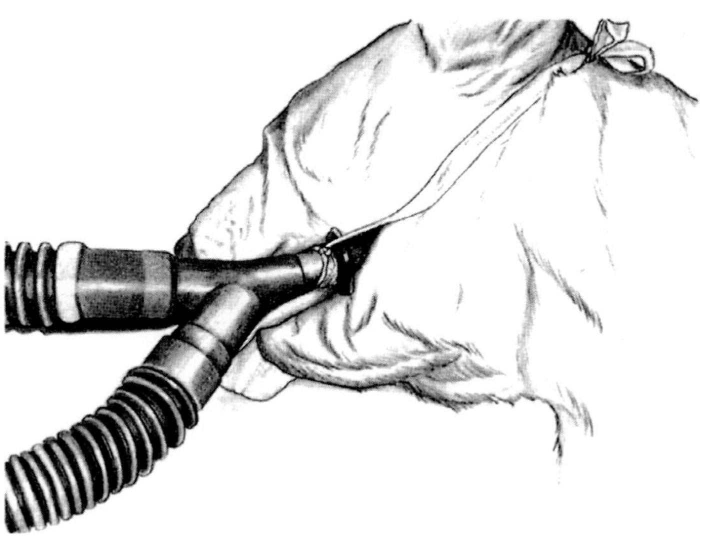

Figure 17-5 Endotracheal tube tied in place.

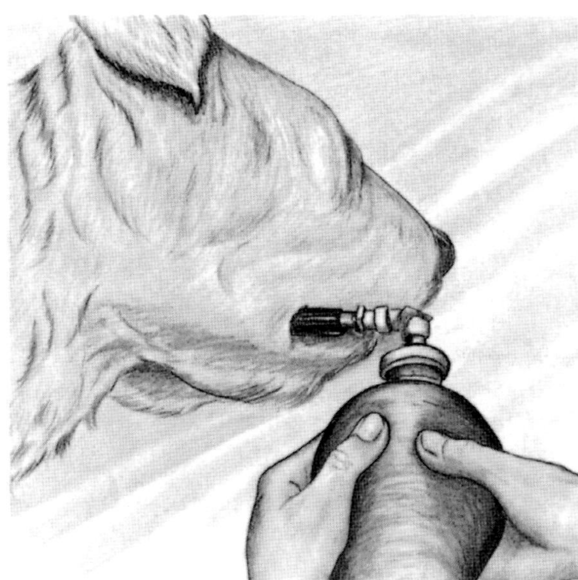

Figure 17-6 Manual ventilation with an Ambu bag.

Technical Action	Rationale/Amplification
11. Connect endotracheal tube to inhalation anesthesia machine, Ambu bag, or respirator when required.	**11.** The Ambu bag is used for manual ventilation of an animal in respiratory arrest (Fig. 17-6).
12. Inflate cuff of endotracheal tube with sufficient air to seal area between tube and trachea (Fig. 17-7).	**12.** Inflate cuff to an air seal of 20 cm H_2O in dogs and 12–15 cm H_2O in cats. Overinflation of the cuff can cause tracheal inflammation and necrosis. If more than 5 mL of air is needed to inflate the cuff in a dog (or 2 mL in a cat), replace endotracheal tube with one of larger diameter. A leak should be heard around the tube when one is manually ventilating an animal with more than twice its tidal volume. This leak will act as a "safety valve" and protect the lungs from overinflation.
13. While animal is intubated, observe frequently for: **a)** Kinking of endotracheal tube due to malpositioning of neck.	**13.** Indications of adequate ventilation include normal pink color of mucous membranes and clear lung sounds on auscultation. It is

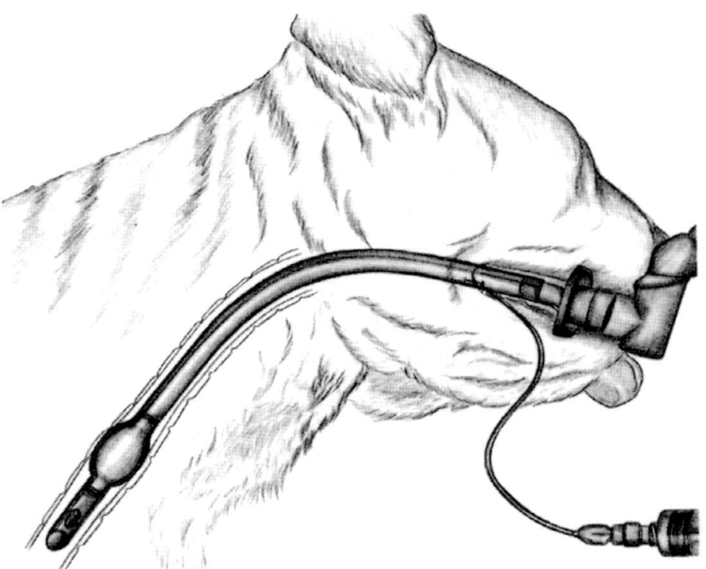

Figure 17-7 Inflating cuff of endotracheal tube.

Technical Action	Rationale/Amplification
b) Obstruction of endotracheal tube with secretions. **c)** Biting of endotracheal tube (because of return of reflexes). **d)** Twisting of endotracheal tube.	sometimes necessary to remove secretions by tracheal suctioning through the endotracheal tube. An animal must be observed closely while regaining consciousness so that it does not bite through the endotracheal tube and aspirate it. Disconnect the tube from the breathing circuit when manipulating or changing position to avoid twisting or pulling on the tube, which can cause tracheal tears.
14. When procedure requiring anesthesia is completed, turn off inhalant anesthetic, but continue delivery of oxygen until animal is ready to be extubated.	**14.** In low-risk patients with good breathing patterns and little potential for airway obstruction, it is acceptable to stop the flow of oxygen and permit them to breathe room air for several minutes before extubation.
15. Loosen tie on tube as reflexes begin to return.	**15.** Loosening the anchoring ties permits rapid removal of the endotracheal tube when the animal begins to swallow.

Technical Action	Rationale/Amplification
16. Deflate cuff and remove tube (extubate) when swallowing reflex has returned.	**16.** Avoid deflating cuff until the animal is ready to extubate. The cuff provides protection from aspiration until the patient's swallowing reflex returns. The animal's mouth and airway should be evaluated for foreign material prior to deflating cuff and extubation. Removing an endotracheal tube with an inflated cuff is traumatic to the trachea and larynx and should be avoided.
17. Position animal with head, neck, and tongue extended and continue to observe until animal is fully conscious.	**17.** In the semiconscious state following anesthesia, an animal can die as a result of airway obstruction. Brachycephalic breeds (e.g. English bulldog, Boston terrier) are particularly susceptible to airway obstruction during anesthesia recovery. We recommend that shortnosed dogs be recovered *in sterna recumbency only.* Careful monitoring for obstruction after the endotracheal tube is removed is essential, because many of these dogs will partially or completely obstruct their upper airway shortly after extubation. Be prepared to reintubate immediately.

CHEST TUBE PLACEMENT

Chest tube placement is the insertion of a flexible catheter into the pleural cavity.

Purposes

1. To remove fluids or air continuously or repeatedly from the chest
2. To infuse certain medications into the chest

Specific Indications

1. Pneumothorax
2. Pleural effusion

Complications

1. Leakage of room air into chest tube with resulting pneumothorax
2. Pleural inflammation or infection
3. Puncture of intercostal artery
4. Laceration of lung with resulting hemothorax or pneumothorax
5. Laceration of heart or great vessels

Equipment Needed

- Sterile chest tube: rubber or soft vinyl urethral catheter, or commercial chest tube 14 F, or larger
- Cotton
- Clipper with No. 40 blade
- Skin preparation material (see Chapter 16)
- Drugs and equipment for general anesthesia, or 2% lidocaine for local anesthesia in critically ill animals
- Cap and mask
- Sterile surgical equipment:
  - Drapes
  - Gown
  - Surgeon's gloves
  - Gauze sponges
  - Scalpel blade and handle
  - Scissors
  - Two curved hemostats
  - Suture material: monofilament, nonabsorbable
  - Three-way stopcock and catheter adapter
  - Straight hemostat
  - 60-mL syringe
- Bandaging material:
  - Sterile gauze sponges
  - Antimicrobial ointment
  - Gauze bandage
  - Adhesive tape (2-inch-wide) or elastic adhesive bandage

Restraint and Positioning

General anesthesia is preferred for the maintenance of strict asepsis during chest tube placement. If the animal's critical condition precludes general anesthesia, the area for chest tube placement, including the pleura, is infiltrated with 2% lidocaine. The animal should be positioned in lateral recumbency.

Procedure

Technical Action	Rationale/Amplification
1. Clip and surgically prepare skin over lateral thorax from fifth to ninth intercostal spaces (see Chapter 16).	**1.** Failure to cleanse the skin thoroughly before chest tube insertion can result in infection.
2. If general anesthesia cannot be used, infiltrate skin, subcutaneous tissue, intercostal muscles, and pleura with 2% lidocaine.	**2.** A total of 2–5 mL of lidocaine may be needed to provide adequate local anesthesia.
3. Don cap, mask, sterile gown, and gloves. Place sterile drapes around chest tube insertion site.	**3.** Strict attention to asepsis is recommended.
4. Cut additional holes in chest tube, if necessary. Seal end of chest tube with catheter adapter and three-way stopcock.	**4.** It is advantageous to have several holes in the tube to decrease the chance of blockage of the tube with secretions. The chest tube should be sealed during insertion to prevent room air from entering the chest.
5. Make small incision in skin at level of mid-thorax over eighth or ninth intercostal space.	**5.** The skin incision should be two intercostal spaces caudal to the intended insertion site of the chest tube.
6. Using curved hemostat, tunnel cranially through subcutaneous tissue to sixth or seventh intercostal space (Fig. 17-8).	**6.** The subcutaneous tunnel is made with the hemostat by gentle blunt dissection. The tunnel must be wide enough to accommodate a second hemostat and a chest tube.
7. Force closed hemostat into thoracic cavity, keeping close to cranial edge of seventh or eighth rib (Fig. 17-9).	**7.** The intercostal arteries are located along the caudal edge of each rib and must be avoided to minimize the chance of severe hemorrhage.

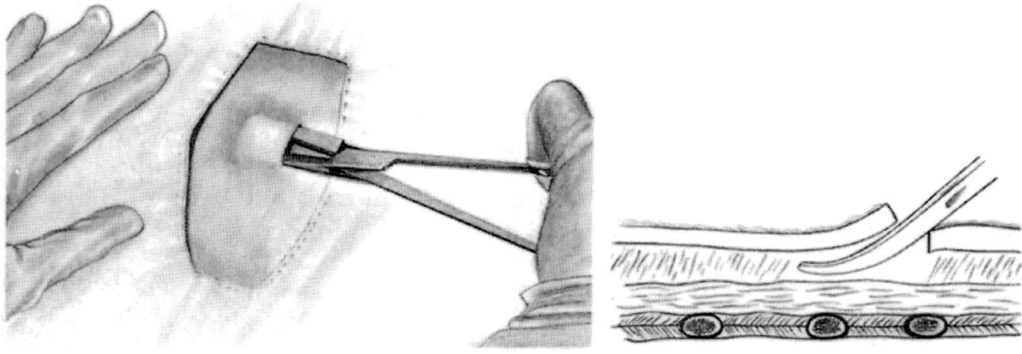

Figure 17-8 Formation of subcutaneous tunnel for chest tube.

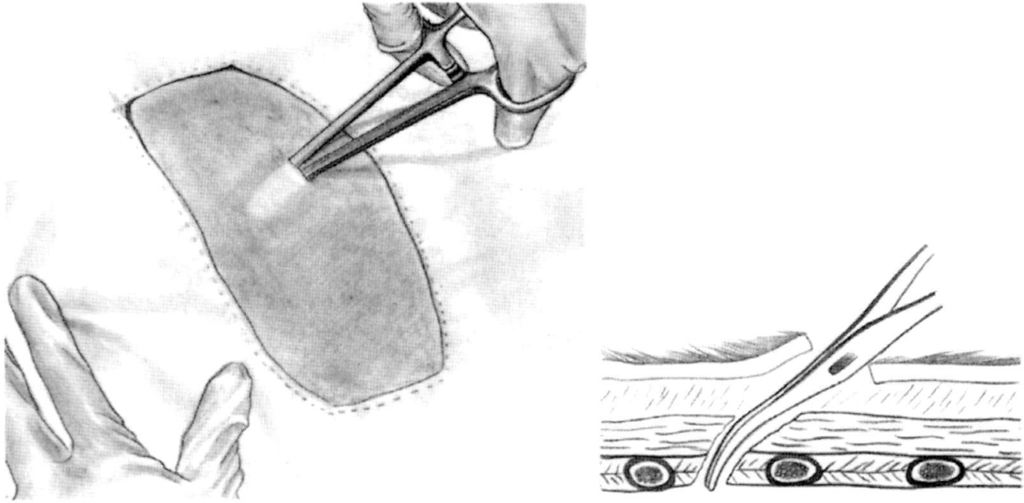

Figure 17-9 Inserting closed hemostat into thorax.

Technical Action

8. Spread jaws of hemostat and leave in place.
9. Place tip of chest tube between jaws of second curved hemostat. Advance second hemostat through subcutaneous tunnel so that tube tip just enters thoracic cavity (Fig. 17-10A).
10. Open jaws of second hemostat and manually advance chest tube well into thoracic cavity (Fig. 17-10B).
11. Remove hemostat that held tube first, then hemostat that was used to create subcutaneous tunnel.
12. Hold sponge over subcutaneous tunnel while aspirating chest tube with 60-mL syringe (Fig. 17-11).
13. Place suture through skin edges around exit point of chest tube from skin (Fig. 17-12A).

Rationale/Amplification

8. Spreading the jaws of the haemostat prevents the pleura and intercostal muscles from occluding the puncture site.
11. Open the jaws of the second hemostat just enough to prevent it from pulling the tube back out of the chest. Once the tube is properly in place through the thoracic wall and pleura, remove the first hemostat.
12. If no fluid or air can be aspirated, the tube should be advanced or withdrawn slightly until patency is ensured.

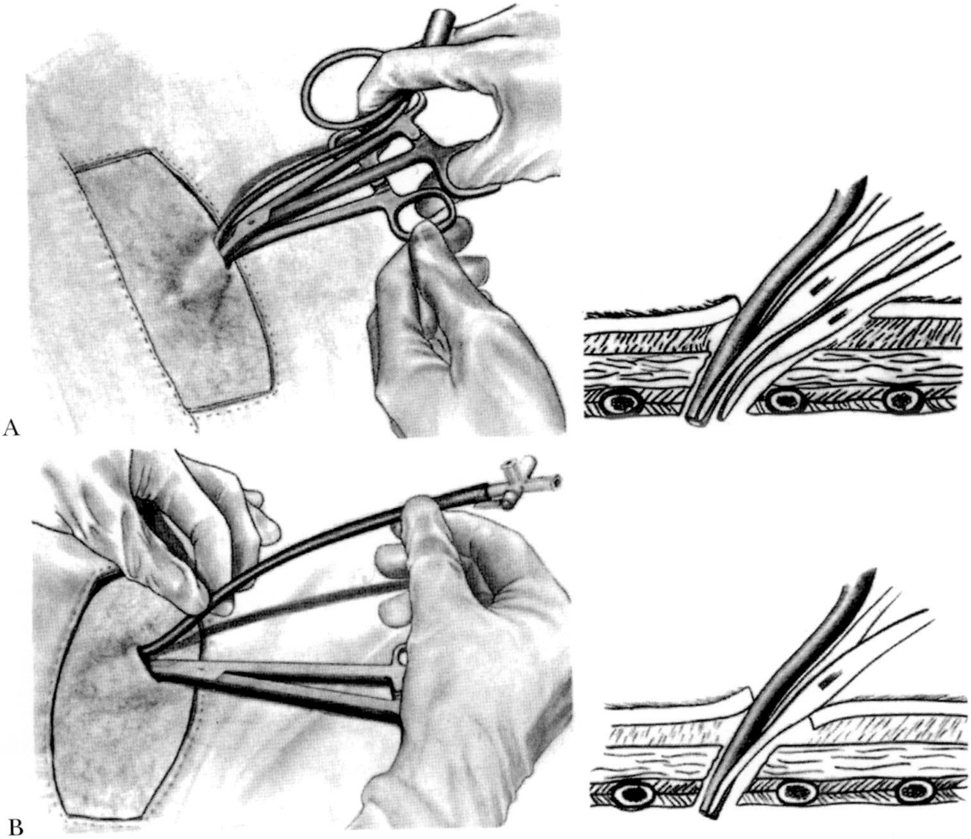

A

B

Figure 17-10 (A) Advancing second hemostat (with tip of tube clamped in jaws) through tunnel created by first hemostat. (B) Sliding chest tube between open jaws of lower haemostat and into pleural space.

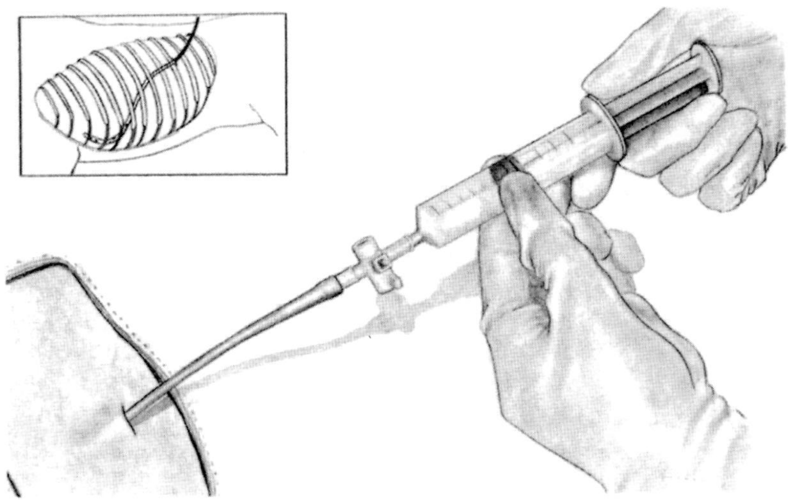

Figure 17-11 Aspirating chest tube to ensure correct placement.

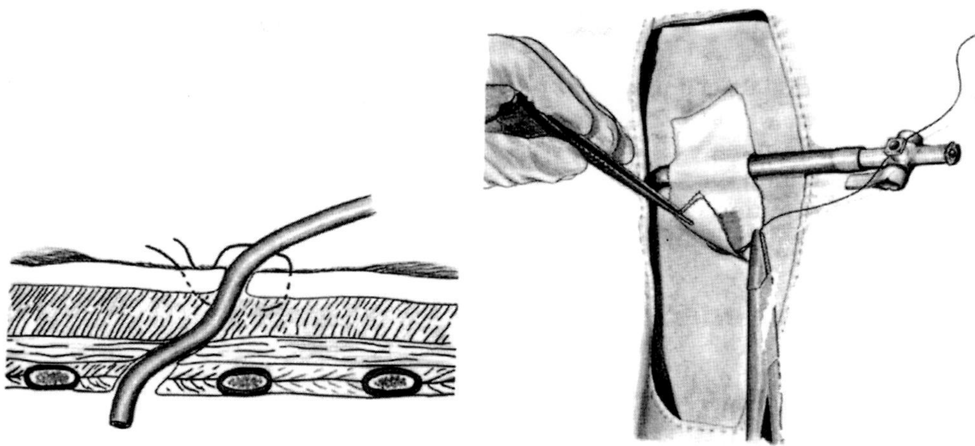

Figure 17-12 (A) Suture around exit point of chest tube. (B) Adhesive tape "butterfly" around chest tube sutured to skin.

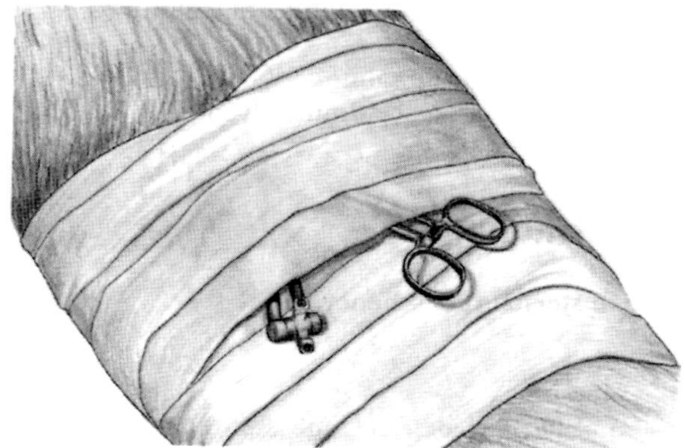

Figure 17-13 Bandage covering chest tube and jaws of hemostat.

Technical Action	Rationale/Amplification
14. Make adhesive tape "butterfly" around chest tube and suture butterfly to skin with simple interrupted sutures (Fig. 17-12B).	**14.** The adhesive tape helps to anchor the chest tube in position.
15. Place antimicrobial ointment and sterile gauze sponge over skin incision.	
16. Bandage chest tube in place by completely encircling thorax with gauze and adhesive tape or elastic adhesive bandage.	**16.** The bandage must permit the animal to breathe easily, but it should be secure.
17. Place straight hemostat on chest tube proximal to stopcock, and incorporate jaws of hemostat into bandage (Fig. 17-13).	**17.** The hemostat is additional protection against iatrogenic pneumothorax should the stopcock become dislodged.

Technical Action	Rationale/Amplification
18. Aspirate chest tube at prescribed intervals, moving animal into various positions if necessary.	**18.** Do not leave an animal with a chest tube in place unattended. Note date, time, volume and appearance of material aspirated, initials, and comments in animal's medical record.

OROGASTRIC INTUBATION

Orogastric intubation is the placement of a tube that extends from the oral cavity into the stomach.

Purposes

1. To administer medication and certain radiographic contrast materials
2. To remove stomach contents
3. To perform gastric lavage (see Chapter 18)
4. To administer nutrients (e.g. to puppies and kittens)

Complications

1. Administration of materials into respiratory tract due to incorrect placement of tube
2. Esophageal trauma
3. Gastric irritation
4. Gastric perforation

Equipment Needed

- Stomach tube:
  - 12 F rubber urethral catheter for kittens and puppies
  - 18 F rubber urethral catheter for adult cats and dogs up to 40 lb.
  - Foal stomach tube for dogs >40 lb.
- Speculum:
  - Commercial canine mouth speculum or roll of 2-inch-wide adhesive tape
  - 1-inch-wide wooden dowel with center hole for cats
- Adhesive tape or ballpoint pen for marking stomach tube
- Lubricating jelly
- Syringe containing 5 mL of sterile saline
- Syringe or funnel for material to be administered

Restraint and Positioning

Restrain the animal in sternal recumbency. Do not attempt to pass an orogastric tube with an animal in lateral recumbency.

Procedure

Technical Action / **Rationale/Amplification**

1. Premeasure stomach tube by holding it next to animal. When tip is at level of last rib, mark point on tube at oral opening with felt pen or adhesive tape (Fig. 17-14).

   When premeasuring the tube, one must follow the curvature of the neck in order to accurately estimate the length of the esophagus.

2. Moisten tip of stomach tube with lubricating jelly.

   Lubrication of the tube helps to minimize the possibility of esophageal trauma while the tube is passed.

3. Insert speculum into animal's mouth and hold animal's jaws closed on speculum.

   Some cats object so strenuously to this procedure that it cannot be performed without anesthesia. Nasogastric intubation should be considered for such cats.

4. Pass lubricated stomach tube through speculum and advance to premarked point (Fig. 17-15). If possible, advance tip of tube past larynx while animal is exhaling.

   Inability to pass the tube to the premeasured length may indicate that:
   a) It has been inserted into the trachea.
   b) There is an obstruction in the esophagus, or
   c) Gastric volvulus has occurred, preventing entry of the tube into the stomach.

5. Check proper placement of stomach tube as follows:
   a) Palpate tube within neck.
   b) Smell end of tube for gastric odors.
   c) Blow into tube while assistant auscults stomach for gurgling.
   d) Administer 5 mL of sterile saline through stomach tube and observe for cough.

   If the tube is in the esophagus, two tubes (the stomach tube and the trachea) should be palpable in the neck. If there is any evidence that the tube has been inserted into the trachea, remove the tube and reinsert it.

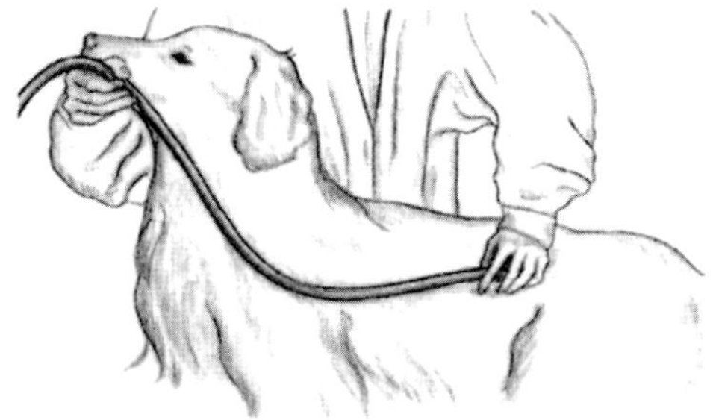

Figure 17-14 Pre-measuring length of stomach tube required for animal.

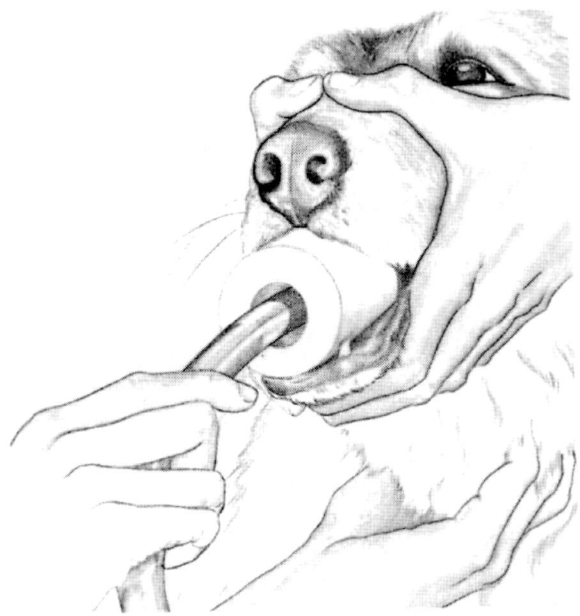

Figure 17-15 Inserting lubricated stomach tube through mouth speculum.

Technical Action	Rationale/Amplification
6. Administer materials prescribed or remove gastric contents. Then administer 5–15 mL of water to flush tube.	**6.** If orogastric intubation is performed on an unconscious animal, a cuffed endotracheal tube should be inserted before passing the stomach tube. This will prevent aspiration of any material regurgitated around the tube.
7. Before removing tube, seal end of tube with thumb.	**7.** Plugging the open end will help to prevent leakage of any material remaining in the tube into the pharynx as the tube is removed.
8. Note in animal's medical record that procedure was performed.	**8.** Note date, time, procedure, any materials removed or administered, initials, and comments.

NASOGASTRIC INTUBATION OF THE CAT

Nasogastric intubation is the placement of a tube that extends through an external naris, the nasal cavity, pharynx, and esophagus, and into the stomach. This procedure is of practical use mainly in the adult cat because of the relatively short nasal passage in that species. The procedure cannot be performed on kittens or on any cat with an obstruction of the nasal cavity.

Purposes

1. To administer medication and radiographic contrast materials
2. To administer nutritional supplements and water

Complications

1. Administration of materials into the respiratory tract
2. Esophageal trauma
3. Gastric irritation

Equipment Needed

- Nasogastric tube: Infant feeding tube or 21-gauge butterfly catheter (winged infusion set) with needle assembly cut off
- Topical ophthalmic anesthetic
- Lubricating jelly
- Syringe with 1 mL of sterile saline
- Syringe for material to be administered
- Bandaging material if catheter is to remain in place:
  - Gauze, 2 inches wide
  - Adhesive tape or elastic adhesive bandage, 2 inches wide
- Injection cap

Restraint and Positioning

The cat is held in a sitting position or in sternal recumbency by an assistant.

Procedure

Technical Action	Rationale/Amplification
1. Instill four or five drops of topical ophthalmic anesthetic into one nostril (Fig. 17-16).	1. The cat may sneeze at first.
2. Wait 2–3 minutes; then instill two or three more drops of topical ophthalmic anesthetic into same nostril.	2. During instillation of the topical ophthalmic anesthetic into the nostril, the cat's head should be positioned with its nose toward the ceiling.
3. Apply a small amount of lubricating jelly to tip of nasogastric tube.	3. Lubrication of the tube helps to minimize irritation to the nasal cavity, esophagus, and stomach during passage of the tube.

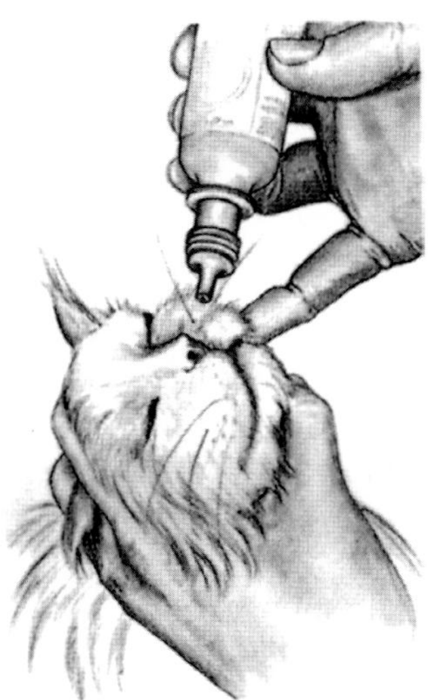

Figure 17-16 Instilling topical ophthalmic anesthetic into cat's nostril.

Technical Action	Rationale/Amplification
4. Hold cat's head with one hand and use other hand to insert tube into ventromedial aspect of anesthetized nostril (Fig. 17-17).	**4.** The cat can feel the pressure of the tube and may resist the procedure slightly.
5. Advance tube approximately 20–25 cm.	**5.** If the tube is difficult to pass, try rotating it gently before advancing it farther.
6. Check proper placement of nasogastric tube by instilling 1 mL of sterile saline into tube.	**6.** If the cat coughs, it should be assumed that the tube is in the trachea and the tube should be removed and reinserted. Vigorous laryngeal reflexes in cats usually prevent inadvertent intubation of the trachea.
7. Administer prescribed materials and flush nasogastric tube with 1 or 2 mL of water.	
8. Bandage catheter in place to side of cat's neck if repeated nasogastric intubation is anticipated and cat will tolerate leaving tube in place (Fig. 17-18).	**8.** Severely debilitated cats usually will tolerate long-term placement of the tube. The end of the catheter should be covered to prevent aspiration of air into the cat's stomach.
9. Before removing tube, seal end of tube with thumb or finger.	**9.** Plugging the end of the tube helps to prevent leakage of any material remaining in the tube into the pharynx as the tube is removed.
10. Note in animal's medical record that procedure was performed.	**10.** Note date, time, procedure, any materials administered, initials, and comments.

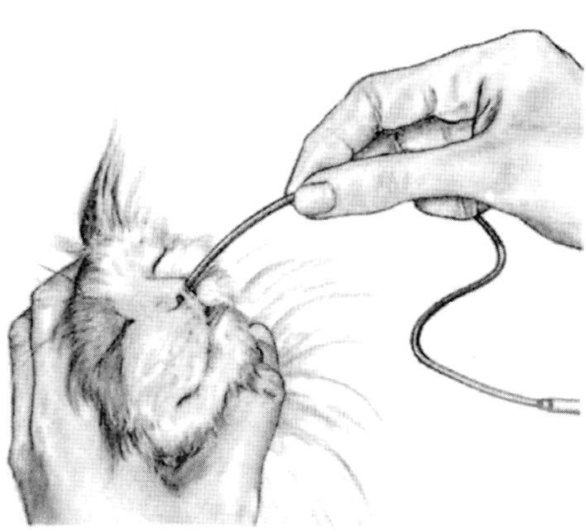

Figure 17-17 Inserting nasogastric tube into cat's nostril.

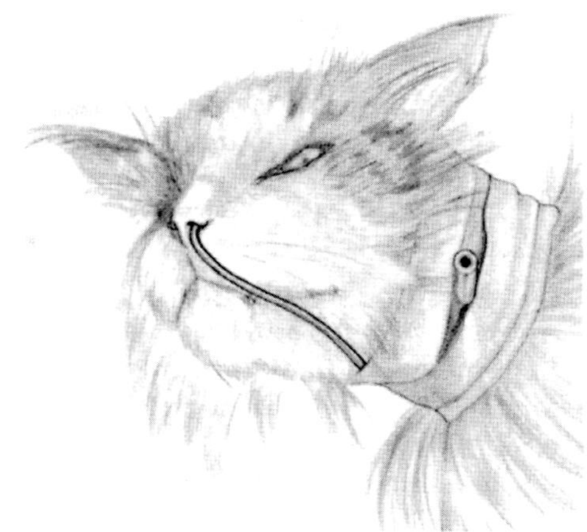

Figure 17-18 Nasogastric tube bandaged in place.

ESOPHAGOSTOMY TUBE PLACEMENT

An *esophagostomy tube* is the placement of a tube through the skin of the neck to the caudal esophagus.

Purpose

To administer nutrients and medications orally over days or weeks to an animal that is unable or unwilling to eat because of debilitation, oral lesions, or head trauma, but whose gastrointestinal tract is functioning normally.

Complications

1. Vomiting or regurgitation
2. Aspiration pneumonia
3. Esophagitis or esophageal perforation
4. Distension of stomach with air
5. Gastritis

Equipment Needed

- Sterile esophagostomy tube: Soft flexible polyurethane or red rubber feeding tube:
  - 10–12 F for cat or small dog
  - Up to 22 F for large dogs

- Commercial mouth speculum for dog or cat
- Clipper with No. 40 blade
- Anesthetic drugs
- Skin preparation materials (see Chapter 16)
- Sterile surgical equipment:
  - Surgeon's gloves
  - Scalpel blade and handle
  - Carmalt curved forceps
  - Suture material
  - Scissors
  - Gauze sponges
- Bandaging material:
  - Sterile gauze sponges
  - Gauze bandage
  - Adhesive tape, 1-inch-wide
  - Adhesive tape or elastic adhesive bandage

Restraint and Positioning

General anesthesia is needed for placement of an esophagostomy tube. The animal is positioned in right lateral recumbency.

Procedure

Technical Action	Rationale/Amplification
1. Clip and surgically prepare skin on left side of animal's neck (see Chapter 16).	
2. Place speculum in animal's mouth.	**2.** A mouth gag facilitates passage of the tube through the mouth and pharynx.
3. Measure distance from mid-cervical esophagus to last rib. Measuring from tip to open end, mark tube at appropriate length.	
4. Pass curved Carmalt forceps through mouth and proximal esophagus to midpoint of cervical esophagus.	
5. Direct forceps laterally toward left side of neck until tip of forceps jaws can be seen (Fig. 17-19).	
6. Make a small incision through skin and through wall of esophagus over tip of forceps (Fig. 17-20).	**6.** The esophageal incision should be as small as possible, just enough for the tip of the forceps to protrude.
7. Push forceps through incision.	

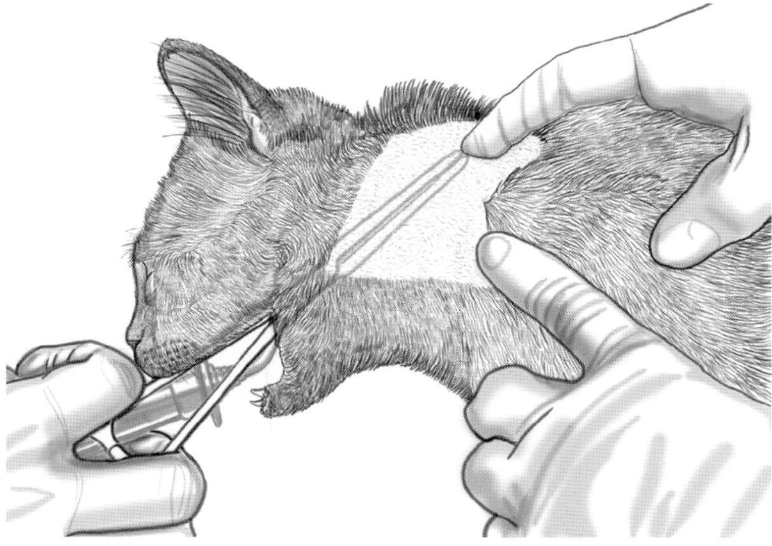

Figure 17-19 Passing forceps through mouth and into cervical esophagus.

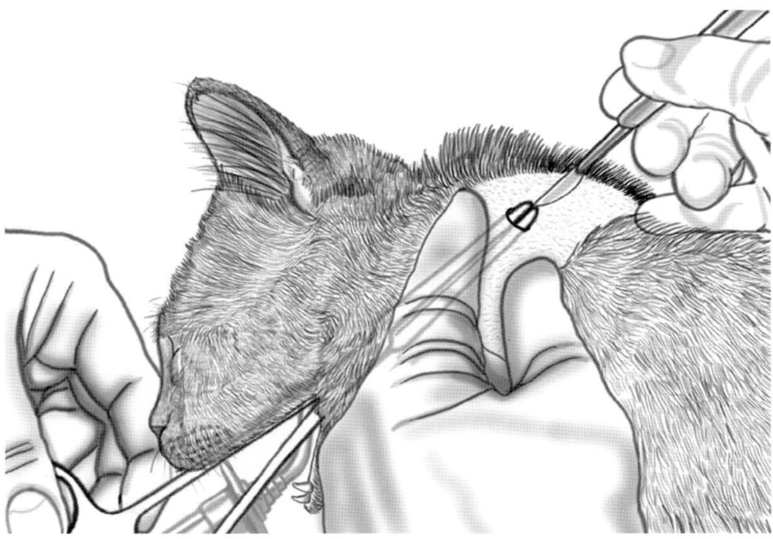

Figure 17-20 Incising skin over forceps jaws.

Technical Action	Rationale/Amplification
8. Grasp tip of esophagostomy tube with forceps and pull up through mouth (Fig. 17-21).	
9. Direct tip of tube aborally down esophagus to predetermined length (Fig. 17-22).	**9.** Push tube with fingers or forceps through mouth until it slides easily down esophagus.

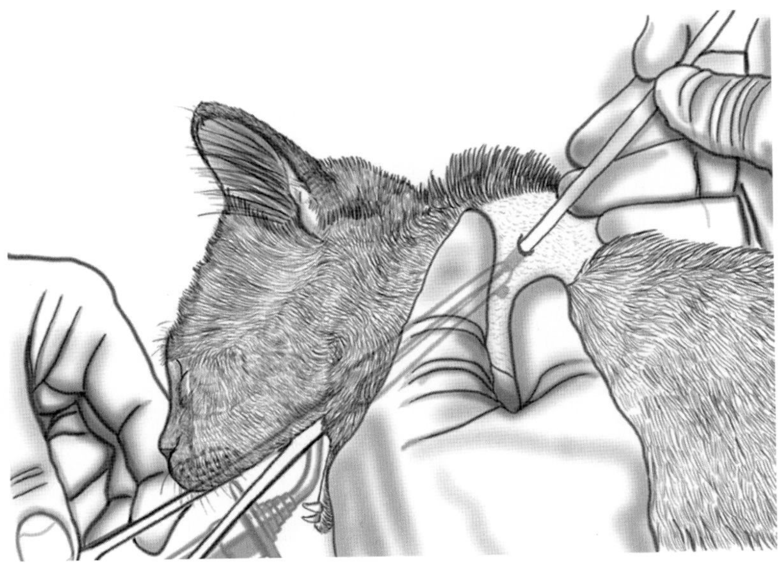

Figure 17-21 Grasping esophagostomy tube with forceps.

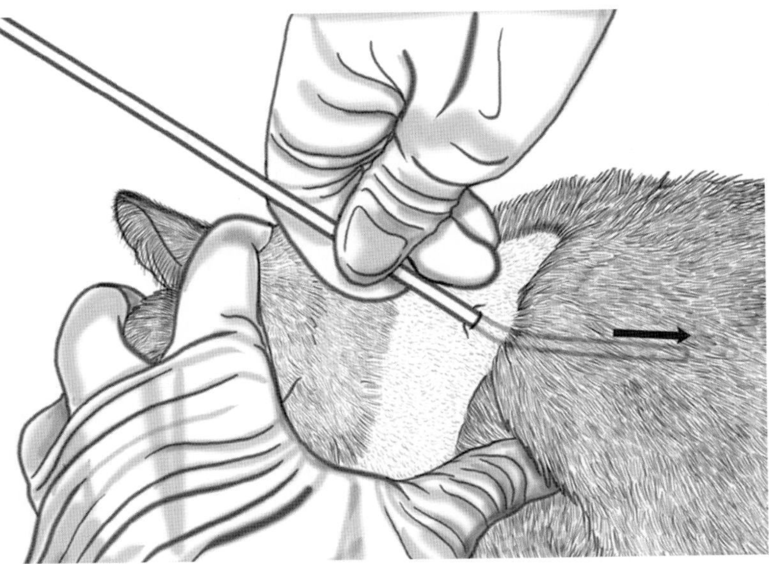

Figure 17-22 Directing esophagostomy tube aborally down esophagus.

Technical Action	Rationale/Amplification
10. Secure tube to cervical skin using an overlapping, interlocking suture (Chinese finger trap) pattern (Fig. 17-23).	

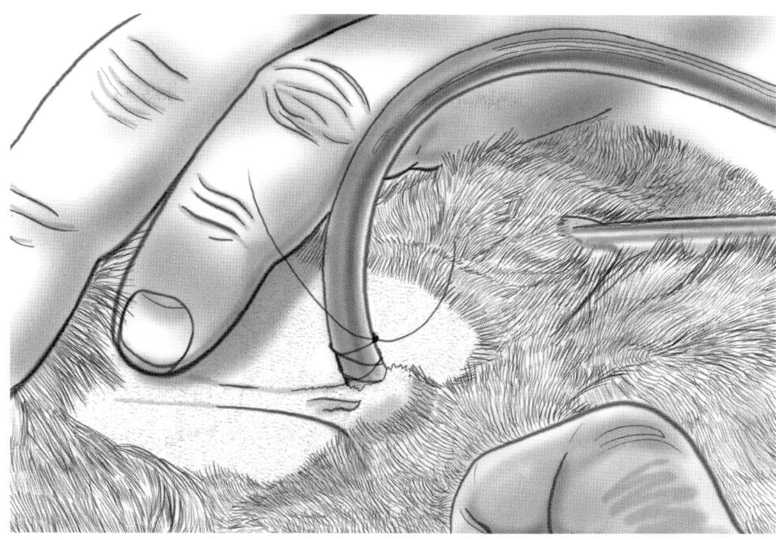

Figure 17-23 Esophagostomy tube sutured in place using finger trap suture pattern.

Technical Action	Rationale/Amplification
11. Place sterile gauze sponge over skin incision.	
12. Bandage tube in place by encircling neck completely with gauze and adhesive tape or elastic adhesive bandage, leaving 4–6 cm protruding from bandage (Fig. 17-24).	**12.** An Elizabethan collar should be placed if the animal attempts to scratch at the bandage frequently.
13. Make a lateral radiograph of thorax to ensure correct position of esophagostomy tube (Fig. 17-25).	**13.** Potential malpositioning problems include advancing the tube too far, knotting it within stomach, or doubling the tube back on itself.
14. When animal is fully awake, test animal's tolerance of feeding through esophagostomy tube by administering small amounts of water every hour.	**14.** Some animals may vomit or regurgitate initially. If this problem persists, the esophagostomy tube should be removed and an alternative method of alimentation instituted.
15. If animal does not regurgitate or vomit, proceed with nutritional program at prescribed intervals.	**15.** The tube should be flushed with 2–6 mL of water before and after each use and plugged between feedings.

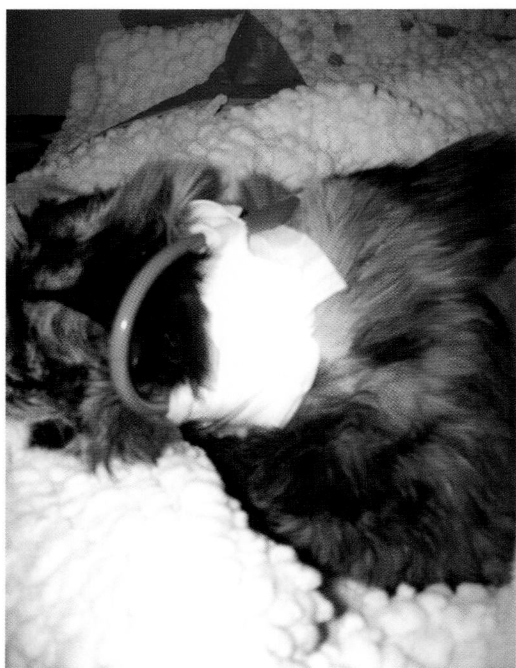

Figure 17-24 Bandage covering esophagostomy tube. Photo courtesy of C Knightly.

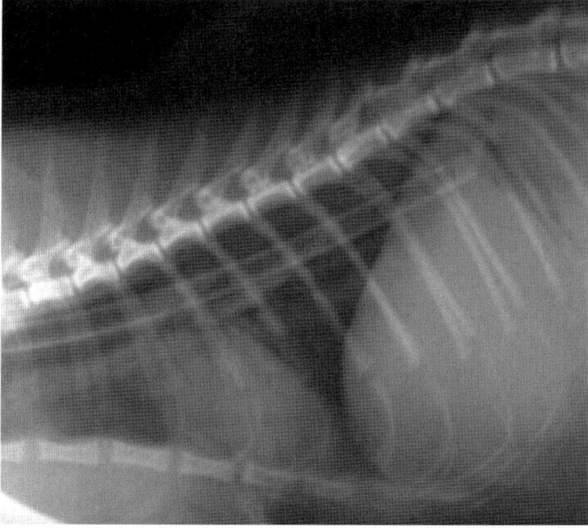

Figure 17-25 Radiograph showing proper position for caudal end of esophagostomy tube.

PERCUTANEOUS GASTROSTOMY TUBE PLACEMENT

A *percutaneous gastrostomy tube* is placed such that it extends through the skin and left cranial abdominal wall into the body of the stomach.

Purpose

To administer nutrients and medications orally over days or weeks to an animal that is unable or unwilling to eat because of debilitation, oral lesions, head trauma, or esophageal disorders, but whose gastrointestinal tract is functioning normally.

Specific Indications

1. Feline hepatic lipidosis
2. Oropharyngeal neoplasia
3. Maxillary or mandibular fractures
4. Oral reconstructive surgery
5. Esophageal masses or foreign bodies
6. Severe pharyngitis

Complications

1. Vomiting or regurgitation
2. Aspiration pneumonia
3. Distension of stomach with air
4. Gastritis
5. Dislodgement of tube leading to fistula formation or peritonitis
6. Infection
7. Pressure necrosis at stoma site

Equipment Needed

- Malecot (18–20 F) or French-pezzar mushroom-tip (18–24 F) catheter
- Sovereign intravenous catheter (18 g, 1½ in.)
- 80 cm (or longer) stainless steel or nylon suture material (00 or 0)
- Rigid vinyl stomach tube of appropriate size and length, with flared or rounded end, or Eld percutaneous gastrostomy tube applicator (Fig. 17-26)
- Clipper with No. 40 blade
- Anesthetic drugs and equipment for general anesthesia
- Skin preparation materials (see Chapter 16)
- Sterile surgical equipment:
  - Surgeon's gloves
  - Scalpel blade and handle
  - Kelly or Crile curved hemostat
  - Needle holder
  - Curved or straight suture needle
  - Suture material: monofilament, nonabsorbable
  - Scissors
  - Gauze sponges

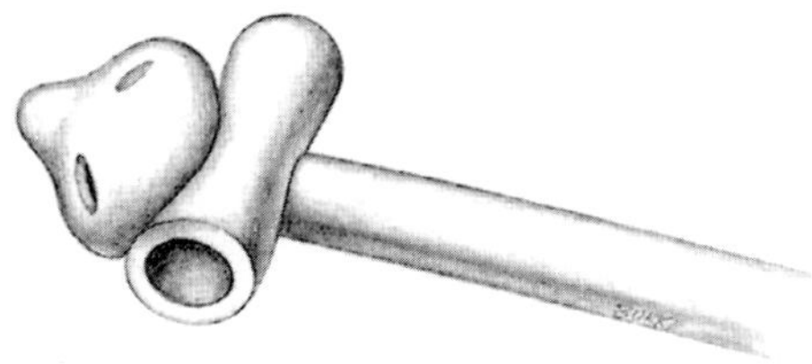

Figure 17-26 Prepared flange and distal end of French-pezzar mushroom-tip catheter (gastrostomy tube).

- Bandaging material:
  - Sterile gauze sponges
  - Antimicrobial ointment
  - Gauze bandage
  - Adhesive tape (1-inch-width)
  - Elastic adhesive bandage (2–6-inch-width)
- Stopper for gastrostomy tube (e.g. male IV catheter adapter)

Advance Preparation of Gastrostomy Tube

Technical Action	Rationale/Amplification
1. Flange preparation and placement (Malecot catheter): **a)** Cut off 3 cm of open (distal) end of catheter with scissors. **b)** Divide this segment into two pieces 1.5 cm (inner and outer flanges). **c)** Cut 3-mm holes on opposite sides of each piece. **d)** Thread distal (cut) end of catheter through holes in inner flange; slide flange toward proximal end of catheter so that flange nearly touches mushroom tip (Fig. 17-26). **e)** Retain second flange for later use. **f)** Cut distal end of catheter to form a sharp bevel point (Fig. 17-32). **g)** Measure length of tube from mushroom tip to 2 cm below bevel.	**1.** The Malecot catheter has an open mushroom-tip design but is much less rigid than the French-pezzar-type catheter. It will frequently dislodge if an inner flange is not used. When the procedures recommended here are followed, the authors have found it to be a reliable gastrostomy tube. The bevel at the end is to permit the catheter to be forced into the wide end of the plastic Sovereign catheter.
2. Flange preparation and placement (French-pezzar mushroom-tipped catheter): **a)** Cut off 1.5 cm of open (distal) end of catheter with scissors.	**2.** The French-pezzar mushroom-tipped catheter has a relatively closed design but is much more rigid than the Malecot catheter. It will rarely dislodge; an inner flange is not

Technical Action	Rationale/Amplification
b) Cut 3-mm holes on either side of 1.5-cm piece (outer flange). **c)** Retain this flange for later use—an inner flange is not needed for this catheter. **d)** Cut distal end of catheter to form a sharp bevel point (Fig. 17-32). **e)** Measure length of tube from mushroom tip to 2 cm below bevel.	needed. The bevel at the open end permits the catheter to be forced into the wide end of the plastic Sovereign catheter.
3. Orogastric tube preparation (not needed if using Eld device):* **a)** Use an open flame to slightly flare and smooth distal end of thick vinyl stomach tube. **b)** Measure length of tube needed to reach stomach by laying tube along animal's side with rounded end 1–2 cm caudal to last rib. **c)** Mark tube with adhesive tape at tip of muzzle. Cut off excess tube. **d)** Put tube in freezer for approximately 30 minutes before beginning procedure.	**3.** Rounding the edge minimizes trauma to the esophagus and stomach during introduction of the tube. Premeasurement helps in determining when the stomach has been entered. The total length of the tube should be only 20–30 cm longer than the premeasured distance from nose to last rib. Do not remove the tube from the freezer until you are ready to pass it into the animal.

*NOTE: *In keeping with the central thesis of this book, we describe a very successful technique that requires very little extra equipment; however, several other methods may be used. Fiber optic endoscopy is used preferentially for large dogs. We recommend purchasing a commercially available percutaneous gastrostomy tube introducer (Eld device) (Fig. 17-27) for cats and small dogs. This handy device*

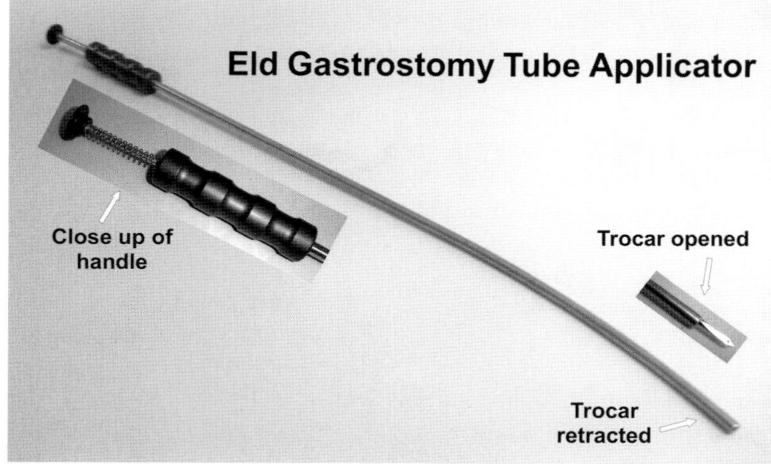

Figure 17-27 Eld percutaneous gastrostomy tube applicator.

is used in place of the orogastric tube, percutaneous catheter puncture, and rigid introducer line. The Eld method is described at the end of the tube procedure.

Restraint and Positioning

General anesthesia is needed for placement of a gastrostomy tube. An endotracheal tube with inflated cuff is used to provide an airway for inhalation anesthesia and protection against aspiration of stomach contents or accidental trauma to the larynx or trachea. The animal is positioned in right lateral recumbency.

Orogastric Tube Method for Line Capture

Technical Action	Rationale/Amplification
1. Clip and surgically prepare skin over left lateral abdominal wall (see Chapter 16).	
2. Place mouth speculum between right upper and lower canine teeth.	**2.** A mouth gag facilitates passage of the tube through the mouth and pharynx.
3. Lubricate rounded end of hardened (frozen) stomach tube, introduce it into animal's mouth and gently advance it down esophagus to level of cardia.	**3.** The tube should pass easily to the level of the cardia.
4. Rotate tube counterclockwise while gently advancing in order to pass cardia with minimal trauma.	**4.** A gentle 90–135-degree rotation usually results in the tube's slipping through the cardia.
5. Turn tube back clockwise and advance tube until it can be visualized through abdominal wall 1–2 cm caudal to last rib.	**5.** Rotating clockwise allows the tube to curve naturally within the stomach.
6. Wiggle and rotate tube until tip lies against stomach and abdominal wall approximately one-third of distance between epaxial muscles and ventral midline (Fig. 17-28).	**6.** In most cases, the end of the tube will be seen easily.
7. Grasp end of tube in one hand.	
8. Make 2–3-mm skin incision directly over lumen of stomach tube.	**8.** Do not penetrate subcutis, peritoneum, or stomach with the scalpel blade.
9. After passing needle tip through skin incision, puncture abdominal and stomach walls with over-theneedle Sovereign catheter (Fig. 17-29).	

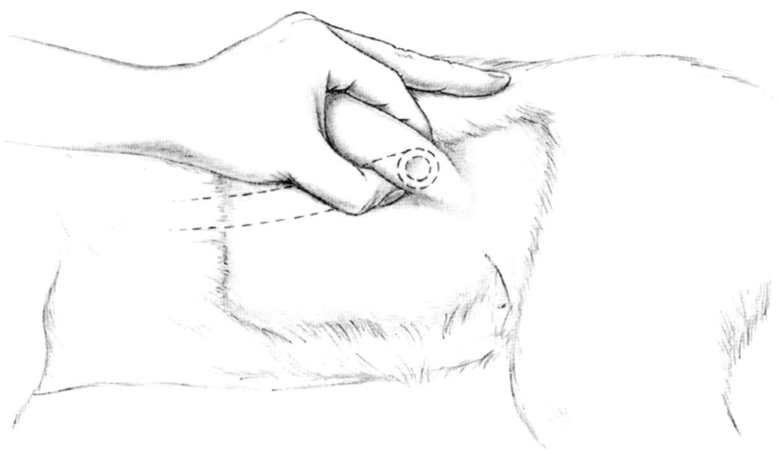

Figure 17-28 Locating the end of rigid stomach tube at left lateral abdominal wall.

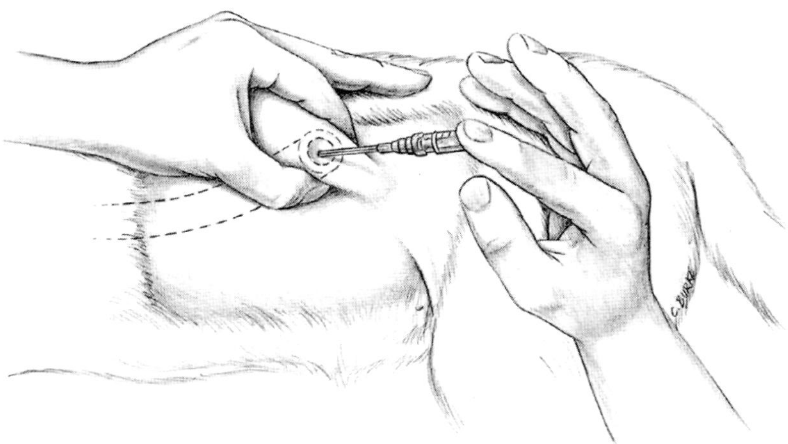

Figure 17-29 Placement of Sovereign catheter through abdominal wall, stomach wall, and into lumen of stomach tube.

Technical Action	Rationale/Amplification
10. Remove needle, leaving plastic catheter inside stomach tube lumen.	**10.** The needle is no longer needed.
11. Thread long, rigid suture (introduction line) through catheter and advance it through stomach tube until end is seen at mouth end of tube (Fig. 17-30).	**11.** Stainless steel usually works best because it is least likely to kink or double back within the tube. The suture material should be at least 20 cm longer than the stomach tube.

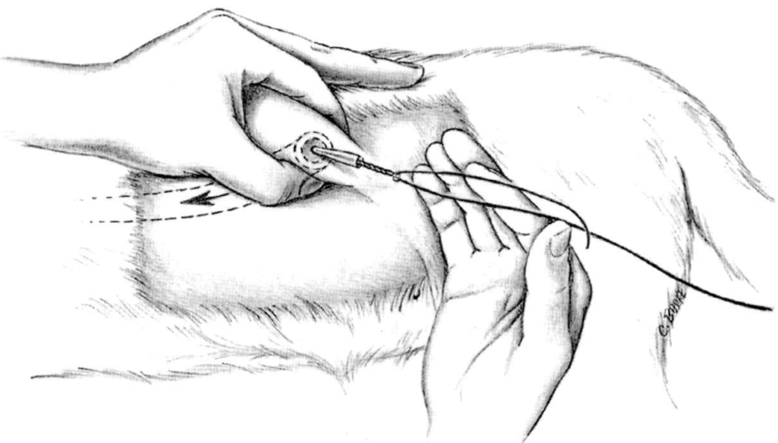

Figure 17-30 Threading introduction line retrograde through Sovereign catheter and stomach tube.

Technical Action	Rationale/Amplification
12. Carefully remove plastic catheter from stomach tube lumen by sliding it over end of introduction line near left lateral abdominal wall skin incision. Place clamp on abdominal end of introduction line.	**12.** Be careful not to pull the introduction line back out of the mouth.
13. Remove stomach tube over oral end of introduction line by applying steady traction.	**13.** The clamp on the abdominal end of the line should prevent it from being pulled back into the stomach.
14. Cut off excess introduction line at oral end.	**14.** Only 20–30 cm are needed for attaching the rubber catheter (gastrostomy tube).

Alternate Method for Line Capture Using Eld Device (for Cats and Small Dogs)

Technical Action	Rationale/Amplification
1. Clip and prepare skin over left lateral abdominal wall for surgery (see Chapter 16).	
2. Place mouth speculum between right upper and lower canine teeth.	**2.** A mouth gag facilitates passage of the tube through the mouth and pharynx.
3. Lubricate tip of percutaneous gastrostomy tube introducer (Eld device).	

Technical Action

4. With trocar point retracted and its distal end curve directed ventrally, slide Eld device over tongue into animal's pharynx.
5. Rotate device one quarter turn counterclockwise while gently advancing past cricopharyngeal area. While directing handle of Eld device slightly laterally, gently advance it down esophagus to level of cardia.
6. Turn device clockwise while passing through cardia and advance tube until it can be visualized through abdominal wall 2–3 cm caudal to last rib.
7. Rotate device back and forth until tip lies against stomach and abdominal wall approximately one-third of distance between epaxial muscles and ventral midline.
8. Palpate carefully to be sure that spleen is not trapped between stomach and abdominal wall.
9. With Eld device pressed firmly against abdominal wall, advance trocar point through stomach and abdominal wall by pushing trigger button against spring until button touches handle.
10. Thread about 20–30 cm of long suture (introduction line) through hole in trocar point (Fig. 17-31).

Rationale/Amplification

4. The curve of the device facilitates easy passage through the mouth and pharynx.
5. The Eld device should pass easily to the level of the cardia.
6. A gentle 90–135-degree rotation usually results in the device slipping through the cardia.
7. Rotating clockwise allows the device to curve naturally toward the greater curvature of the stomach. The distal end of the device is readily identified.
8. If the spleen is lanced by the trocar, severe hemorrhage will occur.
9. Hold the trocar trigger firmly. Do not let the trocar retract until it has been threaded.
10. Only 20–30 cm are needed for attaching the rubber catheter (gastrostomy tube).

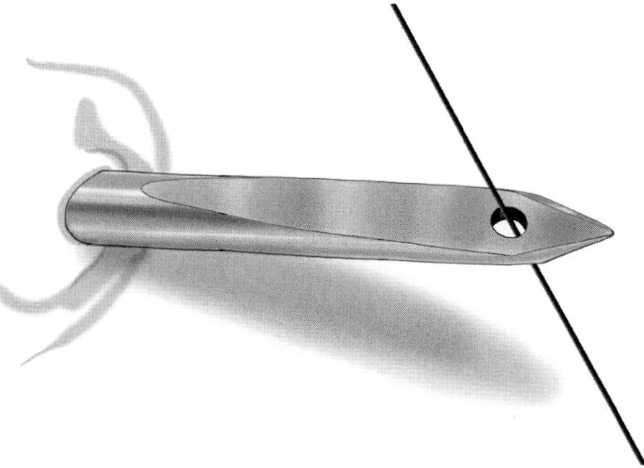

Figure 17-31 Trocar point of Eld percutaneous gastrostomy tube applicator advanced through stomach and abdominal wall, with introduction line passed through hole.

Technical Action	Rationale/Amplification
11. Release trigger button to retract trocar into stomach lumen.	**11.** The suture material will be pulled into the stomach lumen.
12. Withdraw entire device from stomach, esophagus, and pharynx by applying steady traction until end holding suture exits mouth.	**12.** Pull steadily until the introduction line is out of the mouth.
13. Clamp forceps to abdominal end of introduction line.	**13.** Attaching the forceps prevents the end of the introduction line from being pulled into the stomach.
14. Expose trocar again by pushing in on trigger button and remove introduction line from trocar hole.	**14.** After the oral end of the introduction line is retrieved, the Eld device is no longer needed.

Placement of Percutaneous Gastrostomy Tube

Technical Action	Rationale/Amplification
15. Thread tip of plastic Sovereign catheter over oral end of introduction line.	**15.** The narrow tip should be oriented toward mouth.
16. Attach suture needle to oral end of introduction line.	**16.** A straight or curved suture needle or a hypodermic needle may be used to place a suture in the rubber tube.
17. Attach open, beveled end of gastrostomy tube (Malecot or French-pezzar catheter) to introduction line with mattress suture (Fig. 17-32).	**17.** Use several throws to be sure the knot is secure.
18. Carefully force bevel tip of rubber tube into large end of plastic Sovereign catheter. Pull on introduction line until end of rubber tube fits snuggly inside catheter.	**18.** When fitted properly, no cuff of rubber catheter should extend outside the plastic Sovereign catheter.
19. Advance catheter/tube assembly through mouth, esophagus, and stomach by applying steady traction on abdominal end of introduction line.	**19.** Be sure that the catheter/tube assembly passes through the mouth and pharynx smoothly.
20. Catheter will emerge through skin incision first, followed by rubber tube (Fig. 17-33).	
21. As soon as rubber tube is visible, grab it with forceps and pull it through incision.	**21.** Grasping it with forceps helps to prevent the tube from retracting into the stomach.

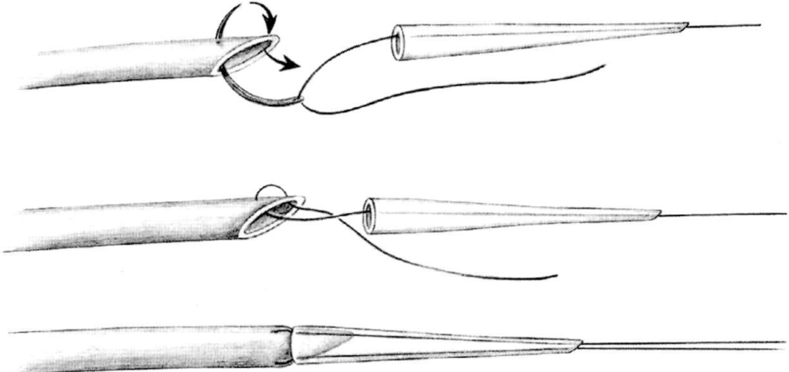

Figure 17-32 Suturing introduction line to beveled end of gastrostomy catheter.

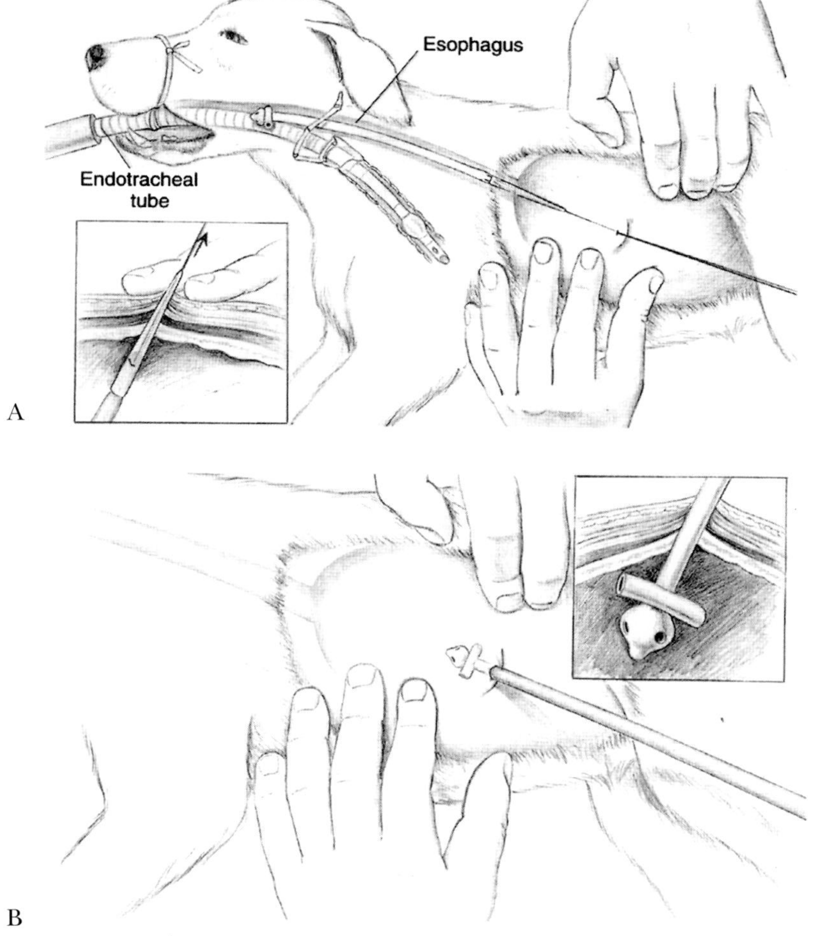

Figure 17-33 Catheter/tube assembly being pulled through (A) mouth and esophagus, and (B) stomach and abdominal walls.

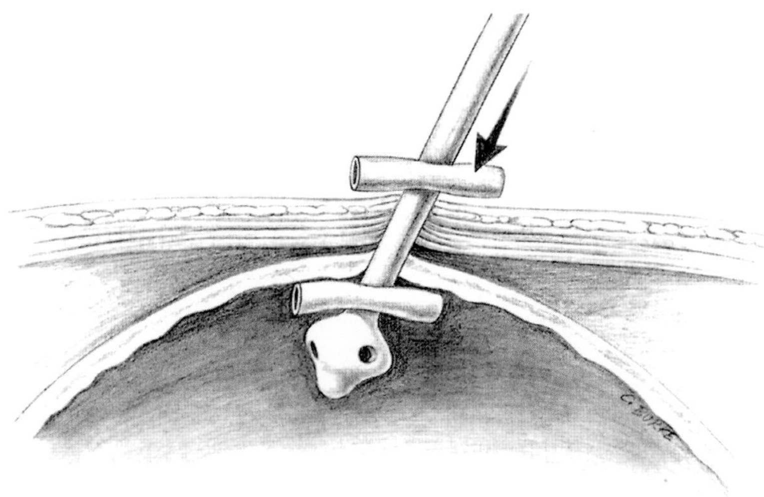

Figure 17-34 Inner and outer flanges in place against stomach mucosa and skin, respectively.

Technical Action	Rationale/Amplification
22. Cut catheter and introduction line with scissors 2 cm below bevel tip.	**22.** By cutting it 2 cm from the bevelled end, its length can be used to determine its position within the stomach.
23. Gently pull rubber tube through abdominal wall until slight resistance is felt.	**23.** When resistance is felt, the inner flange is usually at its desired position, that is, lightly contacting the stomach mucosa. Check position by measuring the length of the tube from skin to distal tip. It should be 2 cm shorter than the original measured length (see **Advance Preparation of Gastrostomy Tube —** Technical Action, step 2e).
24. Slip holes of saved outer flange over end of tube and slide down to skin (Fig. 17-34).	**24.** The external flange is used for suturing the tube to skin, regardless of which type of catheter is used.
25. Insert plug into open end of tube.	**25.** Plugging the end prevents stomach contents from soiling the skin and bandage.
26. Suture external flange to skin.	**26.** Nylon simple interrupted sutures are adequate for securing the tube.
27. Apply antimicrobial ointment and sterile gauze sponge over skin incision.	**27.** Use of antiseptic technique helps to prevent infection at the stoma site.

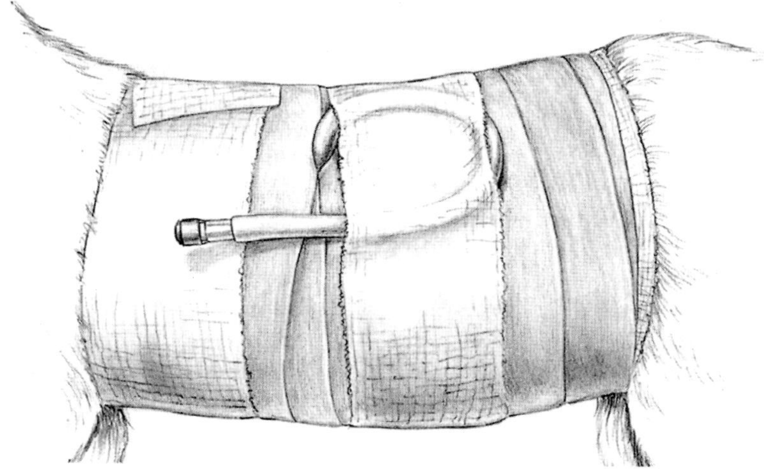

Figure 17-35 Full abdominal bandage showing plugged end of gastrostomy tube emerging dorsally.

Technical Action	Rationale/Amplification
28. Bandage gastrostomy tube in place by encircling abdomen completely with gauze and elastic adhesive bandage, leaving 2–3 cm of tube protruding from bandage dorsally (Fig. 17-35).	**28.** Be sure not to kink the tube in the bandage. The bandage should be changed weekly or whenever it becomes soiled.
29. When animal is fully awake, test animal's tolerance of feeding by gastrostomy tube by administering small amounts of water every hour.	**29.** Some animals may vomit or regurgitate initially. If this problem persists, the gastrostomy tube should be removed and an alternative method of alimentation instituted.
30. If animal does not regurgitate or vomit, proceed with nutritional program at prescribed intervals.	**30.** The tube should be flushed with 2–6 mL of water before and after each use and plugged between feedings.

Removal of Percutaneous Gastrostomy Tube

Technical Action	Rationale/Amplification
1. Remove bandage carefully to expose entire tube.	
2. Flush tube with water prior to removal.	**2.** Cleaning food and mucus from the tube decreases contamination of the stoma site.
3. Remove sutures from outer flange with suture scissors.	

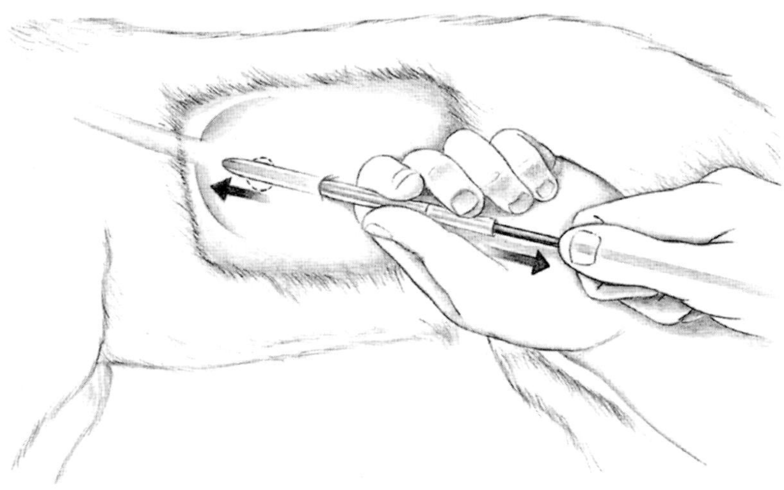

Figure 17-36 Removal of French-pezzar mushroom-tip catheter by stretching tip with intraluminal metal rod.

Technical Action	Rationale/Amplification
4. Slide outer flange up and away from skin far enough to view stoma site.	**4.** It is best to be able to see the stoma site while retracting the tube.
5. Clean any discharge or encrusted material away from stoma with moistened cotton-tipped applicator.	
6. *Malecot catheter*: Remove tube simply by pulling steadily on tube until mushroom tip collapses and slips through inner flange. *French-pezzar mushroom-tip catheter*: Insert blunt metal rod (e.g. Steinman pin) that is 5 cm or more longer than gastrostomy tube into lumen of tube until it reaches catheter tip. Then, while pushing pin inward slightly, pull tube out through stoma (Fig. 17-36).	**6.** *Malecot catheter*: The tip of the Malecot catheter is flexible and will slip through the inner flange holes with steady traction. The inner flange remains in the stomach, but it will usually be passed in the feces within a few days. *French-pezzar mushroom-tip catheter*: The rigid metal rod stretches the mushroom-shaped tip into an eggshaped tip. Traction will then allow removal through the stoma with minimal discomfort to the animal.
7. Clean stoma site and rebandage for several days to avoid soiling.	**7.** The stoma will usually retract and close within 10–14 days. Meanwhile, it is best to cover the site to prevent escaping stoma contents from soiling the animal's coat or the owner's possessions.

Bibliography

Armstrong PJ, Hardie EM: Percutaneous endoscopic gastrostomy: A retrospective study of 54 clinical cases in dogs and cats. J Vet Int Med 4: 202–206, 1990

Bistner SI, Ford RB: Kirk and Bistner's Handbook of Veterinary Procedures & Emergency Treatment, 6th edition. Philadelphia, WB Saunders, 1995

Bojrab MJ, Ellison GW, Slocum BS, eds: Current Techniques in Small Animal Surgery. 4th edition. Baltimore: Williams & Wilkins, 1998

Bright RM: Percutaneous endoscopic gastrostomy. Vet Clin N Amer: Sm Animal Pract 23(3): 531–545, 1993

Bright RM, Okrasinski EB, Pardo AD, Ellison GW, Burrows CF: Percutaneous tube gastrostomy for enteral alimentation in small animals. Compendium Cont Educ Pract Veterinarian 13(1): 367–372, 1991

Crowe DT, Devey JJ: Esophagostomy tube placement and use for feeding and decompression: Clinical experience in 29 small animal patients. J Am Anim Hosp Assoc 33: 393–403, 1997

DeBowes LJ, Coyne B, Layton CE: Comparison of French-pezzar and Malecot catheters for percutaneously placed gastrostomy tubes in cats. JAVMA 202(12): 1963–1965, 1993

Dodman NH, Seeler DC, Court MH: Aging changes in the geriatric dog and their impact on anesthesia. Comp Contin Educ for Prac Vet 6(12): 1106–1112, 1984

Ford RB: Nasogastric intubation in the cat. Comp Contin Educ for AHT 1(1): 29–33, 1980

Fulton RB, Dennis JS: Blind percutaneous placement of a gastrostomy tube for nutritional support in dogs and cats. J Am Vet Med Assoc 201: 697–700, 1992

Glaus TM, Cornelius LM, Bartges JW, Reusch C: Complications with non-endoscopic percutaneous gastrostomy in 31 cats and 10 dogs: A retrospective study. J Small Anim Pract 39: 218–222, 1998

Harvey CE, O'Brien JA: Management of respiratory emergencies in small animals. Vet Clin North Am 2(2): 243–258, 1972

Ireland LM, Hohenhaus AE, Broussard JD, Weissman BL: A comparison of owner management and complications in 67 cats with esophagostomy and percutaneous endoscopic gastrostomy feeding tubes. J Am Anim Hosp Assoc 39: 241–246, 2003

Kirk RW, Bistner SI: Handbook of Veterinary Procedures and Emergency Treatment, 4th edition. Philadelphia, WB Saunders, 1985

MacIntire DK, Drobratz KJ, Haskins SC, Saxon WD: Manual of Small Animal Emergency and Critical Care Medicine. Philadelphia, Lippincott, 2005

McCurnin DM, Poffenbarger EM: Small Animal Clinical Diagnosis and Clinical Procedures. Philadelphia, WB Saunders, 1991

Morgan RV: Handbook of Small Animal Practice, 2nd edition. New York, Churchill Livingstone, 1992

Salinardi BJ, Harkin KR, Bulmer BJ, Roush JK. Comparison of complications of percutaneous endoscopic versus surgically placed gastrostomy tubes in 42 dogs and 52 cats. J Am Anim Hosp Assoc 42: 51–56, 2006

Chapter 18

Gastric Lavage

If you don't learn from your mistakes, there's no sense making them.
HERBERT V PROCHNOW

Gastric lavage is the flushing and evacuation of stomach contents.

Specific Indications

1. Ingestion of poisonous substances
2. Inadvertent overdosage of medication
3. Gastric dilation

Complications

1. Trauma to the pharynx or larynx
2. Esophageal or stomach damage or perforation
3. Electrolyte abnormalities
4. Hypothermia
5. Aspiration of gastric contents into respiratory tract
6. Inadvertent instillation of fluid into respiratory tract

Equipment Needed (Fig. 18-1)

- Orogastric tube
- Speculum or roll of adhesive tape
- Adhesive tape or ballpoint pen for marking stomach tube

Crow and Walshaw's Manual of Clinical Procedures in Dogs, Cats, Rabbits, and Rodents, Fourth Edition. Edited by Jennifer E. Boyle. Published 2016 by John Wiley & Sons, Inc.
Companion Website: www.wiley.com/go/boyle/manual4e

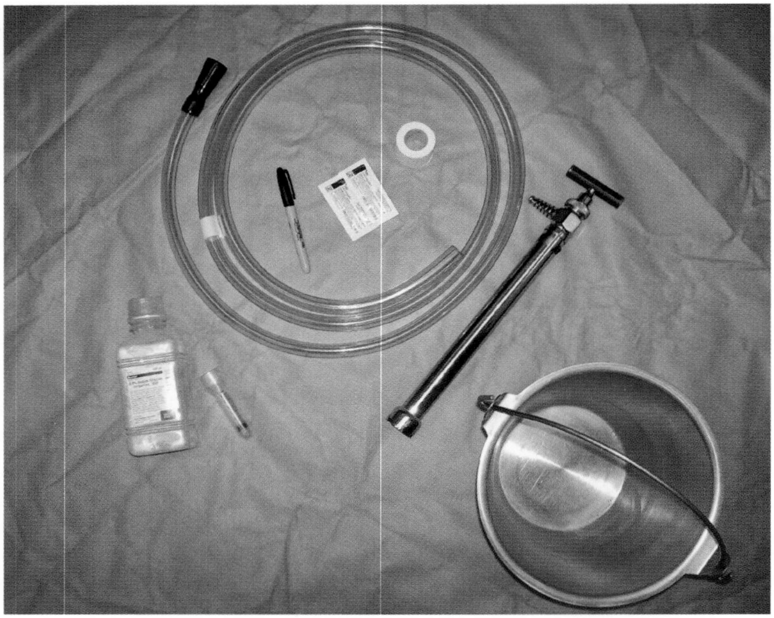

Figure 18-1 Gastric Lavage Equipment. Photo courtesy of C Knightly.

- Lubricating jelly
- Syringe containing 5 mL of sterile saline
- Syringe or funnel for material to be administered
- Warmed (body temperature) water or saline for lavage
- Bucket and manual lavage pump

Restraint and Positioning

The animal is positioned in sternal or right lateral recumbency with head lower than the chest. An agitated patient (e.g. strychnine or metaldehyde poisoning victim) may require general anesthesia, whereas a comatose animal requires no further restraint.

NOTE: *Speed is of great importance. In most instances, gastric lavage is only valuable when performed within 1 hour of toxin ingestion.*

Procedure

Technical Action	Rationale/Amplification
1. Obtain a detailed history and examine label of any suspected toxin, if possible.	1. Several types of poisons or compounds should not be treated by gastric lavage. Their labels generally will indicate same. If in doubt, consult

Technical Action	Rationale/Amplification
	the ASPCA Poison Control Center (888-426-4435).
2. Perform a rapid but thorough physical examination.	**2.** Particular attention to pupillary size and response, swallowing reflexes, and alertness may help in deciding what additional supportive care is needed.
3. Insert endotracheal tube and inflate cuff.	**3.** Sedation or general anesthesia may be required to intubate, unless animal is severely obtunded or unconscious. Endotracheal intubation prevents inadvertent aspiration of stomach contents. See Chapter 17.
4. Pass an orogastric tube. Be sure of its proper position before proceeding.	**4.** See Chapter 17.
5. Evacuate all stomach contents by gravity flow.	**5.** If stomach contents do not empty easily with gravity alone, a siphon effect can be established by filling the tube with water above the head, placing thumb over the tube opening and dropping the tube below the body.
6. Save an aliquot of first collection for possible analysis.	
7. Infuse lavage solution (5–10 mL per kg of body weight) using a stomach pump or funnel.	**7.** This volume should fill the stomach to approximately two-thirds of its maximum volume.
8. Gently undulate/vacillitate the abdomen.	**8.** Mild external agitation of the abdomen may help to dislodge viscous fluids or solid materials adhering to the gastric mucosa.
9. Evacuate stomach contents as in No. 5.	
10. Repeat Nos. 7 through 9 several times.	
11. Infuse antidote or absorbent through tube, if indicated.	**11.** If infusing activated charcoal, wear disposable gloves and wrap a towel around the animal to prevent soiling.
12. Place thumb over end of tube and withdraw tube slowly by applying gentle, steady traction.	**12.** Keep intubated until swallowing reflex is observed. Watch the animal closely for vomiting or regurgitation. Be sure airway is clear of debris before extubating.

Bibliography

Bistner SI, Ford RB: Kirk and Bistner's Handbook of Veterinary Procedures and Emergency Treatment, 8th edition. Philadelphia, WB Saunders, 2006

Burkitt Creedon J and Davis H: Advanced Monitoring and Procedures for Small Animal Emergency and Critical Care. Oxford, Wiley-Blackwell, 2012

Ettinger S, Feldman, E: Textbook of Veterinary Internal Medicine, 6th edition, Volume 1. St. Louis, Saunders, 2005

Hopper K, Silverstein D. Small Animal Critical Care Medicine. St. Louis, Saunders, 2008

Plumb D, Veterinary drug handbook, 8th edition. Oxford, Wiley-Blackwell, 2015

Chapter 19

Transtracheal Wash

You cannot command success, you can only deserve it.
OG MANDINO

Transtracheal aspiration is a diagnostic and occasionally therapeutic procedure involving the placement of a fine catheter through the cricothyroid membrane or interannular membrane of the trachea. * **The following procedure is considered invasive and is typically performed exclusively by veterinarians.**

Purposes

1. To obtain an uncontaminated sputum sample for microbiologic and cytologic studies.
2. To promote coughing in an animal with viscous respiratory secretions
3. To permit instillation of oxygen or drugs into larger lower airways, especially in cases of upper airway obstruction

Specific Indications

1. Chronic cough
2. Productive cough
3. Bronchial and peribronchial radiographic densities

Possible Complications

1. Tracheal laceration and hemorrhage
2. Acute dyspnea
3. Subcutaneous emphysema
4. Pneumomediastinum
5. Iatrogenic infection

Crow and Walshaw's Manual of Clinical Procedures in Dogs, Cats, Rabbits, and Rodents, Fourth Edition. Edited by Jennifer E. Boyle. Published 2016 by John Wiley & Sons, Inc.
Companion Website: www.wiley.com/go/boyle/manual4e

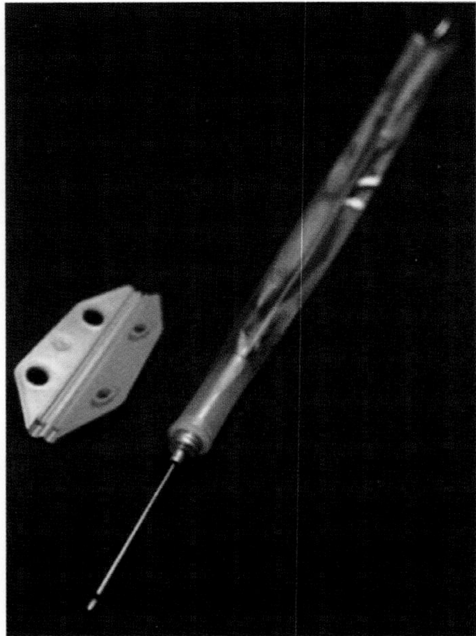

Figure 19-1 Through-the-needle catheter used for transtracheal aspiration.

Equipment Needed

- 14–18-gauge, 20–30-cm long, through-the-needle, intravenous catheter (Fig. 19-1).
- 12-mL or 20-mL syringe filled with sterile physiologic saline solution
- 2% chlorhexidine scrub and 70% alcohol
- Local anesthetic (e.g. 2% lidocaine)
- Sterile gloves

Restraint and Positioning

Physical restraint is usually adequate. Some animals require tranquilization, and local anesthesia is recommended. General anesthesia is contraindicated because the cough reflex is suppressed. The animal is allowed to sit or to lie in sternal recumbency.

Procedure

Technical Action	Rationale/Amplification
1. Extend animal's neck so that nares point toward ceiling.	1. This position facilitates palpation and observation of the ventral aspects of the larynx and trachea.

Technical Action	Rationale/Amplification
2. Prepare skin over cricothyroid membrane or trachea by clipping hair and scrubbing skin in routine manner.	**2.** The cricothyroid membrane is relatively avascular and readily identifiable. This site permits easy access to the tracheal lumen and minimizes trauma to the dorsal tracheal membrane.
3. Inject 0.5 to 0.75 mL of lidocaine 2% into skin and subcutis at puncture site.	**3.** Lidocaine should not be injected into the tracheal wall or lumen.

NOTE: It *is often advisable to use an interannular space near the thoracic inlet to permit passage of the catheter into the carina. Alternatively, a long polyethylene catheter may be introduced through a separate large-gauge needle inserted into the cricothyroid membrane.*

Technical Action	Rationale/Amplification
4. Insert needle into tracheal lumen by puncturing cricothyroid or interannular membrane at a 45-degree angle (Fig. 19-2).	**4.** The needle should be directed caudally toward the thoracic inlet.
5. Advance catheter to its full length (Fig. 19-3).	**5.** The catheter is advanced within the plastic sheath.

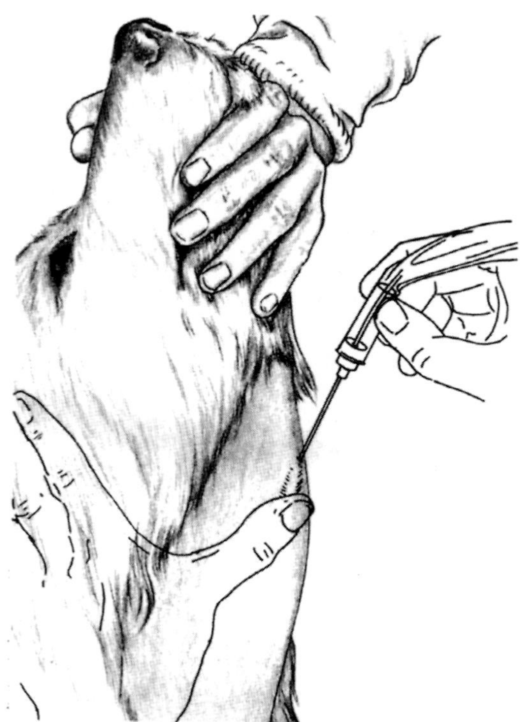

Figure 19-2 Puncturing tracheal or cricothyroid membrane.

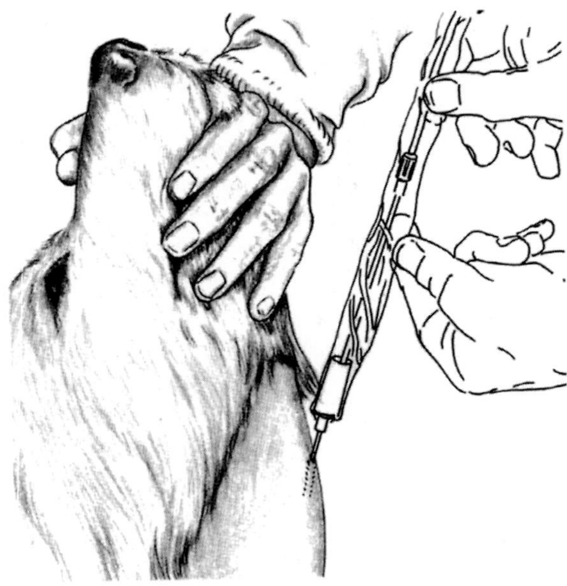

Figure 19-3 Threading catheter through needle into tracheal lumen.

Technical Action	Rationale/Amplification
6. Withdraw needle from trachea, leaving catheter in place (Fig. 19-4).	**6.** A needle guard is secured to prevent severing the catheter inadvertently.
7. Rapidly infuse sterile saline (3–20 mL) through catheter (Fig. 19-5).	**7.** The saline loosens secretions and promotes coughing. Fluid infusion volume should be 0.5 mL/kg of body weight. If little or no coughing is observed after infusion, sharply percuss the chest 2 or 3 times on each side to loosen secretions.
8. While animal is coughing, aspirate secretions and exudates into syringe (Fig. 19-6).	**8.** Do not expect to retrieve all of the infused saline—20% or less of the infused volume is a common yield.
9. Observe patient closely for dyspnea for several minutes before removing catheter.	**9.** If the patient exhibits more severe dyspnea, administer oxygen through the catheter or using an oxygen mask.
10. Transfer contents of syringe to specimen tubes and submit for culture and antimicrobial sensitivity and for cytologic examination.	**10.** Transtracheal aspiration permits sampling from the respiratory tract without contamination from the oropharynx.
11. Remove catheter and apply digital pressure to puncture site for 30 seconds.	**11.** Pressure over the site may prevent excessive bleeding and subcutaneous or mediastinal emphysema.

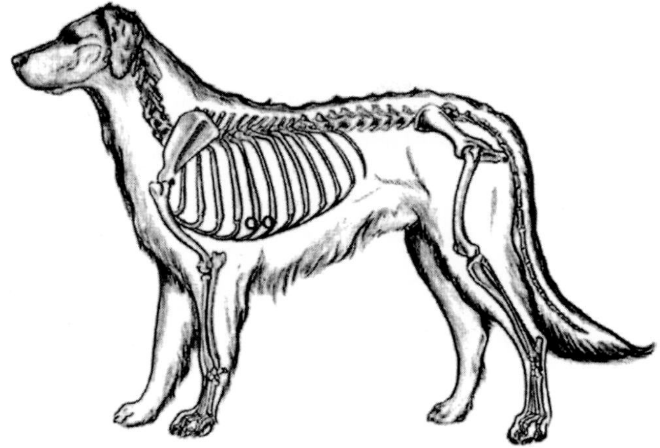

Figure 20-2 Sites for performing pericardiocentesis.

Complications

1. Laceration of myocardium
2. Cardiac dysrhythmias
3. Pneumothorax due to inadvertent laceration of lung

Site

Between the fourth and sixth intercostal spaces of the left hemithorax, slightly ventral to the costochondral junction (Fig. 20-2).

Restraint and Positioning

Minimal restraint is required. The animal is positioned in right lateral recumbency.

ABDOMINOCENTESIS

Specific Indications

1. Abdominal trauma
2. Peritoneal effusion

Complications

1. Perforation of a hollow viscus
2. Laceration of abdominal organs
3. Peritonitis, iatrogenic

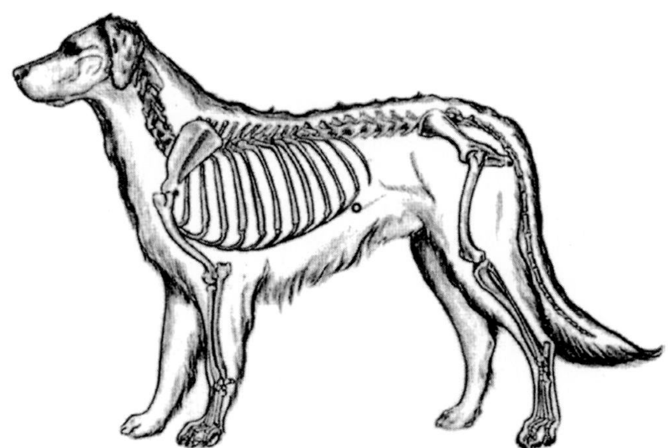

Figure 20-3 Site for performing abdominocentesis.

Site

The site for abdominocentesis is slightly caudal and lateral to the umbilicus (Fig. 20-3).

Restraint and Positioning

The most efficacious and convenient positions are lateral recumbency or standing positions; however, any position that is comfortable for the animal and allows pooling of fluid to the operative site is satisfactory.

CYSTOCENTESIS

Specific Indications

1. Hematuria, dysuria, pyuria
2. Distention of the urinary bladder (when lower urinary tract obstruction cannot be relieved by urethral catheterization)
3. Routine collection of urine for analysis and/or culture

Complications

1. Rupture of bladder, resulting in urine leakage and possible chemical peritonitis
2. Minimal hemorrhage, resulting in contamination of urine by blood

Site

The ventral abdomen just cranial to the pubis is the appropriate site for cystocentesis, even if the bladder can be palpated more cranially (Fig. 20-4).

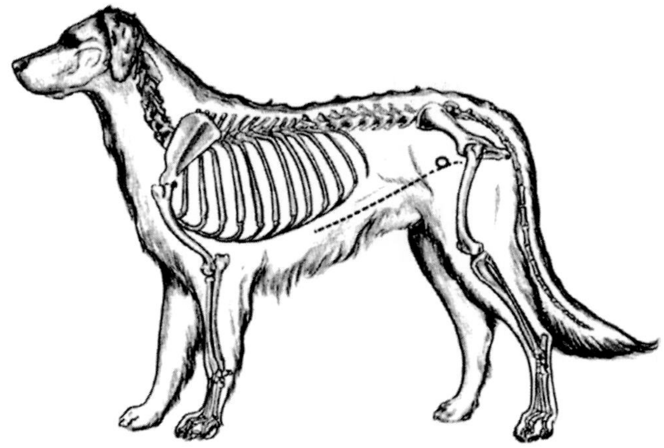

Figure 20-4 Site for performing cystocentesis.

Restraint and Positioning

The animal is placed in dorsal recumbency or in lateral recumbency with the upper leg abducted to expose the inguinal area.

ARTHROCENTESIS

Specific Indications

1. Joint pain
2. Joint distention

Complications

1. Cartilage damage
2. Infectious arthritis, iatrogenic
3. Hemarthrosis, iatrogenic

Site

The preferred sites for arthrocentesis are depicted in Figure 20-5. In each site, carefully avoid superficial blood vessels.

Restraint and Positioning

Because of the possibility of cartilage damage and the discomfort involved, sedation or general anesthesia is recommended.

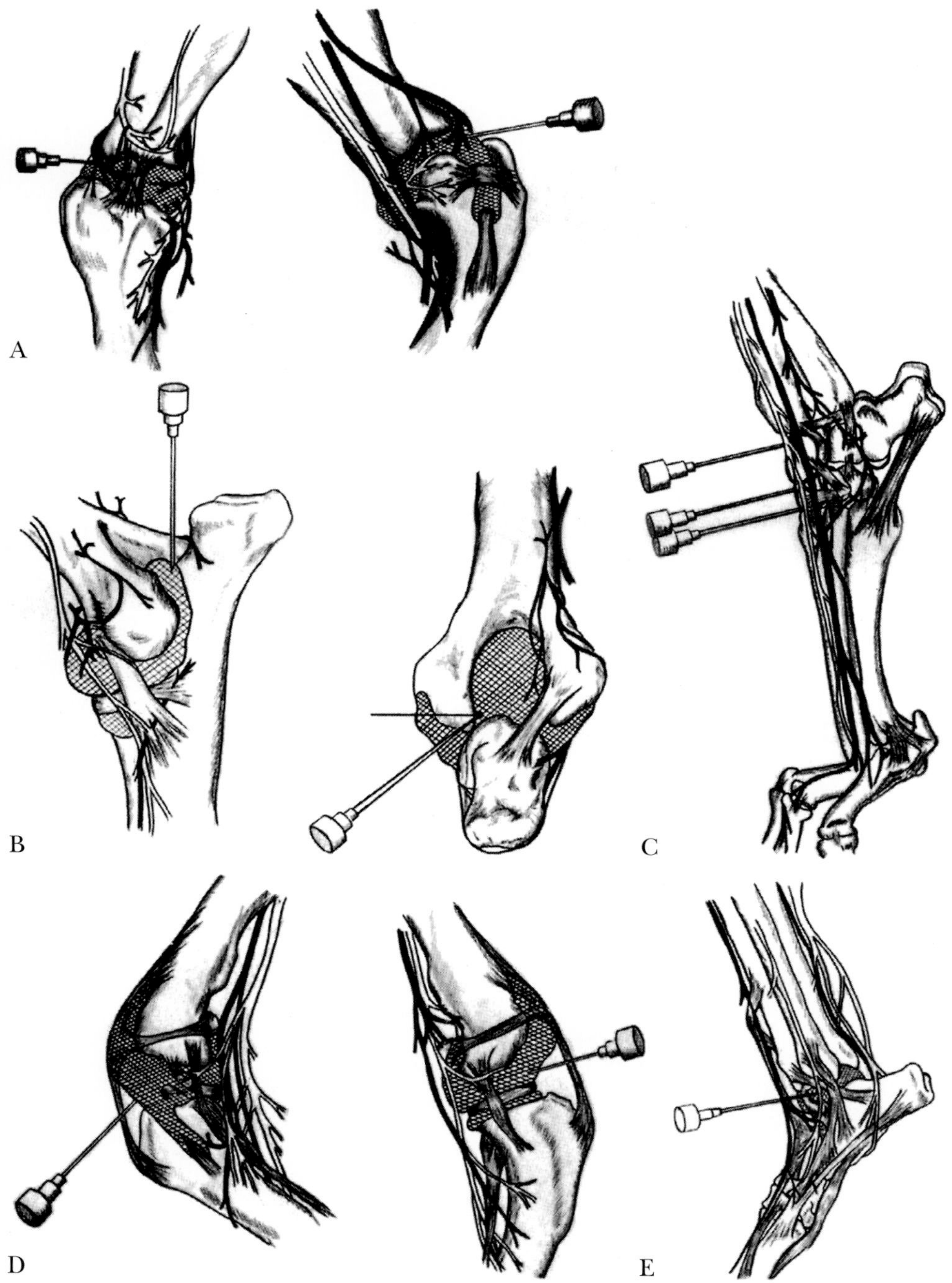

Figure 20-5 Sites for performing arthrocentesis: (A) shoulder, (B) elbow, (C) carpus, (D) stifle, and (E) tarsus.

Equipment Needed

- 22-gauge hypodermic needles (¾–3 ½ inch)
- 3-mL or 6-mL syringe
- Three-way stopcock
- Fluid infusion extension tube

CENTESIS PROCEDURE

Procedure

Technical Action	Rationale/Amplification
1. Clip and prepare operative site for aseptic surgery.	**1.** See Chapter 16. Appropriate prophylaxis of contamination and infection is extremely important.
2. Palpate operative site and instill local anesthetic when indicated.	**2.** Local anesthesia is recommended for thoracentesis and pericardiocentesis; sedation or general anesthesia is recommended for arthrocentesis.
3. Penetrate skin, subcutaneous tissue, and body cavity with one quick motion of sharp needle.	**3.** The needle is attached to an appropriate collection system. • For diagnostic purposes, a 3–10-mL syringe will suffice. • For therapeutic purposes, attach an infusion extension tube, three-way stopcock, and a 60-mL syringe to the cannula. Continue aspiration until no fluid or air is obtained. Record cumulative volume of air or fluid and describe appearance of fluid in animal's record.
4. Remove fluid or air by partial withdrawal of syringe plunger.	**4.** If no fluid or air is obtained, the animal or limb may be moved slightly. If major repositioning is required, the needle should be withdrawn and a second puncture performed.
5. Withdraw needle and syringe quickly after releasing negative pressure.	
6. Transfer sample to specimen containers immediately.	**6.** If fluid is blood tinged, place a portion of the sample in a tube containing an anticoagulant.

Bibliography

Crowe DT: Diagnostic abdominal paracentesis techniques: Clinical evaluation in 129 dogs and cats. JAAHA 20: 223–230, 1984

Ettinger SJ: Pericardiocentesis. Vet Clin N Amer 4: 430–512, 1974
Hardy RM, Wallace LJ: Arthrocentesis and synovial membrane biopsy. Vet Clin N Amer 4: 449–462, 1974
Schall WD: Thoracentesis. Vet Clin N Amer 4: 395–401, 1974
Scott RC, Wilkins RJ, Greene RW: Abdominal paracentesis and cystocentesis. Vet Clin N Amer 4: 413–418, 1974

Chapter 21

Peritoneal Catheterization and Lavage

An old error is always more popular than a new truth.
GERMAN PROVERB

Peritoneal catheterization and lavage involve infusion and recovery of fluids from the peritoneal cavity for diagnostic or therapeutic purposes. * **The following procedures are considered invasive and are typically performed exclusively by veterinarians.**

Purposes

1. To obtain fluid for diagnosis of intra-abdominal disease or injury
2. To infuse medications or fluids into the peritoneal cavity
3. To drain medications or fluids out of the peritoneal cavity
4. To perform peritoneal dialysis in renal failure patients

Specific Indications

1. Peritoneal dialysis for acute oliguric renal failure
2. Acute pancreatitis
3. Urinary tract rupture
4. Ascites
5. Suspected abdominal hemorrhage
6. Suspected septic peritonitis

Complications

1. Catheter incarceration/plugging
2. Puncture of viscus, especially urinary bladder
3. Subcutaneous infusion/leakage of fluids
4. Wound contamination/infection

Crow and Walshaw's Manual of Clinical Procedures in Dogs, Cats, Rabbits, and Rodents, Fourth Edition. Edited by Jennifer E. Boyle. © 2016 John Wiley & Sons, Inc. Published 2016 by John Wiley & Sons, Inc.
Companion Website: www.wiley.com/go/boyle/manual4e

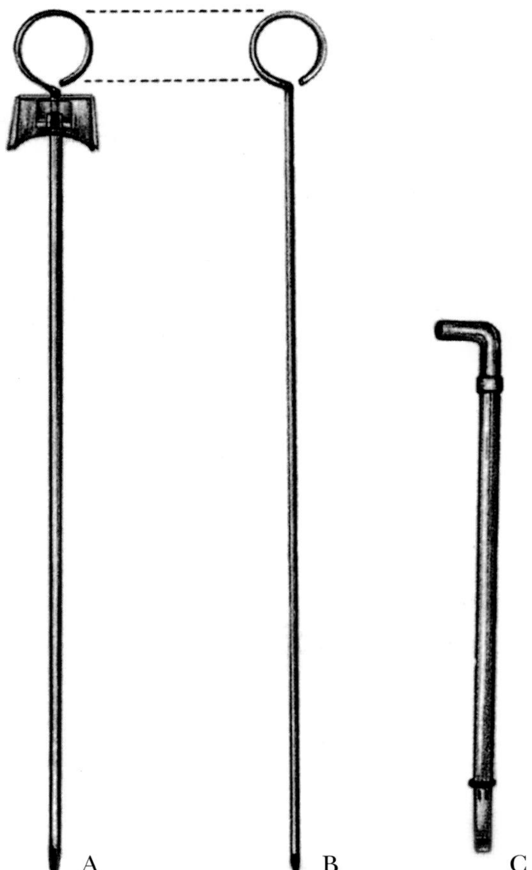

Figure 21-1 Peritoneal catheter set: (A) catheter with trocar/stylet in place, (B) trocar/stylet, and (C) elbow adapter and extender.

Equipment Needed

- Peritoneal catheter set (Fig. 21-1).
- Infusion set or large syringe
- Scalpel blades, No. 11
- Peritoneal dialysis solutions
- Bandaging materials, including gauze and tape

Restraint and Positioning

Before performing peritoneal catheterization, allow animal to urinate, or empty bladder by urethral catheterization. For most animals, local anesthesia is sufficient. A reversible narcotic sedative may be used if necessary. Place the animal in right or left lateral recumbency.

PERITONEAL CATHETERIZATION

Procedure

Technical Action	Rationale/Amplification
1. Clip hair from periumbilical area of ventral abdomen.	1. The area of catheter entry is the midline or paramedian region.
2. Prepare skin for aseptic surgery.	2. See Chapter 16.
3. Make 6–8-mm incision approximately 1 cm caudal to umbilicus.	3. The incision is made either in the ventral midline or slightly paramedian.
4. Drive trocar and catheter through subcutis, abdominal muscles, and peritoneum (Fig. 21-2).	4. Back and forth rotation and a steady thrust are recommended. A popping sensation is usually felt when the trocar penetrates the peritoneum.
5. Direct catheter caudally.	
6. Retract trocar point into catheter and advance catheter 8–10 cm into abdomen.	6. Retraction of the point is essential in order to prevent inadvertent penetration of abdominal organs.
7. Advance remainder of catheter with trocar/stylet still in place (Fig. 21-3).	7. The trocar/stylet acts as a guide to ensure proper catheter advancement.
8. Withdraw trocar/stylet completely and attach elbow adapter and extender to end of catheter (Fig. 21-4).	8. Secure the attachment by wrapping with tape.
9. If catheter apparatus does not have securing wings, apply tape to distal end of catheter, producing a wing on either side of shaft.	
10. Place mattress sutures through each securing wing and through skin (Fig. 21-5).	10. Suturing the catheter to skin prevents unwanted traction on and migration of the catheter.
11. Apply antibiotic ointment to skin at point of catheter entry.	11. Prevention of infection is facilitated by this precautionary procedure.
12. Carefully bandage entire abdomen with gauze and tape or elastic adhesive (Fig. 21-6).	12. Wrap the extender in gauze so that its distal end is both immobile and accessible.

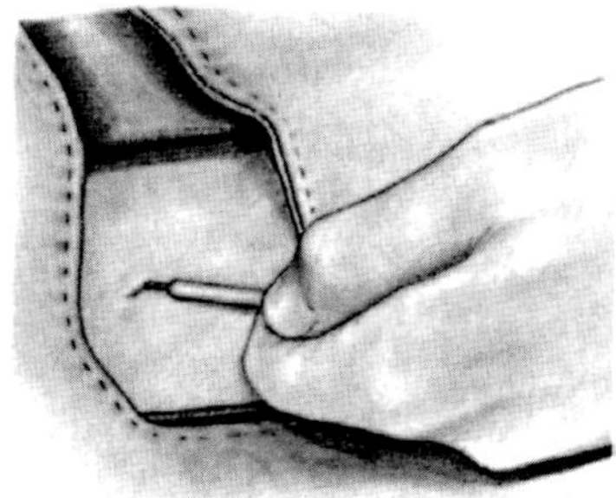

Figure 21-2 Driving trocar and catheter through abdominal wall.

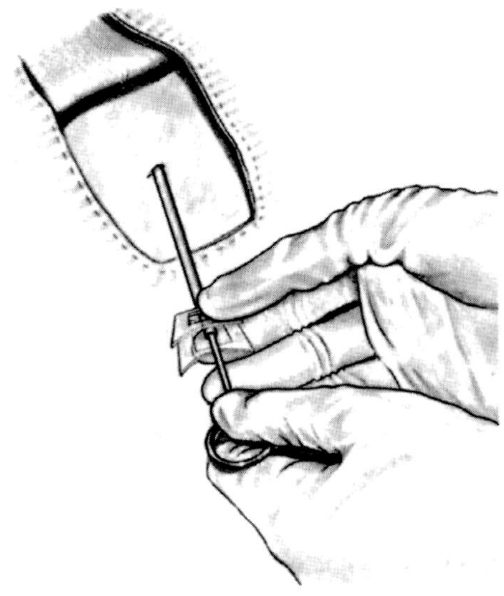

Figure 21-3 Advancing catheter into abdomen.

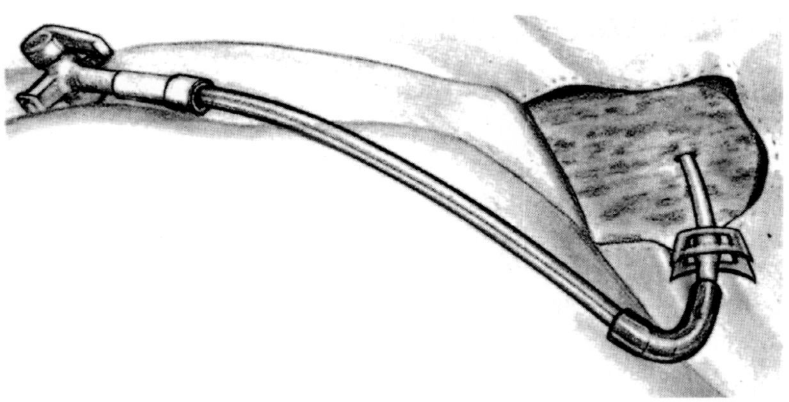

Figure 21-4 Attaching elbow adapter and extender.

PERITONEAL LAVAGE

Procedure

Technical Action	Rationale/Amplification
1. Attach large syringe or infusion set to catheter extender.	
2. Drain any fluid from abdomen by aspiration or gravity flow.	2. Gentle pressure on the abdomen may help in evacuating fluid. Save aliquot for fluid analysis, if indicated.

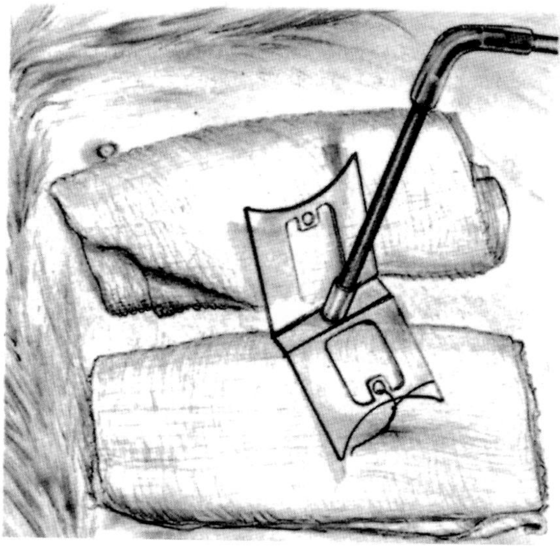

Figure 21-5 Peritoneal catheter sutured to skin.

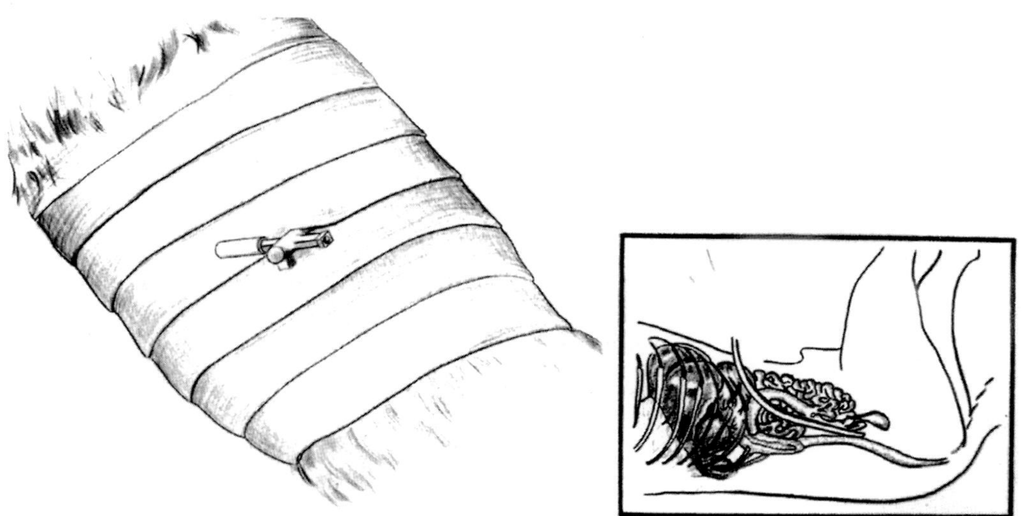

Figure 21-6 Peritoneal catheter bandaged in place.

Technical Action

3. Infuse dialysis solution (30–50 mL/kg of body weight).
4. Jostle abdomen gently with one hand and mix peritoneal cavity contents by rocking animal back and forth.

Rationale/Amplification

3. The abdomen should distend slightly but need not become taut.
4. Leave the dialysis solution in the abdomen for at least 45 minutes to ensure complete osmotic exchange across the peritoneal membrane.

Technical Action	Rationale/Amplification
5. Drain fluid from abdomen by gravity flow.	5. Vigorous suction should not be used because it may result in clogging of the catheter by omentum or mesentery.
6. Repeat Nos. 3 through 5 as frequently as indicated.	6. Repeated or continuous replacements are required for peritoneal dialysis. Single or occasional infusions are used for pancreatitis or peritonitis.
7. Infuse antibacterial solutions through catheter, when indicated.	7. This treatment may be a useful adjunct to systemic therapy for acute pancreatitis or localized peritonitis.
8. If catheter is left in place but not used for infusion or drainage, flush every 4 hours with heparinized saline.	8. Fibrin clots may occlude the many openings in the end of the catheter.
9. Remove or replace catheter after 3 or 4 days.	9. Removal involves cutting the bandage and sutures and withdrawal of the catheter by gentle, steady traction. The short skin incision usually is not sutured, but the abdomen should be bandaged with a sterile dressing for 24–48 hours.

Bibliography

Crowe DT, Crane SW: Diagnostic abdominal paracentesis and lavage in the evaluation of abdominal injuries in dogs and cats: Clinical and experimental investigations. JAVMA 168: 700–705, 1976

Kolata RJ: Diagnostic abdominal paracentesis and lavage: Experimental and clinical evaluations in the dog. JAVMA 168: 697–699, 1976

Parks J, Gahring D, Greene RW: Peritoneal lavage for peritonitis and pancreatitis in twenty-two dogs. JAAHA 9: 442–446, 1973

Chapter 22

Needle Biopsy of Masses and Viscera

The largest room of all is the room for improvement.
WALTER MACKEY

Needle biopsies are procedures for obtaining tissue specimens from viscera and other tissues to establish a histological and/or cytologic diagnosis. * **The following procedures are considered invasive and are typically performed exclusively by veterinarians.**

NOTE: *The procedures described in this chapter represent the author's favored technique for most cases. Because serious hemorrhage may result, coagulation times (PT and PTT) or activated clotting time (ACT) should be performed before proceeding (see Chapter 29). If clotting times are prolonged, biopsies should be delayed or less traumatic procedures should be substituted.*

Most needle biopsy techniques can be used for multiple anatomic locations. For example, fine-needle aspiration of the liver, spleen, kidneys, and prostate are all relatively safe procedures. Transabdominal prostate biopsy is preferred when ultrasound guidance is available. In addition, needle core biopsies can also be used as open techniques during exploratory surgery. Greater exposure of tissue is always desirable if it can be accomplished without adding complications or discomfort for the patient. Appropriate planning of biopsies includes review of all clinical problems before proceeding.

TRANSTHORACIC LUNG ASPIRATION BIOPSY

Transthoracic lung aspiration biopsy is a procedure for establishing a cytologic diagnosis in patients with diffuse lung infiltration or consolidation of one or more lung lobes.

Specific Indications

1. Consolidated or collapsed lung lobe
2. Diffuse interstitial or alveolar pattern of lung infiltration

Crow and Walshaw's Manual of Clinical Procedures in Dogs, Cats, Rabbits, and Rodents, Fourth Edition. Edited by Jennifer E. Boyle. Published 2016 by John Wiley & Sons, Inc.
Companion Website: www.wiley.com/go/boyle/manual4e

Contraindications

1. Severe dyspnea
2. Emphysema or pulmonary bullas
3. Hemorrhagic diatheses

Complications

1. Laceration of lung resulting in pneumothorax or hemorrhage
2. Chest wall puncture resulting in pneumothorax or hemorrhage

Equipment Needed

- 22-g or 25-g, 1½–3½-inch sterile needles
- 6-mL syringe
- Glass microscope slides
- Skin preparation materials

Biopsy Site

Choice of site is determined by radiographic localization of areas of consolidation. In cases of diffuse infiltration of the lungs, the dorsocaudal thorax is often easiest. When the lung lobe to be aspirated is consolidated and in contact with the chest wall, sonography can be helpful in directing the needle. Avoid the caudal edge of a rib space when advancing the needle.

Restraint and Positioning

Sedation and/or local anesthesia is required only for anxious or fractious animals. The animal is positioned in sternal or lateral recumbency to permit maximal exposure of the affected lung.

Procedure

Technical Action	Rationale/Amplification
1. After identifying site for biopsy, clip hair and prepare skin.	1. See Chapter 16.
2. Attach syringe to needle and select exact site for needle penetration.	2. The needle should enter the thorax near the cranial border of a rib to avoid damaging the intercostal vessels.

Technical Action	Rationale/Amplification
3. Using a rapid, fluid motion, thrust needle through skin, subcutis, intercostal muscles, parietal pleura, and lung to depth of lesion or halfway through consolidated lung lobe.	3. Rapid insertion of the needle reduces chances of lacerating the lung.
4. Apply negative pressure (suction) at needle bevel by pulling back on syringe plunger while holding barrel steady.	4. Several brisk excursions of the plunger are made.
5. Partially withdraw needle and then redirect into lung tissue.	5. This step helps to ensure adequate sampling of the diseased lung.
6. Again apply suction by pulling back briskly on syringe plunger.	
7. Release negative pressure by allowing syringe plunger to retract into barrel.	7. By releasing suction, the sample is retained in the needle lumen.
8. Withdraw needle from lung quickly.	8. Again, rapid movements tend to minimize the potential to lacerate the lung.
9. Detach syringe from needle and draw air into barrel of syringe.	
10. Reattach syringe to needle and expel contents of needle lumen onto one or two clean microscope slides.	10. Expulsion should be rapid and forceful. Only a small drop of fluid is obtained in most aspirations.
11. Make smears of aspirated fluid immediately.	11. Push smears or squash preparations are made, depending on the viscosity of the fluid. See Chapter 8 (Figs. 8-4 and 8-5).

Postoperative Care

Hemorrhage is rarely observed, but pneumothorax may occasionally be seen. The animal should be observed for 2–4 hours after biopsy to ensure early detection of pneumothorax. Follow-up radiographs of the thorax are indicated if labored breathing is observed.

PLEURAL BIOPSY

Pleural biopsy is a procedure for establishing a histological diagnosis in patients with pleural thickening or effusion.

Specific Indications

1. Confirmation of cytologic diagnosis of mesothelioma, metastatic carcinoma or sarcoma, or chronic pleuritis
2. Pleural thickening

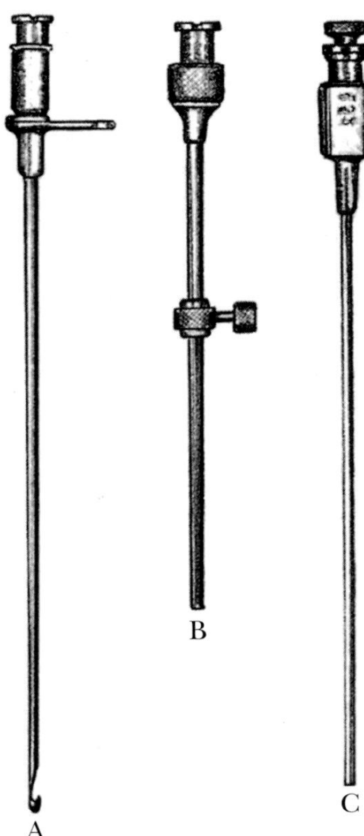

Figure 22-1 Cope needle for pleural biopsy: (A) obturator (with hook), (B) cannula, and (C) stylet.

Complications

1. Laceration of lung resulting in pneumothorax or hemorrhage
2. Chest wall puncture resulting in pneumothorax or hemorrhage

Equipment Needed

- Punch biopsy instrument with hook needle (Cope needle; Fig. 22-1)
- Local anesthetic (e.g. 2% lidocaine)
- Skin preparation materials
- Scalpel blade (No. 11)
- Sterile gloves
- Tissue cassette (Fig. 22-3 D)

Biopsy Site

Choice of site is determined by radiographic localization of areas of pleural thickening. If possible, avoid the cardiac apex/notch area.

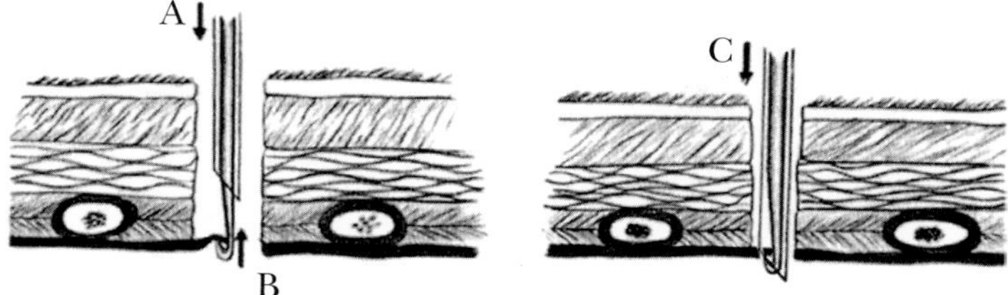

Figure 22-2 Obtaining a pleural biopsy using a Cope needle: (A) Advance obturator while applying lateral pressure. (B) Withdraw obturator until hook catches in parietal pleura. (C) Advance outer cannula into pleural cavity while maintaining light traction on obturator.

Restraint and Positioning

Most animals require some sedation. Cooperative patients may be biopsied using local anesthesia only. Choice of chemical restraint measures should be based on the degree of respiratory insufficiency.

To maximize the space between visceral and parietal pleura, the animal should be positioned so that the biopsy site is uppermost (e.g. mass next to the middle of the right eighth rib, with animal positioned in left lateral recumbency).

Procedure

Technical Action	Rationale/Amplification
1. After identifying site for biopsy, clip hair and cleanse skin. Then inject local anesthetic.	**1.** See Chapter 16.
2. Make a small incision with scalpel blade.	**2.** Incising the skin facilitates insertion of the biopsy needle.
3. Advance biopsy needle (with stylet in place) through incision and intercostal muscles.	
4. Before puncturing pleura to enter thorax, remove stylet from cannula and attach syringe.	**4.** The needle should enter the thorax near the cranial border of a rib to avoid damaging the intercostals vessels.
5. Slowly advance needle with twisting motion until pleural cavity is entered.	**5.** Entry into the pleural space is detected by a sudden change in resistance.
6. Aspirate fluid and retract needle just far enough to prevent further fluid aspiration.	**6.** The cannula is now positioned just outside the pleural cavity.
7. Detach syringe and insert hooked obturator into outer cannula.	**7.** The hook opening is directed dorsally to avoid vessel damage.

Technical Action	Rationale/Amplification
8. Again, slowly advance obturator/ cannula assembly into pleural space while applying pressure in direction of hook opening (Fig. 22-2A).	
9. Slowly withdraw obturator and cannula in unison until hook catches in parietal pleura (Fig. 22-2B).	
10. While applying slight traction on obturator, advance outer cannula, using a rotating motion (Fig. 22-2C), until pleura is severed.	**10.** As the sharpened edge of the outer cannula cuts off the specimen held within the hook, the tension on the obturator will relax.
11. Remove instrument from chest and slide cannula off obturator.	**11.** Working over the biopsy jar prevents inadvertent loss of the specimen.
12. *Assistant:* Open lid of fixative receptacle at appropriate time. Using a sterile hypodermic needle or scalpel blade, transfer specimen immediately to a small tissue cassette before placing it in fixative (Fig. 22-3D).	**12.** Small biopsy tissue samples are placed in a cassette to prevent loss during processing. Once the cassette contains adequate biopsy tissue, it can be immersed in formalin or other fixative solution.
13. If specimen is small or severely fragmented, procedure can be repeated once or twice.	
14. Repeat procedure using same skin incision.	**14.** Direct the hook opening ventrally or cranially during subsequent procedures.

Postoperative Care

Hemorrhage is usually readily controlled by digital pressure. The animal should be observed for 2–4 hours after biopsy to ensure early detection of pneumothorax. Follow-up radiography is recommended.

PERCUTANEOUS LIVER BIOPSY

Percutaneous liver biopsy is a diagnostic technique for establishing a histological diagnosis in patients with suspected diffuse hepatic disease.

In previous editions, we described a technique for liver biopsy using a Menghini needle. Because liver specimens obtained with the Menghini needle are small and often fragment, histopathological interpretation is often very difficult. Consequently, we no longer recommend that procedure. Instead, we strongly recommend using laparoscopy or ultrasound guidance for obtaining liver biopsies. Laparoscopy allows direct visualization of lesions on the liver surface and large pieces of tissue to be obtained; however, the techniques and equipment needed for laparoscopy are beyond the scope of this manual. Consequently, we describe our preferred method of obtaining a core sample with a disposable automatic-trigger needle (see Fig. 22-3).

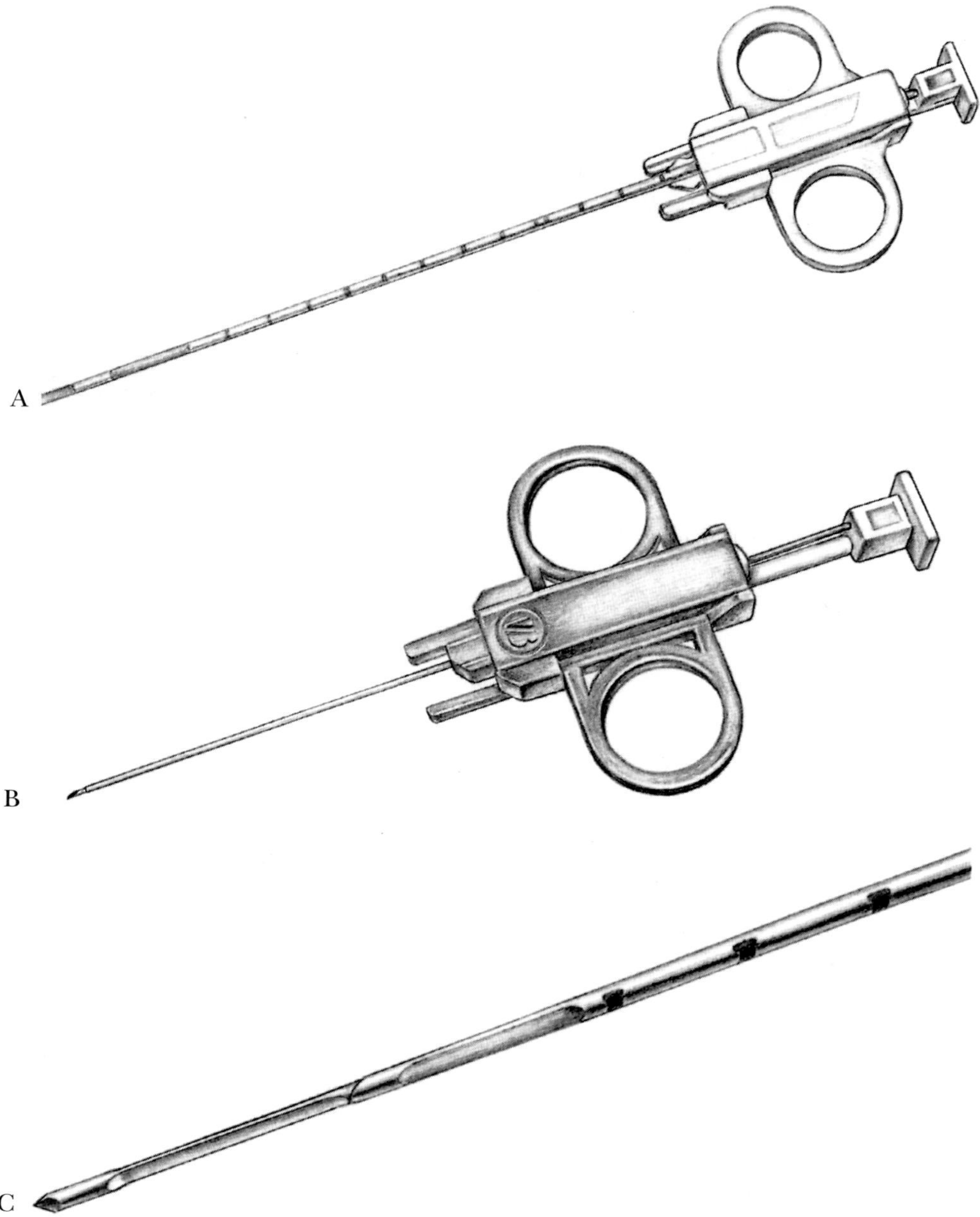

Figure 22-3 (A) Cook needle, (B) Temno needle, (C) close-up side view of obturator tip. (D) Tissues cassettes.

D 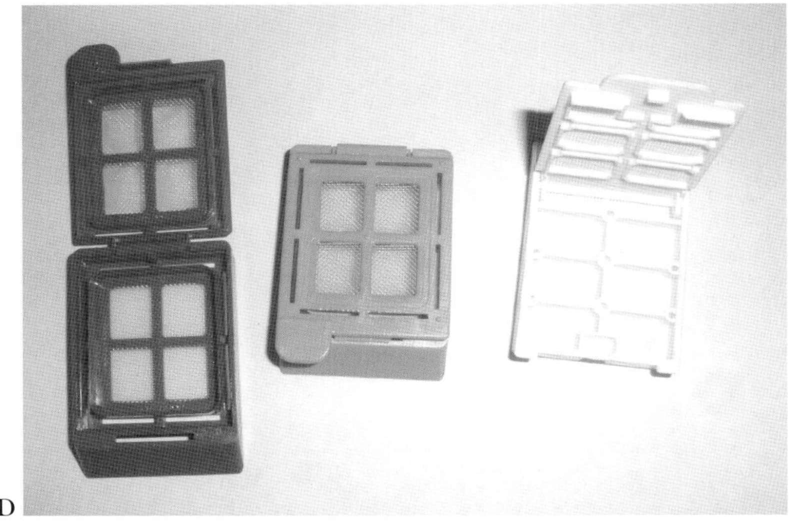

Figure 22-3 *Continued*

Specific Indications

1. Hepatomegaly
2. Hepatic dysfunction (e.g. hypoalbuminemia, icterus, persistently increased serum liver enzyme activities)

Contraindications

1. Abnormal hemostasis
2. Severe circulatory disturbances
3. Extrahepatic biliary obstruction
4. Small liver

Complications

1. Laceration/hemorrhage of viscera, including caudal vena cava, portal vein, liver, spleen, stomach, intestine, pancreas, diaphragm, lung, and heart
2. Puncture of gallbladder/bile peritonitis
3. Iatrogenic infectious peritonitis

Equipment

- Cook or Temno biopsy needles (14–18 g) (Fig. 22-3)
- Scalpel blade (No. 11)

- Local anesthetic (e.g. 2% lidocaine)
- Skin preparation materials
- Sterile gloves
- Tissue cassette (Figure 22-3D)

Biopsy Site/Positioning

If the liver is not palpable, the size and position of the liver should be confirmed by abdominal sonography or radiography. Success of transabdominal percutaneous liver biopsy depends on adequate localization of the liver. Careful direction of the needle is essential; a "hit-or-miss" approach usually is unsuccessful and is associated with marked danger of complications.

Place the patient in dorsal or left lateral recumbency. Introduce the biopsy needle through the ventral abdominal wall between the xiphoid process and either costal arch. Advance the needle dorsolaterally at an angle approximately 30 degrees right or left of the midsagittal plane.

Restraint

Sedation and local anesthesia are adequate for liver biopsy in most dogs and cats. General anesthesia may be necessary in fractious or nervous animals. Needle biopsy of the liver should not be attempted when violent or unpredictable movements prevent localization of the liver. General anesthetics that require liver metabolism or excretion should be avoided in animals with severe liver dysfunction.

Procedure

Technical Action	Rationale/Amplification
Preparatory Phase	**Preparatory Phase**
1. Perform activated clotting time.	**1.** See Chapter 29. If value is normal, proceed. If abnormal, delay procedure until risks have been reassessed.
2. Withhold food for 8–12 hours.	**2.** Fasting decreases stomach size and minimizes the likelihood of inadvertent puncture.
3. Give small amount of fat orally 30–60 minutes before biopsy.	**3.** A fatty meal may induce contraction of the gallbladder, thereby reducing its size and minimizing the chance of inadvertent puncture.
4. Remove ascites by abdominocentesis.	**4.** Distention of the abdomen by fluid may preclude localization of the liver. See Chapter 20, **Abdominocentesis**.

Technical Action	Rationale/Amplification
5. Sedate or anesthetize animal.	**5.** Sedation is essential to minimize discomfort and to prevent the animal from moving during the procedure. Although general anesthesia may accomplish these same goals, many patients needing liver biopsy are poor anesthetic risks.
6. Prepare operative site by clipping hair and cleansing and disinfecting skin in standard manner (see Chapter 16).	**6.** Aseptic technique should be used throughout the biopsy procedure. See Chapter 16.
7. Scrub hands and don surgical gloves using aseptic technique.	**7.** Using aseptic technique is always advisable when introducing a needle into a body cavity.
8. Place all sterile equipment on a sterile surgical towel and cover animal with a fenestrated drape.	**8.** A fenestrated drape helps to prevent contamination of the needle.
9. Prepare needle for use, that is, "load" it by holding cannula handle firmly while pulling out obturator trigger handle until it clicks and locks in place.	**9.** Once the needle is loaded, it is ready for use.
Operative Phase	**Operative Phase**
1. Identify specific liver lobe or lesion within liver to be biopsied by ultrasound or deep palpation.	**1.** If the liver is small or the lesion to be biopsied is too close to the diaphragm, gallbladder, common bile duct, vena cava, or other large blood vessel, another biopsy technique should be used.
2. Inject local anesthetic into skin and parietal peritoneum at proposed biopsy site.	**2.** Even when animal is sedated, we recommend injecting local anesthetic to minimize pain immediately following the procedure.
3. Make a small stab incision with scalpel blade.	**3.** Use a No. 11 or No. 15 scalpel blade.
4. Advance biopsy needle through skin incision, abdominal muscles, and peritoneum toward liver.	**4.** Use gentle, even pressure as the needle is advanced through the abdominal wall.
5. Introduce end of outer cannula, with inner obturator retracted, into liver parenchyma approximately 2 mm (Fig. 22-4A).	**5.** The point of the needle should be directed away from the vena cava, gallbladder, and diaphragm.

Technical Action	Rationale/Amplification
Operative Phase	**Operative Phase**
6. While holding needle handle firmly in one hand, advance inner obturator to its full length by sliding trigger handle smoothly forward (Fig. 22-4B).	**6.** A notch in the obturator accepts the liver tissue to be removed.
7. When trigger button touches outer cannula handle, firmly press spring-loaded trigger button to automatically advance outer cannula (Fig. 22-4C).	**7.** This step cuts off the specimen and protects it within the biopsy notch of the obturator.
8. Quickly but carefully pull entire biopsy needle directly out of liver, abdominal wall, and skin.	**8.** Be careful not to lacerate the liver while retracting the device.
9. Reload needle by holding cannula handle firmly while pulling out obturator trigger handle until it clicks and locks in place.	**9.** It is necessary to reload the device to retrieve the core specimen from the obturator notch.
10. Working directly over biopsy receptacle, advance inner obturator to expose specimen. Do not press trigger button.	**10.** Working over the biopsy jar prevents accidental loss of the specimen. Inadvertent triggering of the device at this time may result in ejection.
11. *Assistant:* Open lid of fixative receptacle at appropriate time. Using a sterile hypodermic needle or scalpel blade, transfer specimen immediately to a small tissue cassette (Fig. 22-3D) before placing in fixative.	**11.** Small biopsy tissue samples should be placed in a cassette to prevent loss during processing. Once the cassette contains adequate biopsy tissue, it is immersed in formalin or other fixative solution.
12. If specimen is small or severely fragmented, procedure can be repeated once or twice.	**12.** Although repeating the procedure adds risk of hemorrhage or other complications, the consequences of not obtaining enough tissue for the pathologist must be considered.

Postoperative Care

Observe the patient for several hours after the procedure to determine whether excessive hemorrhage has occurred. When the specimen is heavily bile stained, particularly careful observation for signs of bile peritonitis should be emphasized to the animal's owner.

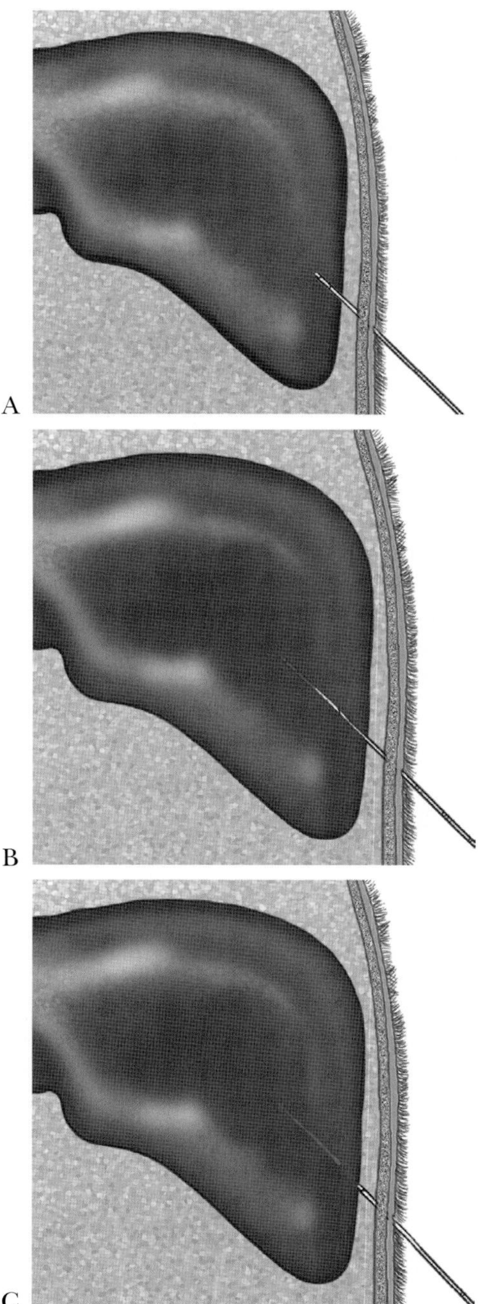

Figure 22-4 Obtaining a liver biopsy using core needle technique: (A) Pierce abdominal wall and advance needle with obturator retracted through peritoneum. Gently explore with needle until capsule or target liver lobe is contacted. Direct needle away from aorta, caudal vena cava, gallbladder, and stomach. (B) Advance inner obturator. (C) Advance outer cannula suddenly by pressing needle's firing button.

Development of signs such as sudden anorexia or vomiting should be pursued vigorously in such cases.

PERCUTANEOUS KIDNEY BIOPSY

Percutaneous kidney biopsy is a procedure for establishing a histological diagnosis in patients with unilateral or bilateral renal disease. It is particularly valuable in obtaining a specimen to predict functional recovery from renal disease.

NOTE: *The technique described here for kidney core biopsy can be readily adapted for performing biopsies of liver, prostate, soft tissue or visceral masses, or other tissues.*

Specific Indications

1. Chronic renal failure
2. Persistent proteinuria (suspect glomerulopathy)
3. Enlarged kidney(s)
4. Small kidney(s)
5. Irregular kidney shape
6. Hematuria of probable renal origin

Contraindications

1. Bleeding/clotting disorders
2. Nonpalpable kidneys

Complications

1. Renal or perirenal hemorrhage
2. Retroperitoneal or intraperitoneal urine leakage

Equipment

- Cook or Temno biopsy needles (16–18 g) (Fig. 22-3)
- Scalpel blade (No. 11)
- Local anesthetic (e.g. 2% lidocaine)
- Skin preparation materials
- Sterile gloves
- Tissue cassette (Figure 22-3D)

Biopsy Sites

Left or right paralumbar fossa

Restraint and Positioning

The animal is held in left or right lateral recumbency. General anesthesia is rarely required, but sedation or tranquilization is recommended.

Prebiopsy Considerations

The patient should be evaluated for coagulation abnormalities. Animals with oliguric or anuric renal failure should be treated with fluids, and adequate urine production should be realized before biopsy is attempted. Intravenous fluids are given during the biopsy procedure and recovery period to prevent decreased renal perfusion.

Procedure

Technical Action	Rationale/Amplification
Preparatory Phase	**Preparatory Phase**
1. Perform activated clotting time.	**1.** See Chapter 29. If value is normal, proceed. If abnormal, delay procedure until risks have been reassessed.
2. Withhold food for 8–12 hours.	**2.** Fasting decreases stomach size and minimizes the likelihood of inadvertent puncture.
3. Remove ascites by abdominocentesis.	**3.** Distention of the abdomen by fluid may preclude localization and immobilization of the kidney. See Chapter 20, **Abdominocentesis.**
4. Sedate or anesthetize animal.	**4.** Sedation is essential to minimize discomfort and to prevent the animal from moving during the procedure. Although general anesthesia may accomplish these same goals, many patients needing kidney biopsy are poor anesthetic risks.
5. Prepare operative site by clipping hair and cleansing and disinfecting skin in standard manner (see Chapter 16).	**5.** Aseptic technique should be used throughout the biopsy procedure. See Chapter 16.
6. Scrub hands and don surgical gloves using aseptic technique.	**6.** Using aseptic technique is always advisable when introducing a needle into a body cavity.
7. Place all sterile equipment on a sterile surgical towel and cover animal with a fenestrated drape.	**7.** A fenestrated drape helps to prevent contamination of the needle.
8. Prepare needle for use, that is, “load” it by holding cannula handle firmly while pulling out obturator trigger handle until it clicks and locks in place.	**8.** Once the needle is loaded, it is ready for use.

Technical Action

Operative Phase

1. Isolate kidney to be biopsied in one hand by deep palpation.
2. Prepare skin of paralumbar fossa overlying kidney in a routine manner; inject local anesthetic into skin at proposed biopsy site.
3. Make a small stab incision with scalpel blade.
4. Advance biopsy needle through incision and retroperitoneal tissue toward either pole of kidney.
5. Introduce end of outer cannula, with inner obturator retracted, through renal capsule approximately 2 mm (Fig. 22-5).
6. While holding needle handle firmly in one hand, advance inner obturator to its full length by sliding trigger handle smoothly forward.

Rationale/Amplification

Operative Phase

1. If the kidney to be biopsied is too small or cannot be held in a fixed position, an open surgical biopsy technique should be used.
2. Even when sedated, we recommend injecting local anesthetic to minimize pain immediately following the procedure.
3. Use a No. 11 or No. 15 scalpel blade.
4. Use gentle, even pressure as the needle is advanced through the abdominal wall.
5. The point of the needle should be directed away from the vena cava and renal pelvis.
6. A notch in the obturator accepts the kidney tissue to be removed.

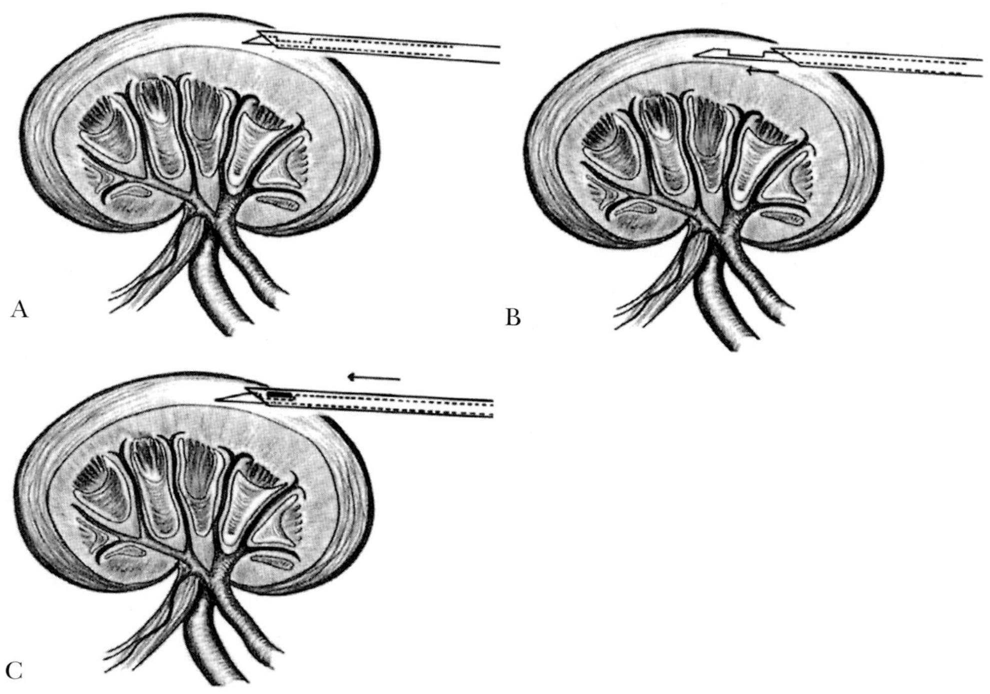

Figure 22-5 Proper position of needle for obtaining a kidney biopsy using a Cook needle.

Technical Action	Rationale/Amplification
Operative Phase	**Operative Phase**
7. When trigger button touches outer cannula handle, firmly press springloaded trigger button to automatically advance outer cannula (Fig. 22-3C).	**7.** This step cuts off the specimen and protects it within the biopsy notch of obturator.
8. Quickly but carefully pull entire biopsy needle directly out of kidney, abdominal wall, and skin.	**8.** Be careful not to lacerate the kidney while retracting the device. Apply firm digital pressure to biopsy site for 3–5 minutes.
9. Reload needle by holding cannula handle firmly while pulling out obturator trigger handle until it clicks and locks in place.	**9.** It is necessary to reload the device to retrieve the core specimen from the obturator notch.
10. Working directly over biopsy receptacle, advance inner obturator to expose specimen. Do *not* press trigger button.	**10.** Working over the biopsy jar prevents inadvertent loss of the specimen. Inadvertent triggering of the device at this time may result in ejection, laceration, or crushing of the specimen.
11. *Assistant:* Open lid of fixative receptacle at appropriate time. Using a sterile hypodermic needle or scalpel blade to remove tissue contained in obturator notch, transfer specimen immediately to a small tissue cassette before placing it in fixative.	**11.** Small biopsy tissue samples should be placed in a cassette to prevent loss during processing. Once the cassette contains adequate biopsy tissue, it is immersed in formalin or other fixative solution.
12. If specimen is small or severely fragmented, procedure can be repeated once.	**12.** Although repeating the procedure adds risk of hemorrhage or other complications, the consequences of not obtaining enough tissue for the pathologist to interpret must be considered.

Postbiopsy Considerations

Many animals have microscopic hematuria for 12–72 hours after the biopsy, whereas only a few have gross hematuria. Severe hemorrhage rarely occurs when proper technique is used.

TRANSPERINEAL PROSTATE BIOPSY

Transperineal prostate biopsy is a percutaneous method of acquiring specimens for histological diagnosis of prostatic disease.

NOTE: *When the prostate is palpably enlarged or is palpable within the abdominal cavity, it is often easier and safer to biopsy the gland using a transabdominal approach.*

Specific Indications

1. Prostatomegaly
2. Prostatic deformity or asymmetry
3. Bloody urethral discharge

Contraindications

1. Prostate not palpable per rectum
2. Fluctuant enlargement of the prostate
3. Bleeding/clotting disorders

Complications

1. Severe intrapelvic hemorrhage
2. Puncture or laceration of rectum, small intestine, urethra, or urinary bladder

Equipment

- Cook or Temno biopsy needles (16–18 g) (Fig. 24-3)
- Scalpel blade (No. 11)
- Local anesthetic (e.g. 2% lidocaine)
- Skin preparation materials
- Sterile gloves
- Tissue cassette (Fig. 22-3-3D)

Biopsy Site

Needle entry is at a point on the skin equidistant between the anal orifice and tuber ischium on the desired side.

Restraint and Positioning

Because of the discomfort produced in digital rectal palpation, heavy sedation or general anesthesia is recommended. If sedation is used, local anesthesia should be added. The animal is positioned in sternal or lateral recumbency, with the tail reflected dorsolaterally.

Procedure

Technical Action	Rationale/Amplification
Preparatory Phase	**Preparatory Phase**
1. Perform activated clotting time.	**1.** See Chapter 29. If value is normal, proceed. If abnormal, delay procedure until risks have been reassessed.
2. Withhold food for 8–12 hours.	**2.** Fasting decreases the likelihood that the colon and rectum will contain large amounts of feces.
3. Evacuate feces from rectum manually or with enema.	**3.** Removing feces from the rectum prevents inadvertent soiling of the perineum during the procedure.
4. Sedate or anesthetize animal.	**4.** Sedation is essential to minimize discomfort and to prevent the animal from moving during the procedure. General anesthesia is rarely needed for prostate needle core biopsy.
5. Prepare perineal region for biopsy by clipping hair and cleansing and disinfecting skin in standard manner (see Chapter 16). Special care is taken to cleanse area because of increased risk of fecal contamination.	**5.** Aseptic technique should be exercised throughout the biopsy procedure. See Chapter 16.
6. Scrub hands and don surgical gloves using aseptic technique.	**6.** Using aseptic technique is always advisable when introducing a needle into a body cavity.
7. Place all sterile equipment on a sterile surgical towel and cover animal with a fenestrated drape.	**7.** A fenestrated drape helps to prevent contamination of the needle.
8. Prepare needle for use, that is, “load” it by holding cannula handle firmly while pulling out obturator trigger handle until it clicks and locks in place.	**8.** Once the needle is loaded, it is ready for use.
Operative Phase	**Operative Phase**
1. Inject local anesthetic in perineal skin, even if sedation is used.	**1.** Even when animal is sedated, we recommend injecting local anesthetic to minimize pain immediately following the procedure.
2. Make 2-mm stab incision in perineal skin with scalpel blade.	
3. Place gloved middle or index finger in rectum and secure prostate against bony pelvis by digital pressure (Fig. 22-6).	**3.** If the prostate is too small or too cranial to be held in a fixed position within the pelvic canal, a transabdominal needle biopsy or open surgical biopsy technique should be used.

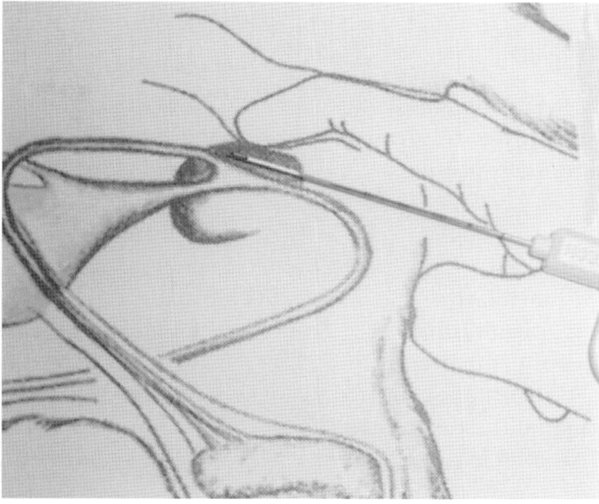

Figure 22-6 Proper position of needle for obtaining a prostate biopsy using a Cook needle.

Technical Action	Rationale/Amplification
Operative Phase	**Operative Phase**
4. Advance biopsy needle cranially through incision and perineum parallel to rectal wall until you can feel tip of obturator touch caudal pole of prostate.	**4.** Use gentle, even pressure as the needle is advanced through the pelvic canal.
5. Introduce end of outer cannula, with inner obturator retracted, into a lobe of prostate approximately 2 mm (Fig. 22-6).	**5.** The point of the needle should be directed away from the spine and rectum.
6. While holding needle handle firmly in one hand, advance inner obturator to its full length by sliding trigger handle smoothly forward.	**6.** A notch in the obturator accepts the prostatic tissue to be removed.
7. When trigger button touches outer cannula handle, firmly press spring-loaded trigger button to automatically advance outer cannula.	**7.** This step cuts off the specimen and protects it within the biopsy notch of obturator.
8. Quickly but carefully pull entire biopsy needle directly out of prostate, pelvic canal, and skin.	**8.** Be careful not to lacerate the prostate or urethra while retracting the device.
9. Reload needle by holding cannula handle firmly, while pulling out obturator trigger handle until it clicks and locks in place.	**9.** It is necessary to reload the device to retrieve the core specimen from the obturator notch.

Operative Phase

Technical Action	Rationale/Amplification
10. Working directly over biopsy receptacle, advance inner obturator to expose specimen. Do not press trigger button.	**10.** Working over the biopsy jar prevents inadvertent loss of the specimen. Inadvertent triggering of the device at this time may result in ejection, laceration, or crushing of the specimen.
11. *Assistant:* Open lid of fixative receptacle at appropriate time. Using a sterile hypodermic needle or scalpel blade, transfer specimen immediately to a small tissue cassette (Fig. 22-3D) before placing in fixative.	**11.** Small biopsy tissue samples should be placed in a cassette to prevent loss during processing. Once the cassette contains adequate biopsy tissue, it is immersed in formalin or other fixative solution.
12. If specimen is small or severely fragmented, procedure can be repeated once.	**12.** Although repeating the procedure adds risk of hemorrhage or other complications, the consequences of not obtaining enough tissue for the pathologist to interpret must be considered.

Postbiopsy Considerations

Frank hematuria may be observed for 1–3 days after prostate biopsy.

NEEDLE CORE BIOPSY OF CUTANEOUS OR SUBCUTANEOUS MASS

Needle core biopsy is a procedure for obtaining tissue from skin or subcutaneous masses to make a histological diagnosis.

Specific Indications

1. Large noncystic dermal masses
2. Subcutaneous masses of varying size and consistency
3. Masses of the neck muscles, thoracic wall, abdominal wall, and peritoneal cavity
4. Masses of the proximal extremities

Contraindications

1. Bleeding/clotting disorders
2. Mast cell tumors

Complications

1. Subcutaneous or intra-abdominal hemorrhage
2. Inadvertent puncture or laceration of viscera

Equipment

- Cook or Temno biopsy needles (14–18 g) (Fig. 22-3 A, B, C)
- Scalpel blade (No. 11 or No. 15)
- Local anesthetic (e.g. 2% lidocaine)
- Skin preparation materials
- Sterile gloves
- Tissue cassette (Fig. 22-3D)

Biopsy Sites

Various

Restraint and Positioning

The animal is held in dorsal, sternal, left lateral, or right lateral recumbency, depending on the location of the mass to be biopsied. Local anesthesia is required, and sedation or tranquilization is recommended.

Prebiopsy Considerations

Unless there is clinical evidence to suspect a coagulopathy, it is usually not necessary to perform coagulation tests for needle biopsies of masses. Because general anesthesia is not generally needed, biopsy of masses does not require overnight fasting.

Procedure

Technical Action

Preparatory Phase

1. If mass being biopsied is intra-abdominal, remove ascites by abdominocentesis.

Rationale/Amplification

Preparatory Phase

1. Hold the mass securely by grasping within the fingers or by pushing it against an immobile surface, for example, bone, fascia, or muscle. If the mass being biopsied is in the abdomen, check for ascites. Distention of the abdomen by fluid may preclude localization and immobilization of the mass.

Technical Action	Rationale/Amplification
2. Prepare operative site by clipping hair and cleansing and disinfecting skin in standard manner (see Chapter 16).	2. Aseptic technique should be exercised throughout the biopsy procedure. See Chapter 16.
3. Inject local anesthetic in intended path of needle.	3. Sedation is recommended to minimize discomfort and to prevent the animal from moving during the procedure. Even when sedated, we recommend injecting local anesthetic to minimize pain immediately following the procedure.
4. Scrub hands and don surgical gloves using aseptic technique.	4. Using aseptic technique is always advisable when introducing a needle into a body cavity.
5. Place all sterile equipment on a sterile surgical towel and cover animal with a fenestrated drape.	5. A fenestrated drape helps to prevent contamination of the needle.
6. Prepare needle for use, that is, "load" it by holding cannula handle firmly while pulling out obturator trigger handle until it clicks and locks in place.	6. Once the needle is loaded, it is ready for use.
Operative Phase	**Operative Phase**
1. Isolate mass to be biopsied in one hand by deep palpation.	1. If the mass to be biopsied is too small or cannot be held in a fixed position, an excisional or incisional biopsy technique should be used instead.
2. Apply additional disinfecting scrub.	2. Grasping the mass often introduces a chance of contamination.
3. Make a small stab incision with scalpel blade.	3. Use a No. 11 or No. 15 scalpel blade.
4. Advance biopsy needle through incision and into outer edge of tumor.	4. Use gentle, even pressure as the needle is advanced through the skin.
5. Introduce end of outer cannula, with inner obturator retracted, through renal capsule approximately 2 mm.	5. The point of the needle should be directed away from the center of large (>5 cm) masses to avoid sampling a necrotic central core.
6. While holding needle handle firmly in one hand, advance inner obturator to its full length by sliding trigger handle smoothly forward (Fig. 22-7).	6. A notch in the obturator accepts the tissue to be removed.

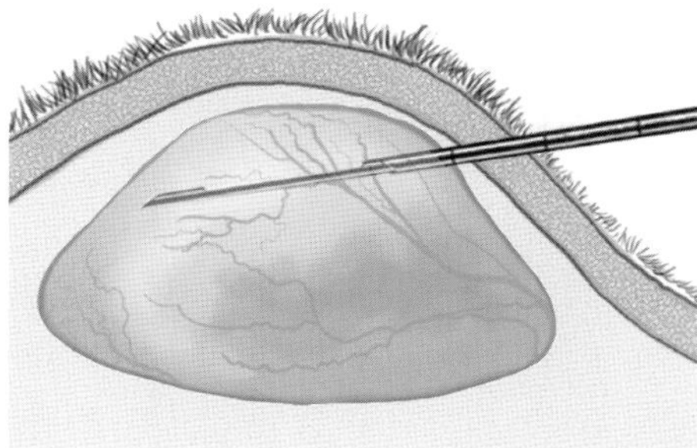

Figure 22-7 Suggested position of needle for obtaining a subcutaneous mass biopsy using a Cook needle.

Technical Action

Operative Phase

7. When trigger button touches outer cannula handle, firmly press spring-loaded trigger button to automatically advance outer cannula (Fig. 22-3C).
8. Quickly but carefully pull entire biopsy needle directly out of mass and overlying skin.
9. Reload needle by holding cannula handle firmly while pulling out obturator trigger handle until it clicks and locks in place.
10. Working directly over biopsy receptacle, advance inner obturator to expose specimen. Do not press trigger button.
11. *Assistant:* Open lid of fixative receptacle at appropriate time. Using a sterile hypodermic needle or scalpel blade, transfer specimen immediately to a small tissue cassette (Fig. 22-3D) before placing it in fixative.
12. The procedure can be repeated several times, unless marked hemorrhage is noted.

Rationale/Amplification

Operative Phase

7. This step cuts off the specimen and protects it within the biopsy notch of the obturator.
8. Be careful not to lacerate the mass or adjacent structures while retracting the device.
9. It is necessary to reload the device to retrieve the core specimen from the obturator notch.
10. Working over the biopsy jar prevents accidental loss of the specimen. Inadvertent triggering of the device at this time may result in ejection, laceration, or crushing of the specimen.
11. Small biopsy tissue samples should be placed in a cassette to prevent loss during processing. Once the cassette contains adequate biopsy tissue, it can be immersed in formalin or other fixative solution.
12. Although repeating the procedure adds risk of hemorrhage or other complications, the consequences of not obtaining enough tissue for the pathologist to interpret must be considered.

Postbiopsy Considerations

Many biopsy sites will appear bruised for 12–72 hours after the biopsy. Severe hemorrhage rarely occurs when proper technique is used.

Bibliography

Berquist TH *et al.*: Transthoracic needle biopsy. Mayo Clin Proc 55: 475–481, 1980

Leeds EB, Leav I: Perineal punch biopsy of the canine prostate gland. JAVMA 154: 925–934, 1969

McEvoy RD, Begley MD, Antic R: Percutaneous biopsy of intrapulmonary mass lesions. Cancer 51: 2321–2326, 1983

Michel RP, Lushpihan A, Ahmed AN: Pathologic findings of transthoracic needle aspiration in the diagnosis of localized pulmonary lesions. Cancer 51: 1663–1672, 1983

Roudebush P, Green RA, Digilio KM: Percutaneous fine-needle aspiration biopsy of the lung. JAAHA 17: 109–115, 1981

Weaver AD: Transperineal punch biopsy of the canine prostate gland. J Small Anim Pract 18: 573–577, 1977

Chapter 23

Urohydropropulsion

Success is simply a matter of luck. Ask any failure.
EARL WILSON

Urohydropropulsion is a therapeutic procedure for removal of foreign material (e.g. uroliths) from the urethra of male dogs.

Specific Indication

Lower urinary tract obstruction by foreign bodies or uroliths.

Equipment

- Sterile flexible urethral catheter of appropriate gauge
- 20 mL or 35 mL syringe
- Sterile physiologic saline
- Examination glove
- Lubricating jelly

Restraint and Positioning

Administer an antispasmodic drug, for example phenoxybenzamine, before proceeding, if possible. The operation requires placing one finger in the rectum. Sedation or tranquilization is recommended. At least two persons are required for this procedure. The dog is held in lateral recumbency and the prepuce is retracted as described for urethral catheterization.

Crow and Walshaw's Manual of Clinical Procedures in Dogs, Cats, Rabbits, and Rodents, Fourth Edition. Edited by Jennifer E. Boyle. Published 2016 by John Wiley & Sons, Inc.
Companion Website: www.wiley.com/go/boyle/manual4e

Procedure

Technical Action	Rationale/Amplification
1. Pass a sterile flexible catheter through urethral orifice proximally to point of obstruction; then withdraw it approximately 2 cm.	**1.** See Chapter 12. A large-gauge catheter should be used to ensure a tight fit.
2. Attach syringe containing physiologic saline to open end of catheter.	**2.** Lubricants such as mineral oil may be added if desired.
3. Place operator's lubricated, gloved finger in rectum and occlude lumen of pelvic urethra by applying digital pressure through ventral rectal wall.	
4. Compress external urethral orifice around catheter using thumb and forefinger.	**4.** The lower urethra and syringe are now a closed system.
5. *Assistant:* Inject saline rapidly until a rebound of syringe plunger occurs (Fig. 23-1).	**5.** The urethra will be maximally dilated at this time.

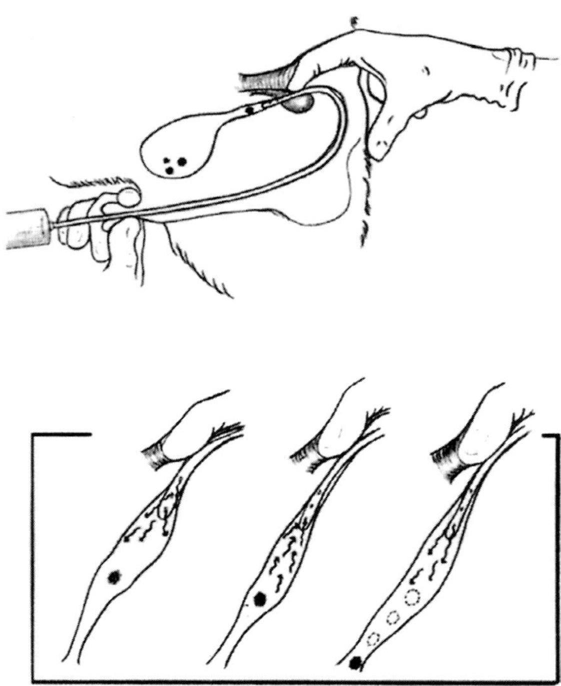

Figure 23-1 Schematic representation of forces and fluid flow during urohydropropulsion.

Technical Action

6. *Operator:*
   a) For a foreign body or large calculus too large to pass through os penis, quickly release pressure on proximal urethra.
   b) For a structure or stone small enough to pass through os penis, quickly release external urethral orifice pressure.

7. Repeat infusion and release sequence several times.

8. If no movement of a calculus is apparent after three or four attempts, discontinue procedure.

Rationale/Amplification

6. The sudden release of pressure on the pelvic urethra causes back flow, allowing the obstructing structure to move back toward the urinary bladder. Conversely, the sudden release of external pressure at the urethral orifice causes flow in the opposite direction, allowing the obstructive object to move toward the external urethral orifice.
7. Alternating the direction of urethral fluid flow will sometimes help to free a calculus. Often it is necessary to repeat this procedure several times to force a calculus back into the bladder or to cause it to be voided.
8. Excessive attempts to dislodge calculi or foreign bodies can lead to tearing of the urethral mucosa.

Bibliography

Osborne CA, Low DG, Finco DR: Urohydropropulsion. In Canine and Feline Urology. Philadelphia, WB Saunders, 1972

Chapter 24

Prostatic Massage/ Washing

Only a mediocre person is always at his best.
SOMERSET MAUGHAM

Prostatic massage/washing is a procedure by which prostatic fluid is obtained.

Purposes

1. To examine prostatic secretions microscopically for microorganisms and cellular elements
2. To obtain prostatic secretions for bacteriologic culture and antibiotic sensitivity testing

Specific Indications

1. Pyuria
2. Hematuria
3. Bloody urethral discharge
4. Prostatic asymmetry or distortion
5. Prostatomegaly

Complications

1. Rupture of prostatic abscess
2. Rectal perforation
3. Ascending urinary tract infection

Crow and Walshaw's Manual of Clinical Procedures in Dogs, Cats, Rabbits, and Rodents, Fourth Edition. Edited by Jennifer E. Boyle. © 2016 John Wiley & Sons, Inc. Published 2016 by John Wiley & Sons, Inc.
Companion Website: www.wiley.com/go/boyle/manual4e

Equipment Needed

- Equipment for urinary catheterization of male dog (See Chapter 12):
  - Cotton
  - Skin disinfectant or mild soap
  - Sterile flexible urinary catheter of appropriate size (See Chapter 12, Table 12-1)
  - Sterile gloves
- Sterile containers for two specimens
- Two 5-mL syringes, each containing 5 mL sterile saline

Restraint and Positioning

If the dog shows signs of pain when its prostate is palpated, a sedative should be given prior to prostatic massage. The dog is restrained in a standing position for prostatic massage and washing. If desired, the dog can be placed in lateral recumbency while the urinary catheter is introduced. Two assistants are usually needed for this procedure.

Procedure

Technical Action	Rationale/Amplification
1. Label sterile containers for urine and prostatic fluid.	
2. Advance urinary catheter into urinary bladder and empty urine from bladder.	**2.** See Chapter 12. It is important to premeasure the catheter by holding it in its approximate intraurethral position, near but not touching the dog.
3. Instill 5–10 mL of sterile saline through catheter into urinary bladder, then aspirate this saline into same syringe and place into sterile container.	**3.** Washing the bladder and comparing results with those of the prostatic massage/washing help to identify organisms and cells that are found only in the prostate.
4. Place gloved finger in rectum.	
5. Withdraw urinary catheter so that catheter tip is in portion of urethra distal to prostate.	**5.** Premeasuring the catheter makes it possible to estimate the approximate location of the prostatic urethra. In some dogs, the catheter tip may be palpated as it is moved within the pelvic urethra.
6. Massage prostate with gloved finger in rectum for 1 minute (Fig. 24-1). Ask assistant to collect any fluid that comes out of catheter during massage.	**6.** Vigorous massage should be avoided if prostatic abscess is suspected.

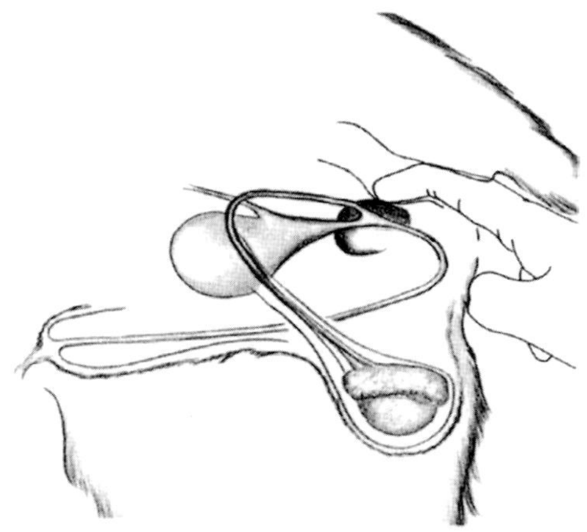

Figure 24-1 Digital massage of prostate transrectally.

Technical Action

7. Instill 5 mL of sterile saline through catheter into urinary bladder, then advance catheter into bladder again and aspirate this saline.
8. Place second aspirate into prostatic fluid container.
9. Submit both specimens for bacteriologic and cytologic evaluation.

Rationale/Amplification

7. Instillation of saline after the massage will enable collection of small amounts of prostatic secretions released during prostatic massage.

9. Specimens should be labeled with date, time, animal identification, and type of specimen.

NOTE: *There is evidence that accurate diagnosis of chronic bacterial prostatitis may be made more readily by analysis of ejaculated semen than from a specimen obtained by the prostatic massage and washing, particularly if the dog has a concurrent urinary tract infection. (See Chapter 25 for semen collection procedure.)*

Bibliography

Barsanti JA, Finco DR: Canine bacterial prostatitis. Vet Clin N Amer 9(4): 679–700, 1979

Barsanti JA, Prasse KW, Crowell WA, Shotts EB, Finco DR: Evaluation of various techniques for diagnosis of chronic bacterial prostatitis in the dog. JAVMA 183(2): 219–224, 1983

Chapter 25

Semen Collection and Artificial Insemination

When love and skill work together, expect a masterpiece.
JOHN RUSKIN

Canine *semen is collected* to evaluate breeding potential or to diagnose suspected prostatic disease or infertility. *Artificial insemination* is a technique used in place of natural breeding for fertile breeding bitches and sires.

SEMEN COLLECTION

Purposes

1. To evaluate spermatogenic capability of proposed sire as part of a prebreeding or prepurchase examination
2. To obtain specimens for culture or cytology from prostate and testicle/epididymis
3. To obtain semen for artificial insemination or cryopreservation

Complications

1. Paraphimosis
2. Physical injury of male or handlers
3. Transmission of venereal infections (e.g. brucellosis)

Equipment

- Artificial vagina (latex rubber cone, with attached sterile graduated centrifuge tube)
- Aqueous lubricating jelly
- Clean, warm glass slides

Crow and Walshaw's Manual of Clinical Procedures in Dogs, Cats, Rabbits, and Rodents, Fourth Edition. Edited by Jennifer E. Boyle. Published 2016 by John Wiley & Sons, Inc.
Companion Website: www.wiley.com/go/boyle/manual4e

Preparation

Attach the collection tube to the latex rubber cone. Lubricate the cone lightly with jelly near its broad end to minimize trauma to the penis and to facilitate removal of artificial vagina after ejaculation.

Restraint

The prospective sire and an estrous bitch are brought together in a quiet room with a floor that is not slippery. Both dogs should be restrained by leash. The male and female may be allowed to play. The male is encouraged to sniff the vulva of the bitch. If the female resists the male's attention by snapping or biting, she should be muzzled and restrained to prevent injury to the male or the handlers. The handler of the estrous bitch should squat or kneel near the female's head and prevent her from biting the male (see Chapter 1). Restraint is particularly important once the male starts to mount.

NOTE: *When semen is collected for diagnostic purposes only, most males do not require a teaser bitch. A docile, anestrous bitch usually will suffice. Inexperienced or shy males may need an estrous teaser to stimulate erection and ejaculation.*

Procedure

Technical Action	Rationale/Amplification
1. When male is ready to mount female, semen collector kneels at male's side.	
2. Stroke male's sheath and penis by applying light digital pressure around mid-shaft portion of penis.	**2.** For inexperienced males or males with diminished libido, repeated and vigorous stroking of the prepuce at the glans/bulbus glandis area may be needed to induce an erection and thrusting of the hips. At this point, the male will usually attempt to mount the female.
3. Once a firm erection occurs, place artificial vagina over end of penis and use cone to gently slide prepuce caudally, enclosing erect penis in rubber cone to a point proximal to bulbus glandis (Fig. 25-1).	
4. Maintain gentle pressure on penis, which is still ensheathed in artificial vagina (Fig. 25-2).	**4.** This step simulates the natural tie.
5. Collect 1–20 mL of ejaculated semen.	**5.** If the semen is to be used for artificial insemination, a total volume of approximately 5 mL of semen is collected. If prostatic disease is suspected, larger amounts should be

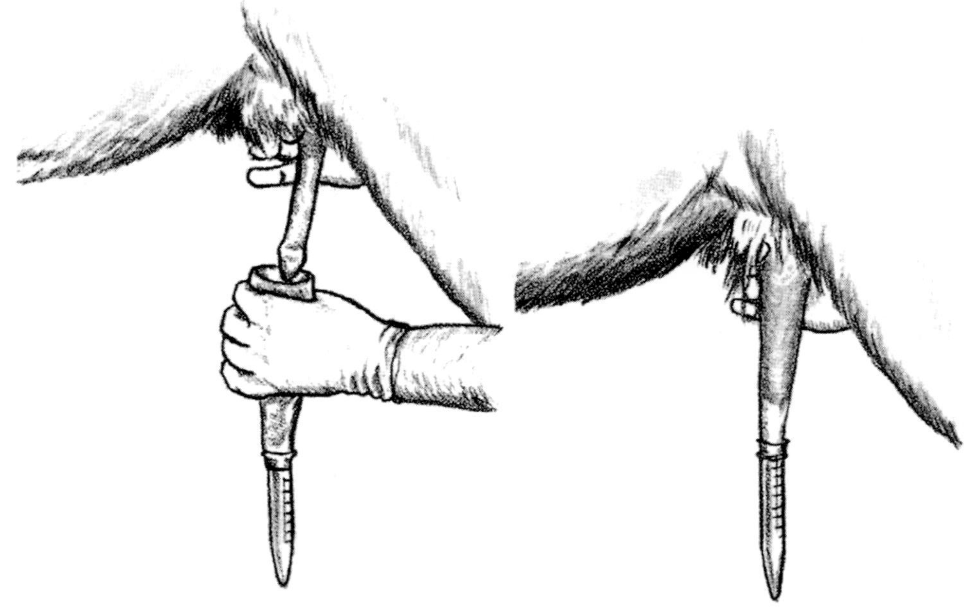

Figure 25-1 Placing artificial vagina over erect penis.

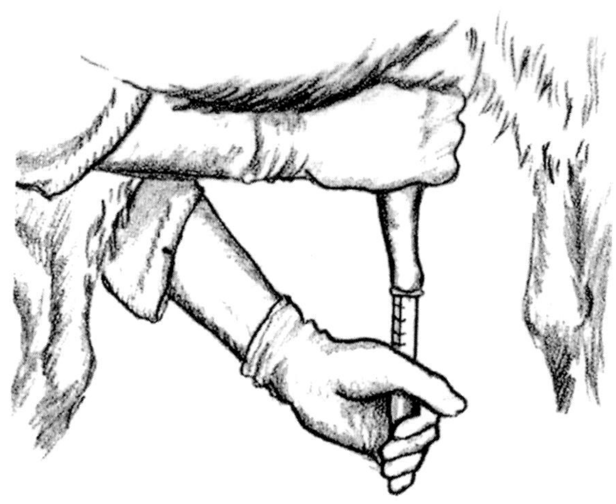

Figure 25-2 Collecting ejaculate.

Technical Action

Rationale/Amplification

collected. If breeding soundness is being tested, the last fraction, which is largely prostatic secretion, should be collected in a separate tube so as not to dilute the sperm-laden fraction.

Technical Action	Rationale/Amplification
6. After collection is complete, carefully remove artificial vagina from shaft of penis.	6. Removal may not be possible in large dogs. If artificial vagina is snug, do not attempt to remove it—let erection subside naturally. Disconnect collection tube and process semen sample. Place a large drop of sperm-rich semen (second fraction) on a prewarmed glass slide; perform semen analysis immediately.
7. Remove teaser bitch from room.	
8. Allow male to rest or walk while erection subsides.	8. Always check male after erection subsides for paraphimosis or trauma to the penis. Never send a dog home until the penis is completely retracted into the prepuce.

ARTIFICIAL INSEMINATION

Purposes

1. To prevent exposure of male to venereally transmitted diseases
2. To breed more than one bitch with one ejaculate
3. To inseminate bitch with frozen, stored semen

Specific Indications

1. Physical abnormality of male or female that prevents intromission
2. Behavioral abnormality of male or female that prevents natural service
3. Geographical separation of sire and dam that precludes natural mating

Complication

Vaginal laceration

Equipment

- Insemination pipette
- Syringe
- Aqueous lubricating jelly
- Semen extender (for shipping fresh chilled semen)
- Specialized equipment for freezing (cryopreservation) of semen

Preparation and Restraint

The bitch to be inseminated is restrained in a standing position. Chemical restraint measures are rarely required. The assistant holds the tail to one side to expose the perineal area (see Chapter 1).

Procedure

Technical Action	Rationale/Amplification
1. Clean vestibule of excess discharge with moistened cotton.	
2. Slide blunt pipette (containing semen) just below dorsal commissure of vulva and through vestibule and vagina to level of cervix.	**2.** The pipette is directed craniodorsally at a 60–75-degree angle from a horizontal plane until it has passed through the vestibule, to avoid contacting the clitoris. Then direct it cranially at a 45-degree angle from a horizontal plane.
3. Elevate bitch's hindquarters by grasping stifles and raising legs off floor (Fig. 25-3).	**3.** This position helps to retain semen at the cervix. If possible, the hindquarters should be elevated for 5 minutes. Most females in heat will readily tolerate this position.
4. Eject semen remaining in pipette by forcing 2–4 mL of air through it with a syringe.	

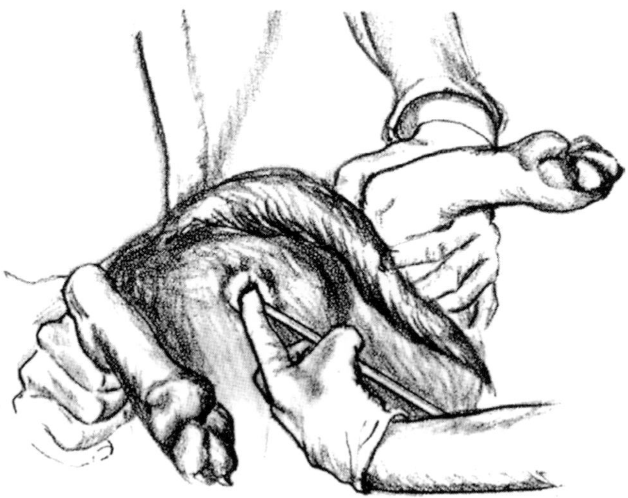

Figure 25-3 Elevating hindquarters of bitch while insemination pipette is inserted.

Technical Action	Rationale/Amplification
5. Gently eject semen from pipette, using a syringe and gravity flow.	
6. Remove pipette as soon as semen is deposited.	**6.** Retention of the pipette causes some discomfort and may cause the bitch to struggle.

Bibliography

Seager SWJ, Platz CC: Artificial insemination and frozen semen in the dog. Vet Clin N Amer 7: 757–764, 1977

Seager SWJ, Platz CC: Collection and evaluation of canine semen. Vet Clin N Amer 7: 765–773, 1977

Chapter 26

Vaginal Examination and Specimen Collection

I hear and I forget. I see and I remember. I do and I understand.

CHINESE PROVERB

Visual and digital examinations of the vaginal mucosa are diagnostic methods essential to a thorough evaluation of the lower female genital tract. Samples are easily obtained for cytology examination and microbiologic study.

Purposes

1. To ascertain the physical characteristics of the mucosal surface of the vagina by inspection and palpation
2. To obtain cytology and microbiologic specimens from the vagina
3. To visualize the urethral orifice for urethral catheterization

Specific Indications

1. Vulvar or vaginal discharge
2. Vulvar swelling or odor
3. Infertility
4. Attraction of males by anestrous or spayed females
5. Estrus determination
6. Dysuria
7. Tenesmus

Crow and Walshaw's Manual of Clinical Procedures in Dogs, Cats, Rabbits, and Rodents, Fourth Edition. Edited by Jennifer E. Boyle. Published 2016 by John Wiley & Sons, Inc.
Companion Website: www.wiley.com/go/boyle/manual4e

Contraindication

The vaginal orifice of dogs less than 10 kg and cats is too small for digital examination.

Complications

1. Vaginal laceration
2. Severe discomfort and/or bleeding, if clitoral membrane present

Equipment

- Sterile examination glove
- Vaginal speculum and light source, anoscope, or proctoscope (adult or pediatric) (Fig. 26-1).
- Sterile, guarded, cotton-tipped applicator (for microbiologic specimen)
- Cotton-tipped applicator (for cytology specimen)
- Aqueous lubricating jelly

Preparation and Restraint

If the perineum is heavily soiled, clean the perivulvar skin and hair thoroughly using mild soap and water. Remove excess vulvar discharge with a moist cotton pledget.

These procedures are best completed with the animal standing. The holder cradles the animal in one arm while raising the tail with the other. It may be advisable to muzzle the dog in some cases.

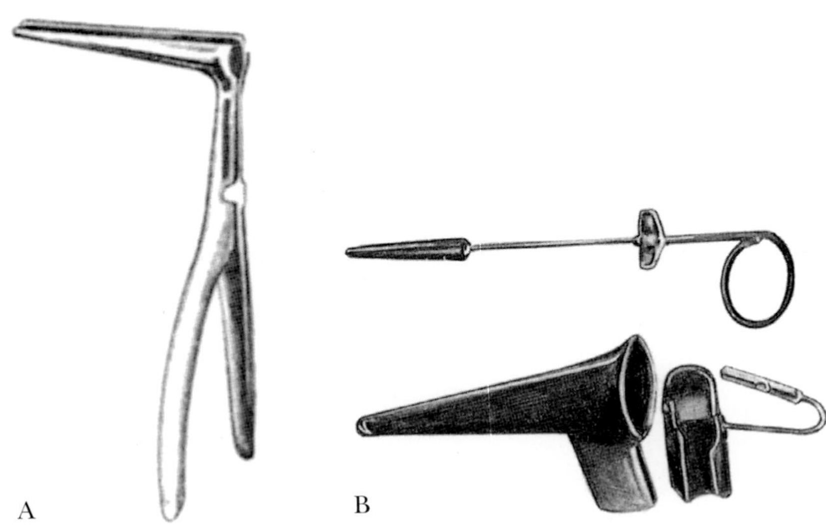

Figure 26-1 Instruments used for vaginal examination: (A) speculum, and (B) anoscope.

Procedure

Technical Action	Rationale/Amplification
Specimen Collection	**Specimen Collection**
1. Grasp vulva gently with thumb and index finger and introduce a guarded, sterile, cotton-tipped applicator stick just below dorsal vulvar commissure into vestibule and direct it along dorsal vaginal wall (Fig. 26-2).	
2. Advance swab tip out of plastic guard.	
3. Move tip from side to side or rotate it. Avoid irritating urethral papilla (orifice), which is located in ventral vaginal wall.	3. These movements of the swab ensure adequate sampling of the vaginal mucosa.
4. Move tip back and forth in cranial and caudal direction.	
5. Pull swab back into guard and remove apparatus from vagina.	
6. Immediately inoculate culture or transport media.	
7. Repeat Nos. 1, 3, and 4 with a standard cotton-tipped applicator to obtain specimen for cytology examination.	
8. Remove swab and immediately roll tip of swab across faces of two or more glass slides.	8. Do not smear the tip on the slide—rolling prevents distortion of vaginal epithelial cells.
9. Allow slides to air dry and stain them immediately.	

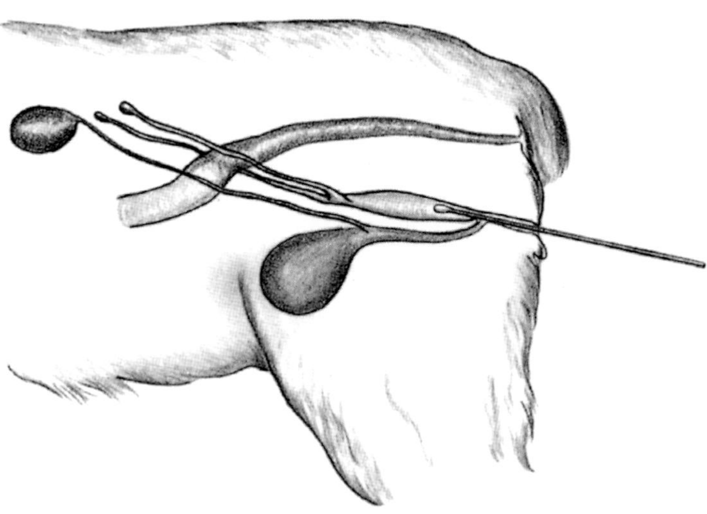

Figure 26-2 Obtaining a swab specimen from the vagina.

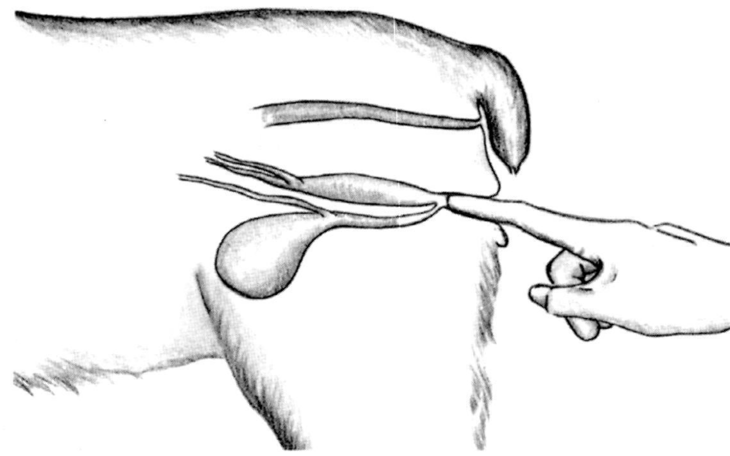

Figure 26-3 Performing digital vaginal examination.

Technical Action	Rationale/Amplification
Digital Examination	**Digital Examination**
1. Grasp vulva with thumb and index finger and gently advance gloved, lubricated index finger of other hand dorsal to clitoral fossa and into vagina (Fig. 26-3).	1. Proper positioning of finger is ensured by introducing it just below the dorsal vulvar commissure and directing it at a 60–75-degree angle to the horizontal plane until the vagina is entered. Do not attempt digital vaginal examination in dogs weighing less than 10 kg or in cats, even if they are anesthetized.
2. Palpate urethral papilla, vaginal wall, cervix, and pelvic bones.	2. Use slow, gentle motions to avoid damage to the fragile mucous membranes.
3. Remove finger slowly and examine it for discharges.	
Visual Examination	**Visual Examination**
1. Grasp vulva with thumb and index finger and introduce speculum into vestibule just below dorsal vulvar commissure. Advance instrument craniodorsally at angle approximately 60–75 degrees from horizontal plane until it passes through vestibule, then direct it forward at approximately 45 degrees from horizontal plane (Fig. 26-4).	1. Be careful not to catch the speculum in the clitoral fossa because this will cause marked discomfort.

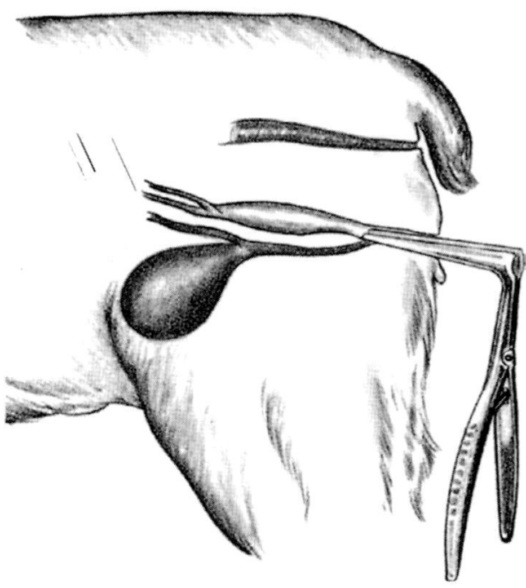

Figure 26-4 Inserting vaginal speculum.

Technical Action

Visual Examination

2. Remove obturator, if anoscope or proctoscope is used; examine all surfaces of vaginal mucosa, proceeding from cranial to caudal. Note appearance of external urethral orifice.
3. Withdraw vaginal speculum slowly, maintaining original directional orientation.

Rationale/Amplification

Visual Examination

2. If abnormalities are noted, a swab for cytology or culture, or a biopsy specimen, is obtained.

Bibliography

Settergren I: Examination of the canine genital system. Vet Clin North Am 1: 103–118, 1971

Chapter 27

Bone Marrow Aspiration and Biopsy

Wonder rather than doubt is the root of knowledge.
ABRAHAM JOSHUA HESCHEL

Bone marrow aspiration and biopsy are diagnostic procedures involving the introduction of a rigid, hollow needle into the marrow-containing, cancellous part of either a long or flat bone. * **The following procedures are considered invasive and are typically performed exclusively by veterinarians.**

Purposes

1. To identify and quantify abnormal cell populations in bone marrow
2. To identify abnormal maturation of hematopoietic stem cell lines
3. To stage certain neoplastic disorders, for example, lymphoma, leukemia, and mast cell tumors

Specific Indications

1. Nonregenerative anemia
2. Thrombocytopenia
3. Persistent leukopenia
4. Atypical cells in blood
5. Monoclonal dysproteinemia
6. Suspected osteomyelitis
7. Suspected non-hematopoietic neoplasia of bone
8. Clinical staging of lymphoma or mast cell tumors

Crow and Walshaw's Manual of Clinical Procedures in Dogs, Cats, Rabbits, and Rodents, Fourth Edition. Edited by Jennifer E. Boyle.
Companion Website: www.wiley.com/go/boyle/manual4e

Complications

1. Bleeding and hematoma formation at operative site, especially when bleeding disorders are present
2. Puncture or laceration of muscles, nerves, or blood vessels
3. Osteomyelitis (iatrogenic)
4. Pain during and after procedure

Equipment

- Bone marrow aspiration needles (Fig. 27-1):
  - 16-gauge Rosenthal needle or Illinois needle for medium-sized or large dogs
  - 18-gauge Rosenthal needle for small dogs and cats
- Jamshidi bone marrow biopsy needles (Fig. 27-2):
  - 12 gauge (adult) for most dogs
  - 14 gauge (pediatric) for small dogs and cats
- Sterile drape or towels
- Sterile gloves
- Antiseptic solutions and gauze sponges
- Local anesthetic (e.g. 2% lidocaine)

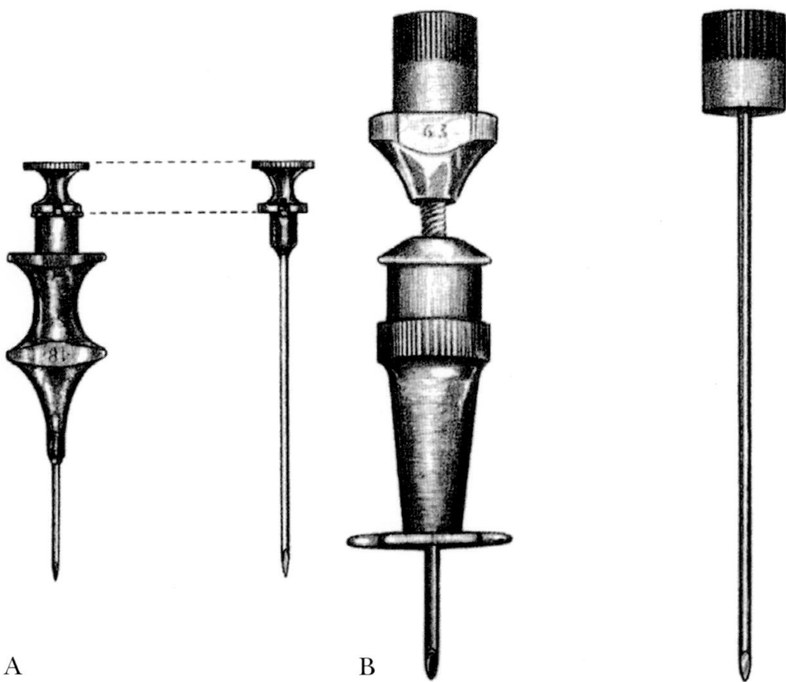

Figure 27-1 Bone marrow aspiration needles: (A) 18-gauge Rosenthal needle with matched stylet, and (B) 16-gauge Illinois needle with matched stylet and depth stop.

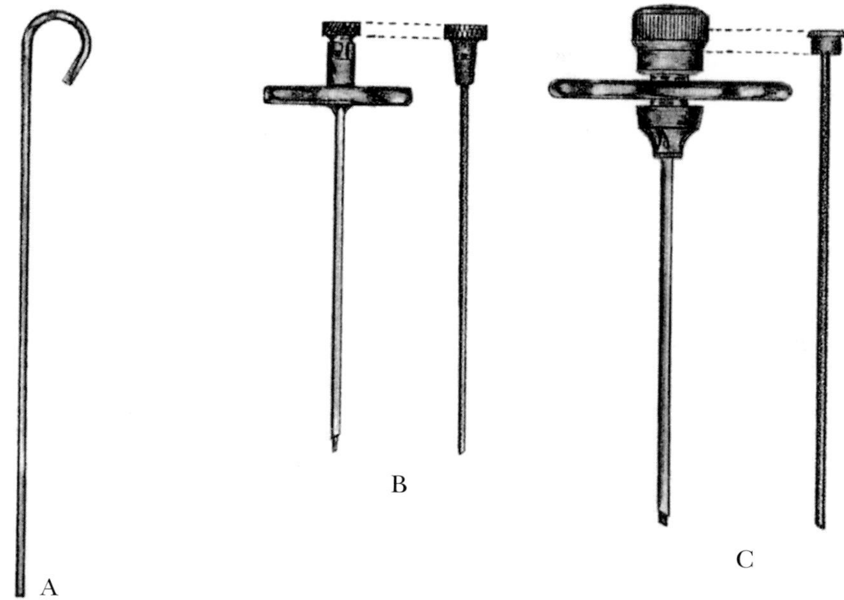

Figure 27-2 Jamshidi bone marrow biopsy needles: (A) specimen expeller, (B) pediatric, and (C) adult.

- Scalpel blade (No. 11)
- Syringes:
  - 6-mL and 20-mL
- Needles:
  - 22 and 25 gauge
- CPDA: citrate phosphate dextrose adenine anticoagulant solution
- Laboratory equipment:
  - Precleaned microscope slides
  - Cover slips
  - Culture tubes (when indicated)
  - Hematocrit capillary tubes or small pipettes
  - Petri dish
- Fixative (formalin or Zenker's fixative)

Preparation

Technical Action	Rationale/Amplification
1. Give tranquilizer, sedative, or general anesthetic as required for comfort and immobilization.	1. Most severely anemic animals do not require systemic chemical restraint.

Technical Action	Rationale/Amplification
2. Restrain animal in appropriate position for site of aspiration or biopsy (see below and Chapter 1).	**2.** Excessive movement may result in contamination of biopsy site, laceration of tissues, or increased pain.
3. Clip hair from operative site, using No. 40 clipper blade. Mark proposed entry site.	**3.** Marking the entry site helps to locate the site for local anesthetic injection after a sterile drape is placed.
4. Prepare skin area for aseptic surgery and cover area with a fenestrated surgical drape.	**4.** See Chapter 16.

ILIAC CREST ASPIRATION AND BIOPSY

Technical Action	Rationale/Amplification
1. Restrain animal in lateral recumbency.	**1.** With an animal that is not anesthetized, two persons are needed for restraint to avoid contamination of the operative site.
2. Locate dorsal iliac crest and mark site for entry (Fig. 27-3A).	**2.** In the obese patient, it is frequently difficult to locate the dorsal iliac crest. Deep palpation will guide the operator.
3. Infiltrate marked area with local anesthetic in skin, subcutis, and periosteum.	**3.** The periosteum is the region of greatest sensitivity.
4. Make 3-mm stab incision in skin.	**4.** A small skin incision facilitates insertion of the large, blunt needle.
5. Advance bone marrow needle (with stylet in place) through incision to contact dorsal iliac crest.	**5.** The tip of the needle (or stylet) is brought into contact with the dorsal iliac crest and directed ventrally, parallel to a sagittal plane.
6. Advance needle by rotation and steady pressure (Fig. 27-4A).	**6.** Avoid unnecessary wobbling by keeping the elbow immobilized while using a pronating and supinating motion of the forearm. Considerable force is often required.
7. Aspiration technique:	**7.** Aspiration technique:
a) When needle penetrates outer cortex of bone, remove stylet.	**a)** There is usually decreased resistance when the marrow cavity is entered.
b) Attach 20-mL syringe and apply negative pressure by forcefully pulling back on syringe plunger (Fig. 27-4B).	**b)** The actual aspiration usually causes considerable discomfort for animals that are not anesthetized.

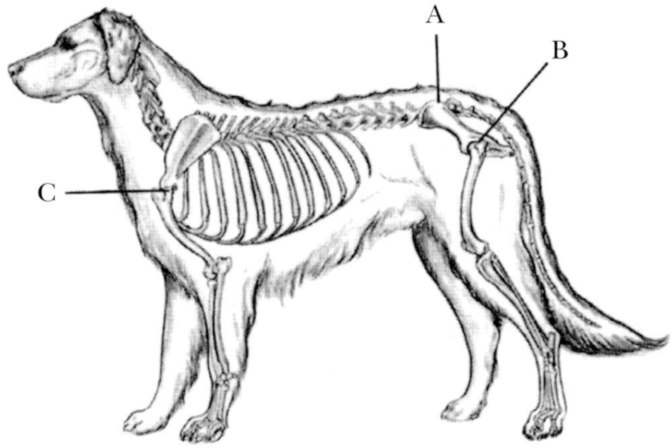

Figure 27-3 Sites for performing bone marrow aspiration or biopsy: (A) iliac crest; (B) trochanteric fossa; (C) head of humerus.

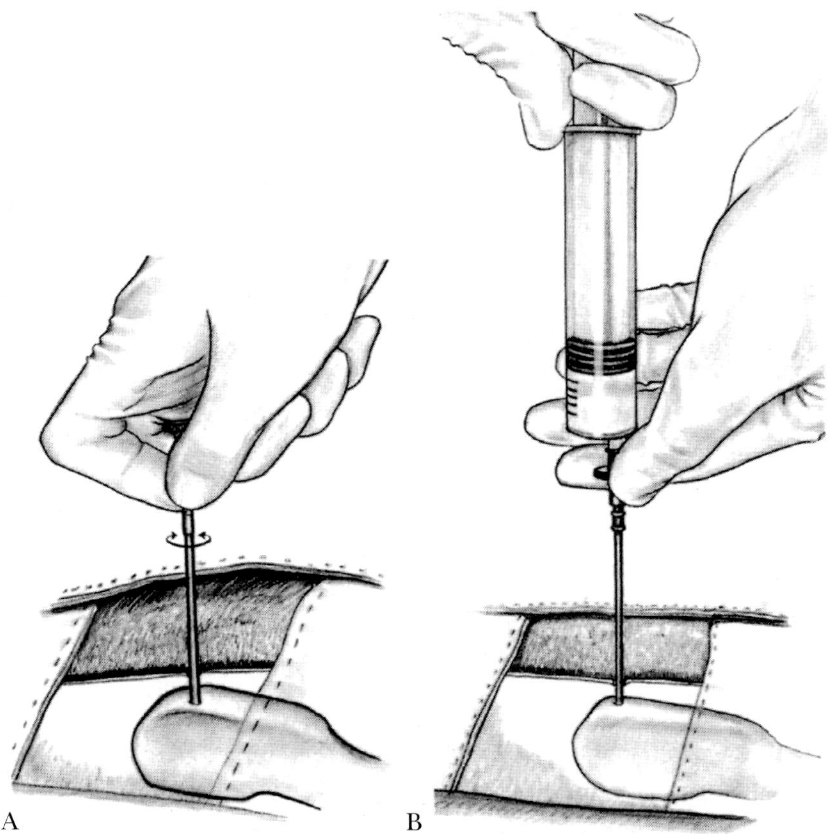

Figure 27-4 Aspiration technique: (A) Advance aspiration needle by applying alternating/rotating motion and steady pressure. (B) Aspirate marrow sample.

Technical Action	Rationale/Amplification
c) Aspirate small volume of bone marrow fluid into syringe.	c) Bone marrow is usually dark red, more viscous than blood, and contains fat particles. Less than 1 mL should be aspirated to avoid excessive dilution of the sample with blood (see alternate technique).
d) Pass syringe to assistant.	
8. *Assistant:* Rapidly touch one or two drops of marrow to surface of 8–10 slides and make thin, even push smears before marrow clots. See Chapter 8 (Fig. 8-4).	8. *Assistant:* The marrow may form a clot in 15–30 seconds, so it is important to make smears quickly.
Alternate Technique	**Alternate Technique**
7. Aspiration technique:	7. Aspiration technique:
a) When needle penetrates outer cortex of bone, remove stylet.	a) There is usually decreased resistance when the marrow cavity is entered.
b) Attach 20-mL syringe containing 2 mL of CPDA solution to bone marrow needle hub.	b) The anticoagulant prevents rapid clotting but does not distort cellular morphology.
c) Apply negative pressure by forcefully pulling back on syringe plunger.	c) The animal may show considerable discomfort during the aspiration.
d) Aspirate 2–3 mL of bone marrow fluid into syringe.	d) A large sample helps in obtaining several bone spicules.
e) Pass syringe to assistant.	e) Pass the syringe aseptically so that the aspiration may be repeated if necessary.
8. *Assistant:* Expel contents of syringe into petri dish. Inspect fluid for cancellous bone spicules. Siphon spicules into capillary tubes and transfer to 8–10 clean glass slides. Make thin, even push smears. See Chapter 8 (Fig. 8-4).	8. *Assistant:* Bone spicules are white or red dense particles, easily distinguished from fat particles. Several spicules can be collected in each capillary tube. Spicules can be transferred to slides by blowing on the other end of the tube or by forcing air through with a tuberculin syringe. Make enough smears to allow for additional stains.
9. Core biopsy technique (Jamshidi needle):	9. Core biopsy technique (Jamshidi needle):
a) When needle and stylet are firmly embedded in bone, remove stylet.	a) The needle should stand in place after the stylet is removed.
b) Advance needle 1–2 cm by gentle rotation and steady pressure (Fig. 27-5A).	b) A comfort knob makes this step easier.

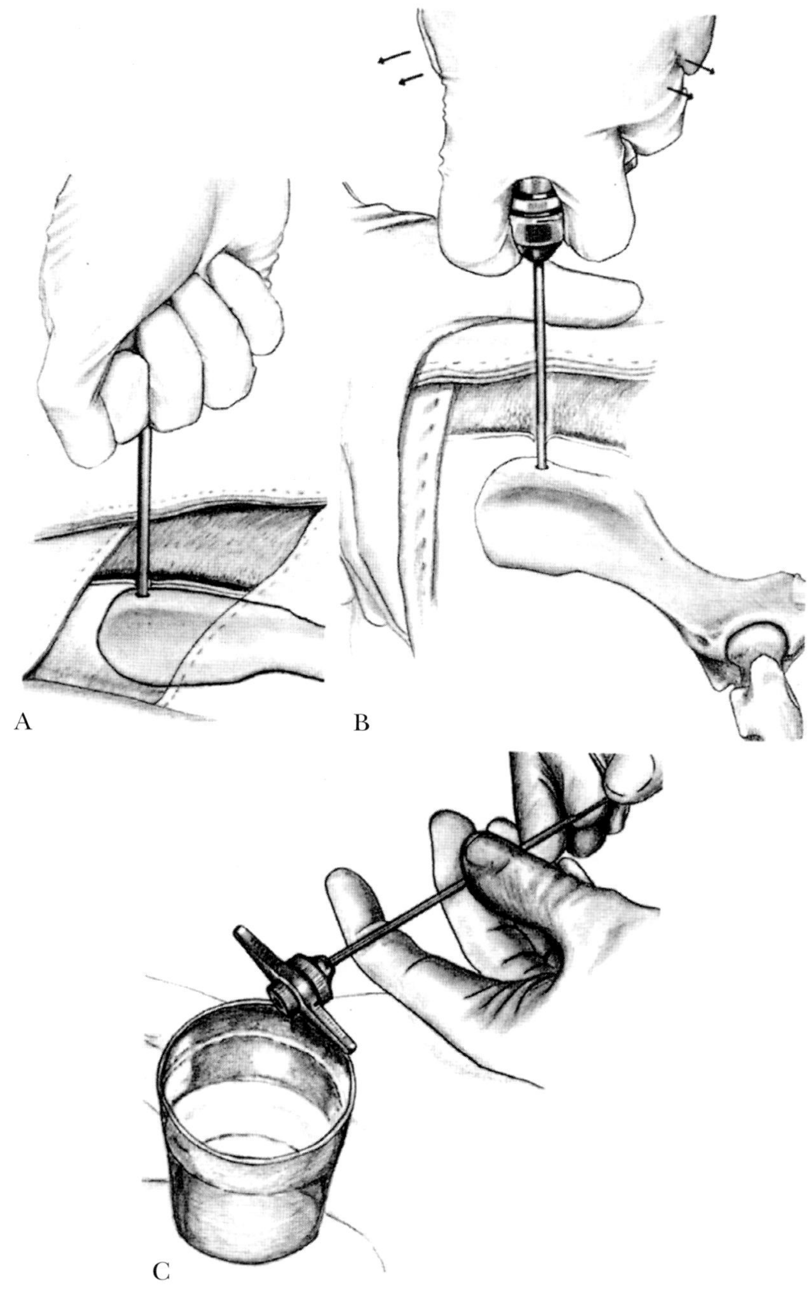

Figure 27-5 Core biopsy technique: (A) Advance biopsy needle by applying alternating/rotating motion and steady pressure. (B) Cut off biopsy sample by alternate, vigorous rotation and gentle wobbling. (C) Remove biopsy by retrograde passage of expeller.

Technical Action	Rationale/Amplification
c) Loosen biopsy sample by alternate rotation and wobbling of needle (Fig. 27-5B).	**c)** Do this gently. Do not bend the needle.
d) Partially withdraw needle, then redirect needle at a slightly different angle and reintroduce it into bone. Repeat rotation and wobbling of needle.	**d)** This repositioning obtains a larger sample and ensures that the specimen is severed from the bone.
e) Remove needle from bone by rotation and steady traction.	
f) Remove biopsy sample from needle using expeller, and place it in appropriate fixative (Fig. 27-5C).	**f)** The expeller is directed retrograde from the tip toward the hub, pushing the specimen out at the broader end. If cytology slides are needed, roll the core of marrow gently across several clean glass slides before transferring the specimen to the fixative jar. Zenker's fixative and formalin are used most frequently.
10. Apply pressure to puncture site until bleeding ceases.	**10.** If thrombocytopenia is present, pressure should be applied to the iliac crest for 3–5 minutes.

TROCHANTERIC FOSSA ASPIRATION AND BIOPSY

Procedure

Technical Action	Rationale/Amplification
1. Locate trochanteric fossa by palpation of greater trochanter (see Fig. 27-3B).	**1.** The fossa is medial and slightly distal to the point of the greater trochanter.
2. Identify trochanteric fossa and mark.	**2.** Orientation is facilitated by cradling the cranial thigh in the palm and extending the thumb along the lateral aspect of the femur. This allows manipulation and restraint of the leg (Fig. 27-6).
3. Infiltrate marked area with local anesthetic in skin, subcutis, and periosteum.	**3.** The periosteum is the region of greatest sensitivity.
4. Make 3-mm stab incision in skin.	**4.** A small skin incision facilitates insertion of the large, blunt needle.
5. Advance bone marrow needle, with stylet in place, through skin and subcutaneous tissue medial to great trochanter and into trochanteric fossa (Fig. 27-6).	**5.** The needle is directed medial to and parallel with the operator's thumb as it lies over the length of the femur.

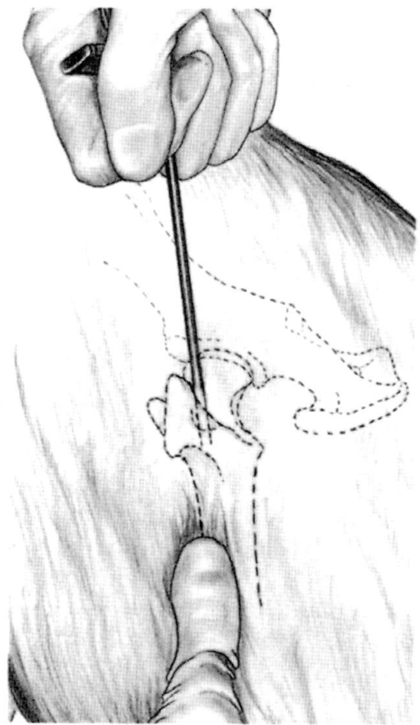

Figure 27-6 Restraint of leg and position of needle for bone marrow aspiration or biopsy from trochanteric fossa.

Technical Action	Rationale/Amplification
6. Advance needle by rotation and steady pressure (Fig. 27-4A).	**6.** Avoid unnecessary wobbling by keeping the elbow immobilized while using a pronating and supinating motion of the forearm. Considerable force is often required.
7. Aspiration technique:	**7.** Aspiration technique:
a) When needle penetrates outer cortex of bone, remove stylet.	**a)** There is usually decreased resistance when the marrow cavity is entered.
b) Attach 20-mL syringe and apply negative pressure by forcefully pulling back on syringe plunger (Fig. 27-4B).	**b)** The actual aspiration usually causes considerable discomfort for an animal that is not anesthetized.
c) Aspirate small volume of bone marrow fluid into syringe.	**c)** Bone marrow usually is dark red, more viscous than blood, and contains fat particles. Less than 1 mL should be aspirated to avoid excessive dilution of the sample with blood (see alternate technique).
d) Pass syringe to assistant.	

Technical Action	Rationale/Amplification
8. *Assistant:* Rapidly touch one or two drops of marrow to surface of 8–10 slides and make thin, even push smears before marrow clots. See Chapter 8 (Fig. 8-4).	**8.** *Assistant:* The marrow may form a clot in 15–30 seconds, so it is important to make smears quickly.
Alternate Technique	**Alternate Technique**
7. Aspiration technique:	**7.** Aspiration technique:
a) When needle penetrates outer cortex of bone, remove stylet.	**a)** There is usually decreased resistance when the marrow cavity is entered.
b) Attach 20-mL syringe containing 2 mL of CPDA solution to bone marrow needle hub.	**b)** The anticoagulant prevents rapid clotting but does not distort cellular morphology.
c) Apply negative pressure by forcefully pulling back on syringe plunger.	**c)** The animal may show considerable discomfort during the aspiration.
d) Aspirate 2–3 mL of bone marrow fluid into syringe.	**d)** A large sample helps in obtaining several bone spicules.
e) Pass syringe to assistant.	**e)** Pass the syringe aseptically so that aspiration may be repeated, if necessary.
8. *Assistant:* Expel contents of syringe into petri dish. Inspect fluid for cancellous bone spicules. Siphon spicules into capillary tubes and transfer to 8–10 clean glass slides. Make thin, even push smears. See Chapter 8 (Fig. 8-4).	**8.** *Assistant:* Bone spicules are white or red dense particles, easily distinguished from fat particles. Several spicules can be collected in each capillary tube. Spicules can be transferred to slides by blowing on the other end of the tube or by forcing air through with a tuberculin syringe. Make enough smears to allow for additional stains.
9. Core biopsy technique (Jamshidi needle):	**9.** Core biopsy technique (Jamshidi needle):
a) When needle and stylet are firmly embedded in bone, remove stylet.	**a)** The needle should stand in place after the stylet is removed.
b) Advance needle 1–2 cm by gentle rotation and steady pressure (Fig. 27-5A).	**b)** A comfort knob makes this step easier.
c) Loosen biopsy sample by alternate rotation and wobbling of needle (Fig. 27-5B).	**c)** Do this gently. Do not bend the needle.
d) Partially withdraw needle, then redirect needle at a slightly different angle and reintroduce it into bone. Repeat rotation and wobbling of needle.	**d)** This repositioning obtains a larger sample and ensures that the specimen is severed from the bone.

Technical Action

Alternate Technique

e) Remove needle from bone by rotation and steady traction.

f) Remove biopsy sample from needle using expeller, and place it in appropriate fixative (Fig. 27-5C).

Rationale/Amplification

Alternate Technique

f) The expeller is directed retrograde from the tip toward the hub, pushing the specimen out at the broader end. If cytology slides are needed, roll the core of marrow gently across several clean glass slides before transferring the specimen to the fixative jar. Zenker's fixative and formalin are used most frequently.

10. Apply pressure to puncture site until bleeding ceases.

10. If thrombocytopenia is present, pressure should be applied to the iliac crest for 3–5 minutes.

HUMERAL HEAD ASPIRATION AND BIOPSY

NOTE. *The head of the humerus is an excellent source of bone marrow in small, anesthetized animals; however, obtaining a sample is more difficult to perform safely in large dogs or unanesthetized animals due to the thick cortex of the proximal humeral metaphysis. Care must be taken to avoid having the needle slip off the hard bone and inadvertently puncture the chest wall or other vital structures.*

Procedure

Technical Action	Rationale/Amplification
1. Restrain animal in lateral recumbency.	**1.** With an animal that is not anesthetized, two persons are needed for restraint to avoid contamination of the operative site.
2. Locate humeral head by palpation. (Fig. 27-3C).	**2.** *Assistant:* Flexes elbow and shoulder joints and rotates the elbow inward towards the body wall, so that the shoulder joint is turned outward. The bony prominence distal to the spine of the scapula and the acromium process is the greater tubercle of the humerus.
3. Infiltrate marked area with local anesthetic in skin, subcutis, and periosteum.	**3.** The periosteum is the region of greatest sensitivity.
4. Make 3-mm stab incision in skin.	**4.** A small skin incision facilitates insertion of the large, blunt needle.

Technical Action

5. Advance bone marrow needle, with stylet in place, through skin and subcutaneous tissue and into the greater tubercle parallel to the long axis of the humerus, aiming for the point of the elbow.

Rationale/Amplification

5. The needle is held in the palm of the hand using a pistol grip, with the heel of the needle in the palm of the hand and the needle being supported by the index finger.

Technical Action

6. Advance needle by rotation and steady pressure (Fig. 27-4A). Once in the medullary cavity the needle should feel firmly lodged and it should not be possible to move the needle from side to side.

Rationale/Amplification

6. It may be difficult to get a purchase in the bone, but with repeated twisting of the needle to and fro with firm pressure the needle tip enters the bone cortex. Now further firm pressure is applied whilst rotating the needle to and fro to advance the needle. *Assistant:* Similarly firm counter pressure needs to be applied by an assistant to stop the animal being pushed off the table.

Technical Action

7. Aspiration technique:
   a) When needle penetrates outer cortex of bone, remove stylet.
   b) Attach 20-mL syringe and apply negative pressure by forcefully pulling back on syringe plunger (Fig. 27-4B).
   c) Aspirate small volume of bone marrow fluid into syringe.
   d) Pass syringe to assistant.

Rationale/Amplification

7. Aspiration technique:
   a) There is usually decreased resistance when the marrow cavity is entered.
   b) The actual aspiration usually causes considerable discomfort for an animal that is not anesthetized.
   c) Bone marrow usually is dark red, more viscous than blood, and contains fat particles. Less than 1 mL should be aspirated to avoid excessive dilution of the sample with blood (see alternate technique).

Technical Action

8. *Assistant:* Rapidly touch one or two drops of marrow to surface of 8–10 slides and make thin, even push smears before marrow clots. See Chapter 8 (Fig. 8-4).

Rationale/Amplification

8. *Assistant:* The marrow may form a clot in 15–30 seconds, so it is important to make smears quickly.

Alternate Technique

Technical Action

7. Aspiration technique:
   a) When needle penetrates outer cortex of bone, remove stylet.
   b) Attach 20-mL syringe containing 2 mL of CPDA solution to bone marrow needle hub.

Rationale/Amplification

7. Aspiration technique:
   a) There is usually decreased resistance when the marrow cavity is entered.
   b) The anticoagulant prevents rapid clotting but does not distort cellular morphology.

Technical Action	Rationale/Amplification
Alternate Technique	**Alternate Technique**
c) Apply negative pressure by forcefully pulling back on syringe plunger.	**c)** The animal may show considerable discomfort during the aspiration.
d) Aspirate 2–3 mL of bone marrow fluid into syringe.	**d)** A large sample helps in obtaining several bone spicules.
e) Pass syringe to assistant.	**e)** Pass the syringe aseptically so that aspiration may be repeated, if necessary.
8. *Assistant:* Expel contents of syringe into petri dish. Inspect fluid for cancellous bone spicules. Siphon spicules into capillary tubes and transfer to 8–10 clean glass slides. Make thin, even push smears. See Chapter 8 (Fig. 8-4).	**8.** *Assistant:* Bone spicules are white or red dense particles, easily distinguished from fat particles. Several spicules can be collected in each capillary tube. Spicules can be transferred to slides by blowing on the other end of the tube or by forcing air through with a tuberculin syringe. Make enough smears to allow for additional stains.
9. Core biopsy technique (Jamshidi needle):	**9.** Core biopsy technique (Jamshidi needle):
a) When needle and stylet are firmly embedded in bone, remove stylet.	**a)** The needle should stand in place after the stylet is removed.
b) Advance needle 1–2 cm by gentle rotation and steady pressure.	**b)** A comfort knob makes this step easier.
c) Loosen biopsy sample by alternate rotation and wobbling of needle.	**c)** Do this gently. Do not bend the needle.
d) Partially withdraw needle, then redirect needle at a slightly different angle and reintroduce it into bone. Repeat rotation and wobbling of needle.	**d)** This repositioning obtains a larger sample and ensures that the specimen is severed from the bone.
e) Remove needle from bone by rotation and steady traction.	
f) Remove biopsy sample from needle using expeller, and place it in appropriate fixative (Fig. 27-5C).	**f)** The expeller is directed retrograde from the tip toward the hub, pushing the specimen out at the broader end. If cytology slides are needed, roll the core of marrow gently across several clean glass slides before transferring the specimen to the fixative jar. Zenker's fixative and formalin are used most frequently.
10. Apply pressure to puncture site until bleeding ceases.	**10.** If thrombocytopenia is present, pressure should be applied to the iliac crest for 3–5 minutes.

Bibliography

Abrams-Ogg A: New Techniques for Bone Marrow Aspiration and Core Biopsy in Dogs and Cats. 64th Convention of the Canadian Veterinary Medical Association, 2012
Perman V, Osborne CA, Stevens JB: Bone marrow biopsy. Vet Clin North Am 4: 293–310, 1974
Schalm OW, Switzer JA: Bone marrow aspiration in the cat. Feline Practice 1: 56–62, 1972
Suter SE, McDonald CE: Personal Communication, 2006
Villiers E: Bone Marrow Aspiration. British Small Animal Veterinary Congress, 2010

Chapter 28

Cerebrospinal Fluid Collection

Good intent does not always result in beneficial outcome.
CARL OSBORNE

Collection and analysis of cerebrospinal fluid (CSF) is one of the most common diagnostic procedures for diseases involving the central nervous system. Collection involves introducing a fine-gauge needle into the subarachnoid space at the cisterna magna or pelvic intumescence to withdraw a small volume of CSF. * **The following procedures are considered invasive and are typically performed exclusively by veterinarians.**

Purposes

1. To obtain CSF for chemical, cytological, and microbiologic analysis
2. To allow injection of radiopaque substances for contrast encephalography and myelography
3. To inject anticancer drugs intrathecally
4. To determine CSF pressure (see note below)

NOTE: *A procedure for measuring CSF pressure was described in the first two editions. Although the technique for that measurement has not changed, CSF manometry is now less frequently done by neurologists due to increased risk of damage to the spinal cord during the attachment and detachment of the manometer and stopcock. Advanced imaging techniques (e.g. myelography, CT, and MRI) are more often used and more reliable in determining the presence of mass lesions within the brain and spinal cord.*

Specific Indications

1. Focal, multifocal, and diffuse dysfunction of the cerebrum, cerebellum, or brain stem, including the following:

Crow and Walshaw's Manual of Clinical Procedures in Dogs, Cats, Rabbits, and Rodents, Fourth Edition. Edited by Jennifer E. Boyle. Published 2016 by John Wiley & Sons, Inc.
Companion Website: www.wiley.com/go/boyle/manual4e

   a) Motor deficits
   b) Sensory deficits
   c) Visual deficits
   d) Cranial nerve deficits
   e) Altered state of consciousness and mentation (e.g. dementia or personality and behavior changes)
   f) Epileptic seizures
2. Myelopathy, resulting in motor or sensory deficits

Contraindications

1. Congenital abnormalities, involving malformations of the foramen magnum, or suspected neural malformations in the region of the cisterna magna
2. Fractures, dislocations, or subluxations of the occipital region of the skull or cranial cervical region, resulting in instability or distortion of the brain stem, medulla, or cervical cord
3. Suspected or anticipated brain herniation
4. Infection of soft tissues overlying the puncture site

Complications

1. No CSF obtained
2. Iatrogenic hemorrhage
3. Contamination of the CSF with blood
4. Herniation of the brain
5. Puncture or laceration of the medulla or cranial cervical spinal cord
6. Infection of the central nervous system
7. Respiratory or cardiac arrest
8. Vestibular dysfunction
9. Paresis/paralysis

NOTE: *Serious complications may result when one is performing a cerebrospinal fluid collection, but problems are not common when proper technique is used and specific contraindications are considered.*

Equipment

- Sterile spinal needles
- Sandbags
- Sterile syringes (preferably glass)
- Sterile tubes
- Sterile drape and gloves

Restraint and Positioning

Collection of CSF is always performed with the animal under general anesthesia. The animal is positioned carefully in sternal or lateral recumbency. Sandbags should be used, when necessary, to ensure symmetrical posture. The lateral position is preferred because it permits collection of fluid without the use of a syringe.

Cisternal puncture is facilitated by ventral flexion of the neck, which increases the dorsal exposure of the foramen magnum. Care must be taken to avoid kinking the endotracheal tube. Use of a wire-reinforced endotracheal tube is recommended. The ears are pulled toward the commissures of the lips (Fig. 28-1).

Lumbar puncture is facilitated by drawing the hind legs forward so that the stifles are adjacent to the animal's umbilicus (Fig. 28-2).

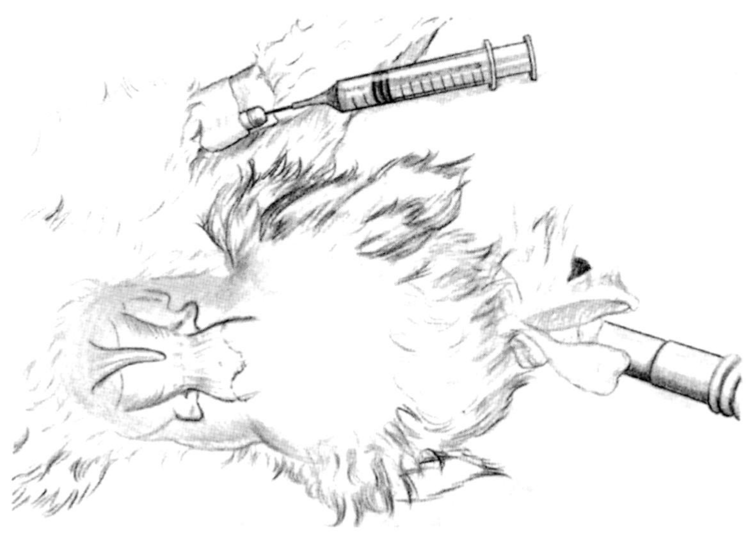

Figure 28-1 Correct positioning of dog for cisternal puncture.

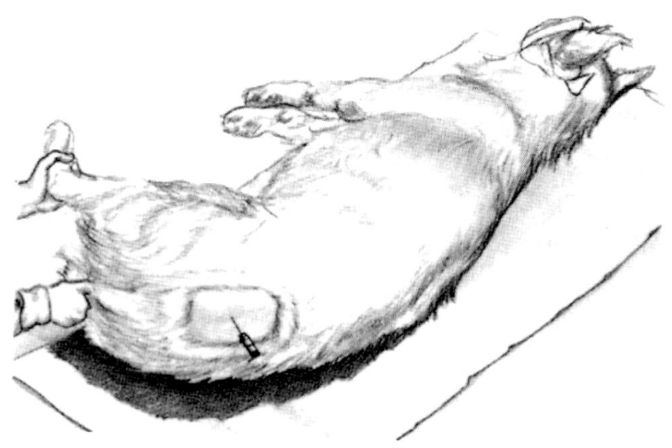

Figure 28-2 Correct positioning of dog for lumbar puncture.

Collection Sites

Cisternal puncture: In most cases, CSF is collected by entering the subarachnoid space at the cisterna magna. This site is particularly useful for suspected lesions of the brain. Anatomic landmarks include the external occipital protuberance, the cranial borders of the wings of the atlas, and the dorsal cervical musculature. When the animal's neck is flexed, a slight depression can be seen or palpated. This depression is the site for needle insertion (Fig. 28-1).

Lumbar puncture: Collection of CSF from the lumbar region is performed less often in small animal practice because the subarachnoid space is narrow at this site. Only small amounts of CSF can be obtained. Lumbar puncture and CSF analysis ordinarily are performed before myelography, usually for evaluation of suspected lesions of the caudal cervical and thoracolumbar segments of the spinal cord. Anatomic landmarks include the dorsal and transverse processes of the lumbar vertebrae, the iliac crests, and the dorsal lumbar muscles (Fig. 28-2).

Cisternal Puncture Procedure

Technical Action	Rationale/Amplification
1. Clip hair from dorsal occipital and cranial cervical regions; prepare skin in a routine manner. Place sterile drape around site.	**1.** See Chapter 16. Attention to asepsis is important in avoiding microbial contamination of the CSF.
2. *Assistant:* **a)** Flex neck ventrally so that animal's chin nearly touches its manubrium (cranial edge of sternum). **b)** Pull ears rostrally toward medial canthi. **c)** Raise muzzle and rotate head so that entire cervical spine forms straight line from skull to shoulder blades.	**2.** *Assistant:* A depression usually is visible when the skin is pulled taut in this manner.
3. *Operator:* **a)** Direct needle (with stylet in place) through skin and underlying tissue starting on midline at point midway between external occipital protuberance and cranial edge of spinous process of axis (C2 vertebra).	**3.** *Operator:* **a)** The distance from skin to cistern magna is variable but is usually between 1 and 3 cm. A 1.5-inch long needle is adequate for cats and a majority of dogs. The needle will often contact the dorsal lamina of the atlas. When this occurs, the needle should be redirected cranially in several small steps until it does not contact bone.
b) Advance needle with moderate force through opening between occiput and atlas (Fig. 28-1) and	**b)** Entry into the subarachnoid space is sensed by a sudden slight loss of tension against the needle.

Technical Action

meninges (dura mater and closely adherent arachnoid membrane).

Rationale/Amplification

With practice, this sensation can be readily felt in most cases. The animal will often jerk or twitch if the parenchyma of the spinal cord is penetrated.

c) Pull stylet out to observe for fluid after passing through individual soft tissue layers.

c) By checking at each tissue interface, there is less chance of advancing the needle too far.

d) When fluid is seen in needle hub, place collection tube below and let CSF drip into tube by gravity flow.

d) A small amount (0.25 mL) is collected for culture, and a larger amount (1–5 mL) is obtained for fluid analysis. Collect as much CSF as possible to permit chemical and cytological evaluation.

e) Replace stylet and remove needle by steady traction.

4. Relax neck and observe animal until normal respiration returns.

4. When the procedure is properly performed, complications are rare, but the animal should be observed carefully for the next 24 hours.

Lumbar Puncture Procedure

Technical Action

1. Clip hair over dorsal lumbosacral region and prepare skin in routine manner. Place sterile drape around site.
2. *Assistant:* Draw hind legs forward until stifles contact ventral abdominal muscles.
3. *Operator:*
   a) Direct needle (with stylet in place) ventrally and cranially through skin, subcutis, and musculature toward dorsal lamina of more caudal vertebra. An angle of 20 degrees from perpendicular to long axis of spine is usually best. Keep needle in mid-sagittal plane by directing it parallel to spinous processes (see Fig. 28-2).
   b) Advance needle with moderate force through opening between vertebrae and meninges (dura

Rationale/Amplification

1. See Chapter 16.
2. *Assistant:* This position tends to open the spaces between the dorsal laminae of the lumbar vertebrae.
3. *Operator:*
   a) Entry point is midway between the dorsal processes of fourth and fifth or fifth and sixth lumbar vertebrae. When bone is contacted (2–8 cm below the skin), the needle is redirected slightly cranially or caudally until the dura mater is contacted.

   b–e) During lumbar puncture, the spinal cord may be punctured, resulting in jerking movement

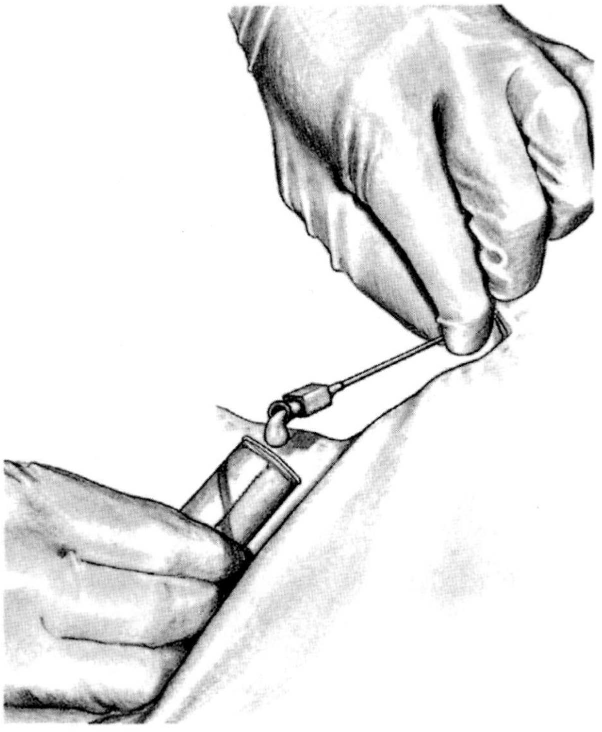

Figure 28-3 Collecting CSF by gravity flow.

Technical Action

mater and closely adherent arachnoid membrane).

c) Remove stylet.

d) When fluid is seen in needle hub, place a sterile tube below needle hub and allow CSF to drip into tube by gravity flow (Fig. 28-3).

e) Replace stylet and remove needle by steady traction.

Rationale/Amplification

of one or both hind limbs. This complication is more likely to occur if a more cranial site is chosen. For this reason, the preferred puncture site is between the spinous processes of the fifth and sixth lumbar vertebrae. If no CSF is obtained, however, remove the needle and reinsert it between the dorsal processes of the fourth and fifth lumbar vertebrae.

Bibliography

Campbell M: Personal communication, 2008

Kay WJ, Israel E, Prata RG: Cerebrospinal fluid. Vet Clin North Am 4: 419–436, 1974

Mohammad-Zadeh LF, Sisson AF: Cerebrospinal Fluid Collection & Analysis, NAVC Clinician's Brief, p. 22. November 2005

Part III

Emergency Procedures

An emergency is a serious situation or occurrence that happens unexpectedly and demands urgent and immediate action. The procedures outlined in this section are often not available in many veterinary practices, but they are common procedures in emergency clinics, specialty centers, and teaching hospitals.

Transfusions of fresh or frozen blood or blood components on a large scale require organization and attention to detail. Keeping an active donor roster and avoiding shortages requires the full-time attention of a dedicated staff member.

Double- and triple-lumen catheters are extremely useful in managing animals in an intensive care unit. They allow continual sampling of blood while maintaining a patent avenue for administration of fluids and intravenous medications. Proficiency in placement requires some practice, but once learned, the technique can be completed in just a few minutes.

Tracheostomy is a technique that must be done very rapidly; consequently, the person with the most experience placing tracheostomy tubes should perform the operation.

Just do it.

NIKE

Chapter 29

Rapid Evaluation of Bleeding and Clotting Disorders

There is nothing so useless as doing efficiently that which should not be done at all.

PETER DRUCKER

Although many tests are available for evaluation of coagulation factors and platelets, the activated clotting time and bleeding time are inexpensive, easy, and require no sophisticated equipment or reagents. Each test can be performed in a few minutes at most veterinary facilities.

BLEEDING TIME

Bleeding time is a clinical evaluation of primary hemostasis. It is the time between the making of a small incision and the moment when bleeding ceases.

Purposes

1. To evaluate platelet function in animals with a normal platelet count
2. To screen animals with hemorrhagic diatheses for von Willebrand's disease

Specific Indications

1. Petechial or ecchymotic hemorrhages
2. Persistent epistaxis, hematuria, or hematochezia

Crow and Walshaw's Manual of Clinical Procedures in Dogs, Cats, Rabbits, and Rodents, Fourth Edition. Edited by Jennifer E. Boyle. Published 2016 by John Wiley & Sons, Inc.
Companion Website: www.wiley.com/go/boyle/manual4e

Contraindications

1. Clinically evident prolonged bleeding (e.g. at venipuncture sites)
2. Severe anemia
3. Severe thrombocytopenia

Complications

1. Prolonged bleeding
2. Infection of incision sites

Equipment Needed

- Tourniquet (pneumatic cuff or rubber strap and hemostatic forceps)
- Stopwatch with sweep second hand
- Filter paper (Whatman No. 1 discs)
- Skin preparation materials:
  - 2% chlorhexidine surgical scrub
  - Sterile gauze sponges (2 inch × 2 inch)
  - 70% alcohol
- Clipper with No. 40 blade
- Template and No. 11 scalpel blade (Fig. 29-1A)
- Simplate-II bleeding time device* (Fig. 29-1B)
- Commercial pet toenail clippers (guillotine or scissors type, Fig. 29-1C)

Restraint and Positioning

Little restraint is needed for most dogs and cats. The animal is held in sternal or lateral recumbency by an assistant.

TEMPLATE BLEEDING TIME

Procedure

Technical Action	Rationale/Amplification
1. Carefully clip hair from 3-inch-square (7.5 cm) area of skin on dorsolateral surface of antebrachium.	1. Even a short-hair coat will prevent proper assessment of the cessation of bleeding. In addition, long hairs may provide an increased chance for wound contamination.

*General Diagnostics, Division of Warner-Lambert Company, Morris Plains, NJ 07950.

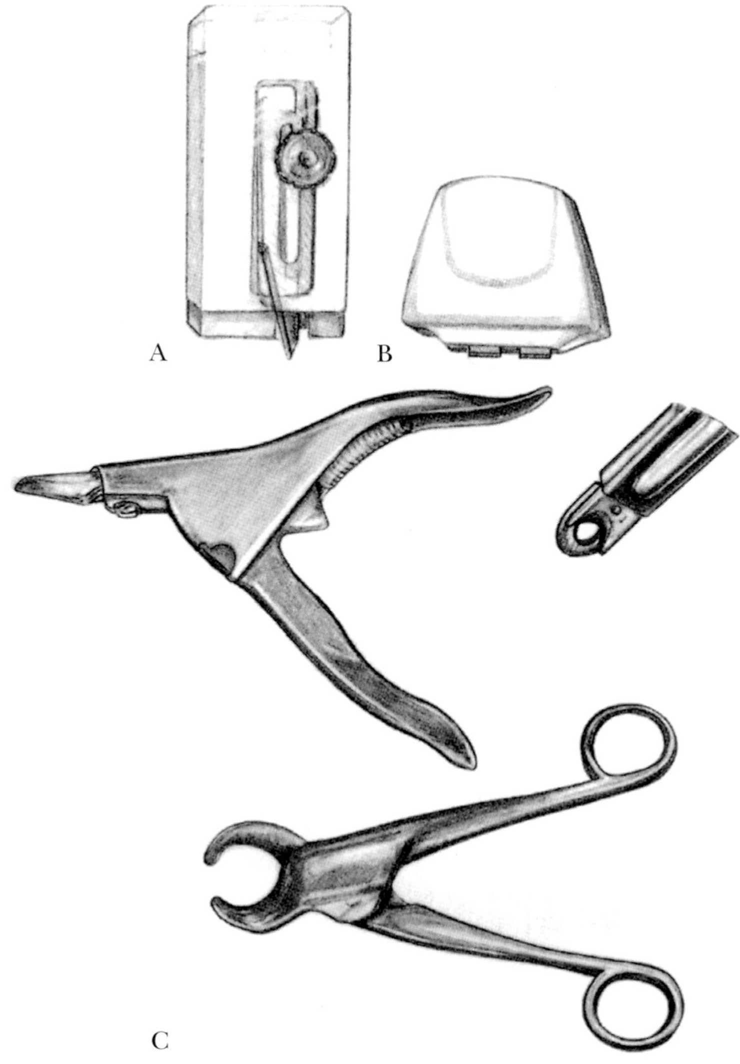

Figure 29-1 Equipment needed for obtaining template and cuticle bleeding time: (A) template and No. 11 scalpel blade, (B) Simplate-II bleeding time device, and (C) guillotine- and scissors-type pet toenail clippers.

Technical Action	Rationale/Amplification
2. Scrub clipped area of skin gently.	**2.** See Chapter 16. Careful clipping and scrubbing is essential to avoid skin irritation, which could result in surface capillary trauma and increased capillary perfusion.

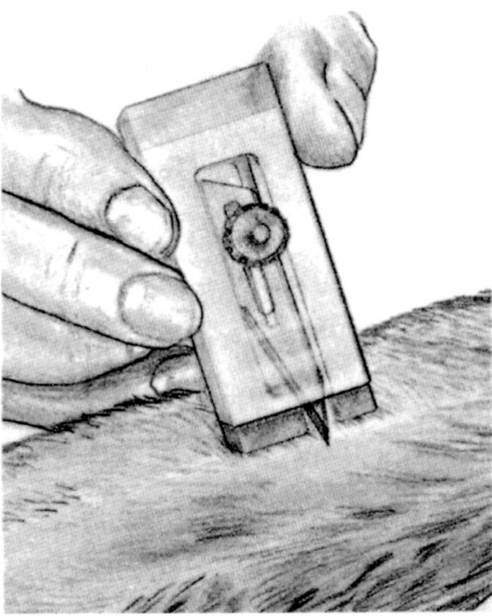

Figure 29-2 Making skin incisions with template and No. 11 scalpel blade.

Technical Action	Rationale/Amplification
3. Apply tourniquet to leg above elbow. Wait 30–60 seconds before proceeding.	**3.** The tourniquet helps to standardize capillary perfusion in the test leg.
4. Make several incisions of uniform depth and length (Fig. 29-2).	**4.** Use either the Simplate-II bleeding time device or a template and No. 11 scalpel blade (Fig. 29-2). Avoid placing the device directly over or near the cephalic vein.
5. Remove incision device and start stopwatch.	**5.** Do not separate incision edges or otherwise disturb the wounds.
6. After 30 seconds, blot the blood droplet that accumulates at incision sites with edge of dry filter paper (Fig. 29-3).	**6.** Bring the edge of the filter paper close to the incisions without touching the wound edges. Rotate the paper between each blotting.
7. Repeat blotting every 30 seconds until blood no longer stains filter paper. Record total elapsed time from incision until cessation of hemorrhage.	**7.** Normal range for template bleeding time in dogs is 4–5 minutes. If incisions bleed different lengths of time, use the longest time obtained. Animals with bleeding disorders frequently bleed longer and more profusely.
8. Remove tourniquet and apply cotton ball or gauze bandage, as for venipuncture.	**8.** See Chapter 2, Nos. 11 to 12. If bleeding persists, consider placing a pressure bandage.

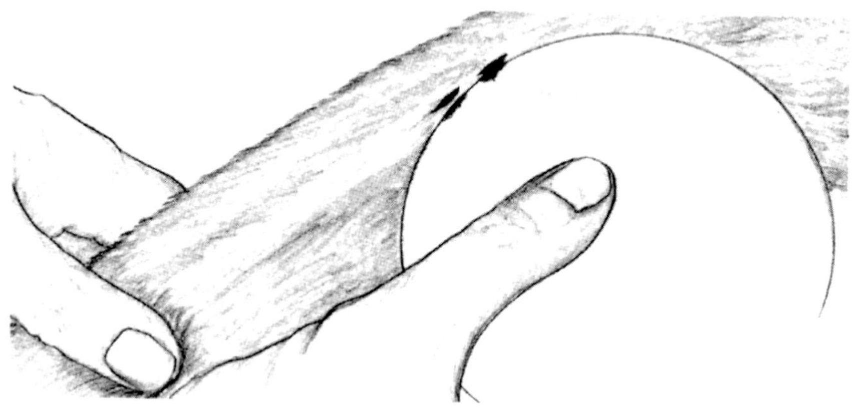

Figure 29-3 Blotting blood droplets with filter paper.

CUTICLE BLEEDING TIME

Procedure

Technical Action	Rationale/Amplification
1. Wipe toenail and blades of toenail clipper with 70% alcohol. Allow to dry for at least 30 seconds.	1. Application of an antiseptic such as alcohol minimizes the possibility of infection of the nail.
2. Clip nail slightly too short to initiate bleeding (Fig. 29-4).	2. See Chapter 11. Darkly pigmented nails should be clipped in small (1 mm) increments until bleeding starts; in white nails, the nail matrix (blood supply) is visible so that an exact clip can be performed.
3. Allow nail to bleed naturally.	3. Do not squeeze foot, toes, or nails. Droplets of blood should not be blotted. Bleeding should stop normally within 2–5 minutes.
4. Repeat Nos. 1–3 on a second nail to recheck results.	4. Bleeding may continue for 15 minutes or more in animals with von Willebrand's disease or other platelet disorders. Hemophiliacs will often stop bleeding after 2–3 minutes, but bleeding will then restart and continue indefinitely.

ACTIVATED CLOTTING TIME

Activated clotting time is a rapid test for evaluating the intrinsic and common coagulation pathways. It is the elapsed time between mixture of whole blood with a surface activator and the development of a fibrin clot.

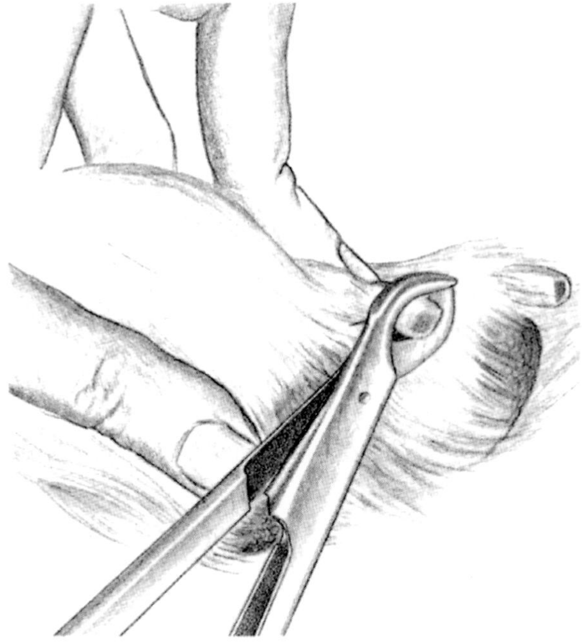

Figure 29-4 Clipping nail to level of blood vessels.

Purposes

1. To aid in the diagnosis of specific coagulation disorders
2. To identify animals with subclinical coagulation disorders before performing invasive or traumatic diagnostic procedures
3. To monitor anticoagulant therapy
4. To evaluate progression or regression of coagulation disorders

Specific Indications

1. Spontaneous subcutaneous hematoma
2. Hemarthrosis
3. Suffusion hemorrhage
4. Prolonged postoperative bleeding
5. Excessive hemorrhage at venipuncture sites

Equipment Needed

- Vacutainer®* holder and needles
- Vacutainer clotting time test tubes containing activator, and standard clot tubes

*Becton, Dickinson and Company, Rutherford, NJ 07070.

- 37°C heating block or water bath
- Stopwatch with sweep second hand

NOTE: *When the procedure is performed in the field, warming the tube in a pocket or in the palm may be substituted for the heating block or bath.*

Restraint and Positioning

The animal is held in sternal recumbency, with forelegs extended forward and ventrally and the neck extended dorsally, as for routine jugular venipuncture (see Chapter 2).

Procedure

Technical Action	Rationale/Amplification
1. Preheat tubes in heating block or bath. Prepare skin and distend jugular vein as for routine venipuncture.	**1.** See Chapter 2.
2. Puncture vein with one smooth stroke of sterile Vacutainer® needle.	**2.** It is essential that the venipuncture be atraumatic to avoid the accumulation of tissue
3. Insert standard clot tube in holder and push tube until needle punctures tube stopper. Collect 2–3 mL of blood.	**3.** Hold Vacutainer® collection assembly firmly throughout procedure to prevent migration of needle and laceration of vein.
4. Disconnect tube from holder while keeping needle within lumen of vein. Discard tube or save for serum tests.	**4.** This first collected sample is used to draw any thromboplastin out of the needle.
5. Insert tube containing activator into holder and puncture stopper with needle.	**5.** Blood normally will appear in vacuum tube immediately.
6. Start stopwatch the instant blood enters tube and continue collection until blood stops flowing into tube.	**6.** Collection normally should be completed within 10–12 seconds.
7. Immediately disconnect tube from holder, gently invert it three times, and place tube in heating block or water bath. *Assistant:* Apply digital pressure to venipuncture site for at least 1 minute.	**7.** Do not shake the tube. Inversion provides adequate mixing of blood with the activator.
8. When stopwatch reads 60 seconds, remove tube from heating block or bath and invert tube gently once	**8.** Observe for clot in tube as blood flows from end to end. If no clot is seen, replace tube in heat source.

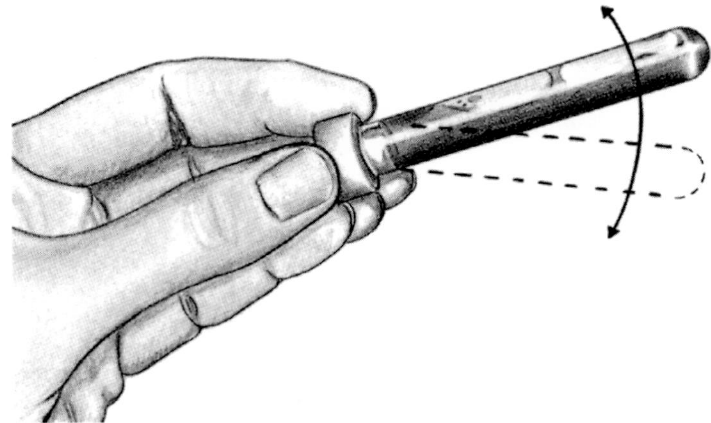

Figure 29-5 Inverting activated clotting time tube to observe for formation of clot.

Technical Action	Rationale/Amplification
(Fig. 29-5). If no clot has formed, replace tube in heating block.	
9. Repeat inversion and replacement every 5 seconds until a clot is formed. At the first sign of a clot, record the elapsed time to the nearest 5 seconds.	**9.** The first sign of a clot is seen as a thickening or sludging effect prior to solid clot formation. Normal activated clotting time in the dog is 60–100 seconds; in the cat, it is 70–120 seconds.

Bibliography

Activated Clotting Time (ACT) Test, Animal Blood Bank® January 18, 2006 (published)

Byars TD *et al.*: Activated coagulation time (ACT) of whole blood in normal dogs. Am J Vet Res 37: 1359–1361, 1976

Dodds WJ: Cuticle Bleeding Time in Bleeding Disorders of Small Animals. Western States Veterinary Medical Association Annual Conference, Las Vegas, February 1983

Middleton DJ, Watson ADJ: Activated coagulation times of whole blood in normal dogs with coagulopathies. J Small Anim Pract 19: 417–422, 1978

Mielks CH: Use of template for bleeding time incisions. Blood 34: 204–206, 1969

Chapter 30

Blood Pressure Measurement

Courage is grace under pressure.
ERNEST HEMINGWAY

Purposes

1. Assess cardiovascular stability in the emergent patient
2. Assist in diagnosing hypotension or hypertension in patients
3. Assess perfusion in debilitated and anesthetized patients
4. Assess vascular fluid overload (CVP)

ARTERIAL BLOOD PRESSURE

Mean arterial blood pressure (MAP) is a function of cardiac output and systemic vascular resistance and is used to assess adequate perfusion. Typically, systolic pressures of 80–140 mmHg, diastolic pressures of 50–80 mmHg and mean pressures of 60–100 mmHg are considered normal in dogs and cats.

Indirect Measurement (Noninvasive)

Restraint and Positioning

If patient is awake, this will require an assistant. Lay patient in lateral or sternal recumbency, if possible. Dorsal recumbency is acceptable in anesthetized patients.

Doppler (Fig. 30-1)

NOTE: *Doppler measures systolic pressure only.*

Crow and Walshaw's Manual of Clinical Procedures in Dogs, Cats, Rabbits, and Rodents, Fourth Edition. Edited by Jennifer E. Boyle. Published 2016 by John Wiley & Sons, Inc.
Companion Website: www.wiley.com/go/boyle/manual4e

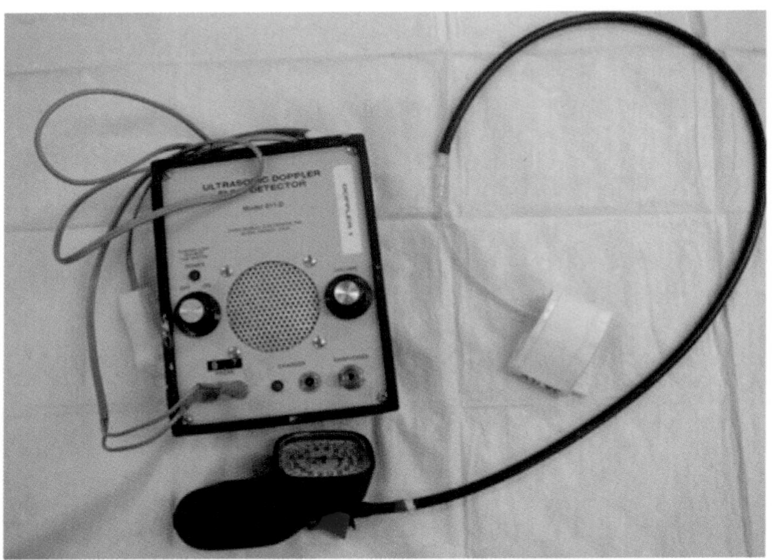

Figure 30-1 Doppler machine with sphygnomanometer and cuff. Photo courtesy of S Epstein.

Complications

1. False low or high reading due to inappropriate sized cuff or poor placement of cuff
2. False high reading due to bent limb
3. Increased blood pressure caused by patient stress during procedure
4. Movement in limbs will cause false values
5. Pronounced arrhythmias and slow heart rates can potentially also cause erroneous results

Equipment needed

- Doppler machine
- Sphygnomanometer
- Measuring tape
- Appropriate sized cuff for patient
- Porous tape
- Ultrasound gel

Procedure

Technical Action	Rationale/Amplification
1. Place patient in lateral or sternal recumbency with limb extended.	1. Cuff must be at level of heart for most reliable measurement; bent limb can cause false high reading; lateral recumbency gives most consistent readings.

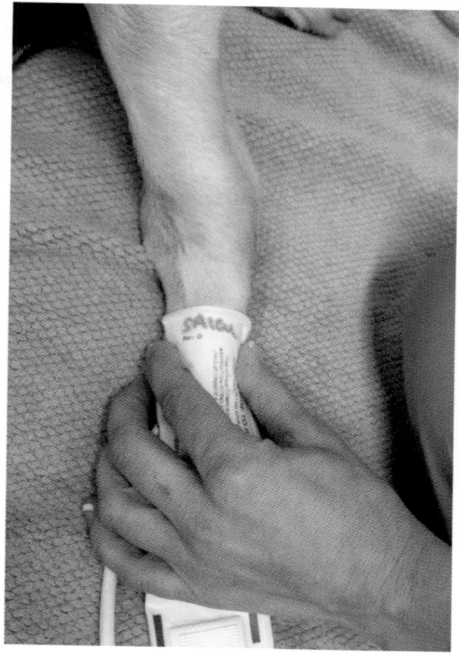

Figure 30-2 Measuring appropriate cuff size. Photo courtesy of S Epstein.

Technical Action	Rationale/Amplification
2. The tail is an alternate site.	2. Any place you can locate a pulse and place a cuff proximal to it is acceptable for obtaining a BP measurement.
3. Shave a small area just proximal to the large central palmar metacarpal/metatarsal pad or base of the tail over the artery.	3. If using the tail, make sure you have room to place the cuff proximal to your shaved area.
4. Measure area in which cuff will be placed and select correct size cuff (Fig. 30-2).	4. Measure circumference of appendage, ideally above carpus/tarsus and below elbow/hock for limbs, multiply by 0.4 for dogs and 0.3 for cats and round up for correct cuff size. A cuff that is too wide will result in lower readings and a cuff that is not wide enough will result in higher readings.
5. Place cuff on limb/appendage at measure site. Velcro snugly but not tight. A small piece of porous tape may be used to secure the cuff.	5. Placing a short strip of tape on the cuff is fine as long as it does not completely encircle the cuff, restricting its ability to inflate.

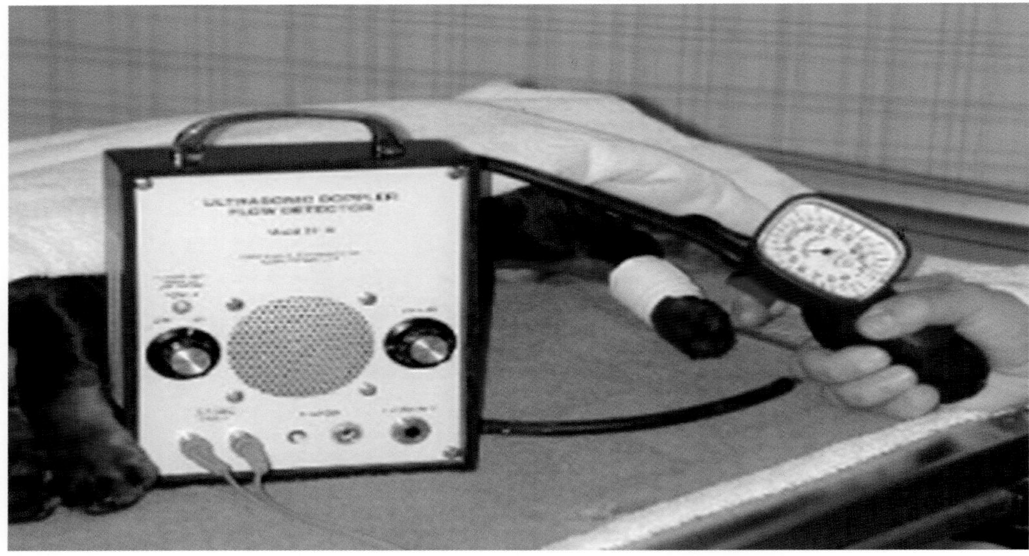

Figure 30-3 Measuring systolic blood pressure using Doppler machine.

Technical Action	Rationale/Amplification
6. Apply ultrasonic gel to sensor and place sensor on shaved area.	**6.** Be sure to use ultrasound specific gel for best results. ECG gel and KY jelly are not meant for use with Doppler.
7. Find a strong signal and gently tape the sensor in place.	**7.** Have tape ready and keep the volume low or use headphones to prevent the patient from being upset by the sound.
8. Pump up the cuff until flow ceases (no sound) and go 20 mmHg or more above that. SLOWLY release the pressure in the cuff. Listen for the first return of flow. This is the systolic pressure. Repeat this several times until you feel confident that the result is repeatable (Figure 30-3).	**8.** Ideally you want to obtain multiple measurements over about 5 minutes, with the later readings generally being more accurate.

Oscillometric (Fig. 30-4)

NOTE: *Oscillometric measures systolic, diastolic, and mean pressures.*

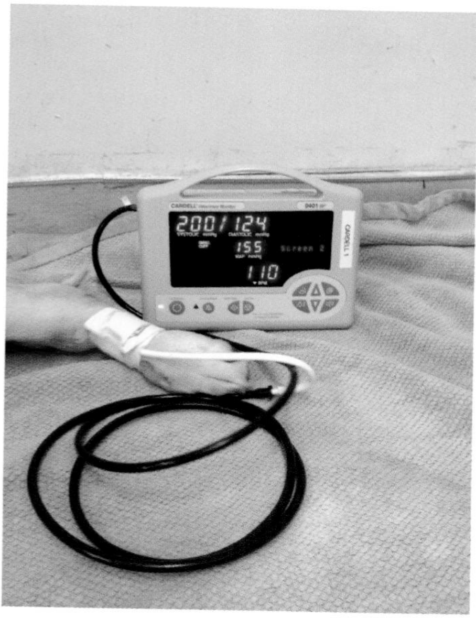

Figure 30-4 Measuring systolic, diastolic and mean blood pressure using oscillometric machine. Photo courtesy of S Epstein.

Complications

1. False low or high reading due to inappropriate sized cuff or poor placement of cuff
2. False high reading due to bent limb
3. Increased blood pressure caused by patient stress during procedure

Equipment Needed

- Oscillometric blood pressure machine
- Appropriate sized cuff for patient
- Porous tape

Procedure

Technical Action	Rationale/Amplification
1. Place patient in lateral or sternal recumbency with limb extended.	1. Cuff must be at level of heart for most reliable measurement; bent limb can cause false high reading; lateral recumbency gives most consistent readings.
2. The tail is an alternate site.	2. Any place you can locate a pulse and place a cuff proximal to it is acceptable for obtaining a BP measurement

Technical Action	Rationale/Amplification
3. Measure area in which cuff will be placed and select correct size cuff (Fig. 30-2).	**3.** Measure circumference of appendage, multiple by 0.4 for dogs and 0.3 for cats and round up for correct cuff size. The cuff can be placed on the front part of the foot, medioproximal to the carpus or to the ventral root of the tail or to the tarsal artery of the hind leg. The cuff can also be placed over the brachial artery on the upper foreleg of small dog breeds and cats.) (A cuff that is too wide will result in lower readings and a cuff that is not wide enough will result in higher readings.)
4. Place cuff on limb/appendage at measure site. Velcro snugly but not tight. A small piece of porous tape may be used to secure the cuff.	**4.** Placing a short strip of tape on the cuff is fine as long as it does not completely encircle the cuff, restricting its ability to inflate.
5. Once initiated, the oscillometric system will automatically inflate and deflate the cuff at a defined rate and will provide a digital readout on the screen. Multiple readings are taken in immediate succession, allowing for a more accurate reflection of blood pressure (Fig. 30-4).	

Direct Measurement (Invasive)

Restraint and Positioning

This method should be used exclusively for anesthetized or moribund patients. Direct arterial blood pressure monitoring is not indicated in active, relatively healthy patients due to possible morbidity from arterial catheter placement and risk of the patient pulling the catheter out or disconnecting the arterial line and causing significant hemorrhage. Animals with arterial catheters must be strictly supervised at all times.

Complications

1. Vascular injury
2. Disconnection
3. Accidental injection of drugs
4. Infection
5. Damage to nearby nerves
6. Inaccurate measurements due to movement

NOTE: *Accidental disconnection can produce rapid exsanguination with the risk of hypotension, shock, and death if not immediately identified. Constant monitoring of the extension tubing and connection points is important to avoid this complication.*

Transducer Technique

Equipment Needed

- Arterial catheter in place
- Freshly mixed heparinized saline bag at 1000u heparin/l
- Appropriate sized pressure sleeve
- Microdrip
- Luer lock 3-way stopcock or Luer lock T-port
- 6–12 inch-length of rigid small diameter pressure tubing
- Pressure transducer
- Appropriate cable for the transducer used
- Blood pressure monitor
- Heparinized saline filled syringe

Procedure

Technical Action	Rationale/Amplification
1. Place arterial catheter.	1. See Chapter 33.
2. Attach the pressure transducer to the patient monitor at the appropriate plug site.	
3. Following attachment, connect 3-way stopcocks to the Luer adapters in the transducer housing.	3. In permanent transducers, two stopcocks are required; in disposable units, only one may be necessary.
4. Leave stopcock "open" to room air and fill the chamber with heparinized saline, being sure that ALL air bubbles are removed.	
5. "Zero" the transducer to the machine by pressing the zero control button on the monitor panel.	5. This adjusts the electronics to provide accurate measurement.
6. Attach the flush infusion device to one stopcock unless it is embedded in the transducer device.	
7. Attach the microdrip IV infusion set to the heparinized IV bag and place in the pressure sleeve.	
8. Pressurize sleeve/bag to 300 mmHg.	8. The heparinized saline bag is pressurized to prevent backwards flow of arterial blood into the tubing.

Technical Action	Rationale/Amplification
9. Prime the 6–12inch-length of rigid IV tubing with heparinized saline and attach to a stopcock to interface the catheter to the transducer.	**9.** Rigid tubing is manufactured specifically for pressure monitoring. Compliant tubing should not be used because it absorbs energy from the fluid transmitting the pressures and returns it to the system with a slight delay, resulting in distortion of the waveform.
10. Turn stopcock off to prevent fluid drainage once the tubing is filled.	
11. A catheter adapter with a side port is flushed with heparinized saline filled syringe with the syringe attached after flushing.	
12. Flush the connecting tubing with saline using the flush device embedded in the disposable transducer or by using a saline filled syringe attached to the stopcock immediately adjacent to the extension tubing.	**12.** Be sure that there are no visible air bubbles following the flush procedure.
13. Attach the connecting tubing to the catheter adapter extension.	
14. Level the transducer at the estimated base of the heart.	**14.** The transducer should be maintained at heart base level (sternum level if in lateral, point of the shoulder if in dorsal or ventral recumbancy) for the most accurate results. The transducer can be taped directly to the patient (if under anesthesia or recumbent), to a sandbag (Fig. 30-5), or to a wall of the patient's cage.
15. Close the line to the patient and open it up to room air using the stopcock.	
16. Press the zero button again to recalibrate the system to the patient.	**16.** The transducer should be zeroed at heart base level (sternum level if in lateral, point of the shoulder if in dorsal or ventral recumbency) for the most accurate results.
17. Close the stopcock to air and open to the patient.	
18. You should see a well-defined wave form on the monitor.	**18.** Systolic, mean and diastolic pressure as well as heart rate are displayed.

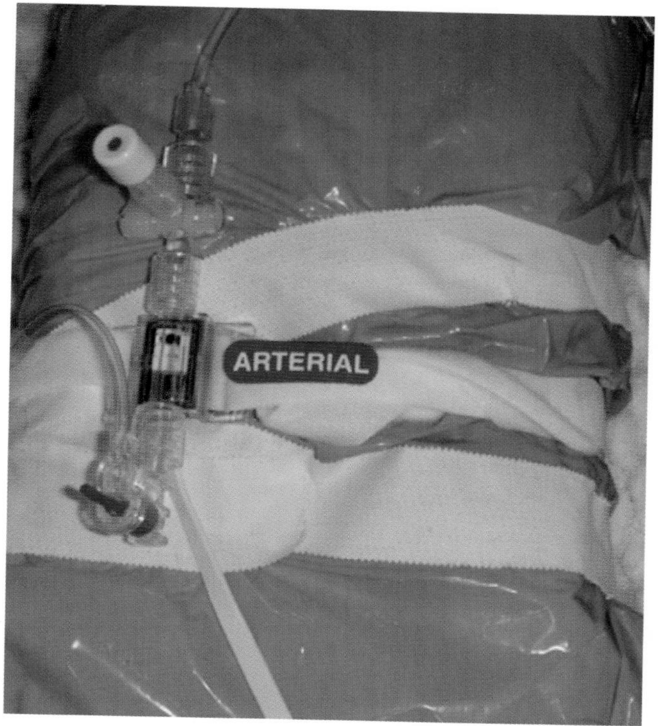

Figure 30-5 Pressure transducer taped to sandbag. Photo courtesy of S Epstein.

Technical Action	Rationale/Amplification
19. If the wave form dampens over time, repeat the flush, being attentive to the total heparin-saline volume used during the procedure	**19.** The fluid line needs to be flushed periodically (and whenever the pulse wave dampens) to avoid clot development at the catheter site. Be aware of cumulative heparinized saline volumes administered while flushing. Large volumes are a concern in small or cardiovascularly compromised animals.

NOTE: *If the flush flows easily but very low pressures register immediately check the arterial catheter site for poor connections/hemorrhage.*

Manometer Technique

Equipment Needed

- Arterial catheter in place
- Freshly mixed heparinized saline bag at 1000u heparin/l

- Appropriate sized pressure sleeve
- Microdrip
- Luer lock 3-way stopcock or Luer lock T-port
- 6–12 inch-length of rigid small diameter pressure tubing
- Aneroid manometer or sphygmomanometer
- Heparinized saline filled syringe

Procedure

Technical Action	Rationale/Amplification
1. Place arterial catheter.	**1.** See Chapter 33.
2. Connect rigid tubing from the catheter to a 3-way stopcock.	
3. Attach the stopcock to the bag of pressurized flush at one port and an aneroid manometer or sphygmomanometer to the third port.	
4. Pressurize the aneroid manometer or sphygmomanometer and close off stopcock to the bag of flush.	**4.** The manometer must be positioned at the level of the right atrium.
5. As the pressure in the manometer decreases, fluid will travel towards the patient.	**5.** Care should be taken to avoid allowing air to enter the arterial catheter.
6. When the pressure reading on the manometer equals the mean arterial pressure, the fluid flow will stop and oscillate gently in the tubing.	**6.** Note that this type of system only measures MEAN pressure.

CENTRAL VENOUS PRESSURE

Central venous pressure (CVP) is a measure of the hydrostatic pressure in the cranial or caudal vena cava as it enters the heart and is considered to be equal to the right atrial pressure. CVP is used to assess patients for overhydration or excess fluid loss and can be used as a guide in volume resuscitation. This can be done by measuring CVP before and after a fluid bolus. Normal CVP in dogs and cats ranges from 0–5 cmH_2O. Values >10 cmH_2O can indicate increased preload. Hypovolemic patients may have negative CVP values.

Complications

1. Clot formation
2. Infection
3. Hemorrhage
4. False high or low readings due to catheter malpositioning

Restraint and Positioning

The patient should be restrained in lateral recumbency and the level of the right atrium (this is usually near the manubrium, the cranial tip of the sternum) identified.

Transducer Technique

Equipment Needed

- Central venous catheter in place
- A bag of crystalloid fluids
- Appropriate sized pressure sleeve
- Fluid extension set
- Luer lock 3-way stopcock or Luer lock T-port
- Pressure transducer
- Appropriate cable for the transducer used
- Blood pressure monitor

Procedure

Technical Action	Rationale/Amplification
1. Place central venous catheter.	1. See Chapter 4. Jugular catheter is preferred, but long, indwelling saphenous catheters can be used. Tip of catheter should be positioned near the right atrium (confirmed by a lateral radiograph).
2. Attach the pressure transducer to the patient monitor at the appropriate plug site.	
3. Attach the fluid administration set to the fluid bag and place in the pressure sleeve.	3. In permanent transducers, two stopcocks are required, in disposable units, only one may be necessary.
4. Connect the administration set to the pressure transducer.	
5. Connect the 3-way stopcock to the patient side of the pressure transducer.	
6. Connect the extension set to the 3-way stopcock.	
7. Pressurize sleeve/bag to 300 mmHg.	7. The fluid bag is pressurized to prevent backwards flow of blood into the tubing.

Technical Action	Rationale/Amplification
8. Run fluid through the pressure transducer and fill the extension set.	
9. Set the pressure transducer at the level of the right atrium.	**9.** The transducer can be taped directly to the patient (if under anesthesia or recumbent), to a sandbag or to a wall of the patient's cage.
10. Attach the extension set to the patient.	**10.** If using a multi-lumen catheter, be sure that the other port(s) are flushed and closed before opening line to patient.
11. Open the stopcock to room air (closed to the patient catheter).	
12. Zero the monitor with the fluid column open to air.	**12.** This adjusts the electronics to provide accurate measurement.
13. Open the stopcock to the extension (patient's catheter).	
14. Wait for a waveform to appear on the monitor and note the numbers that appear, record the lower number in parentheses (Fig. 30-6).	**14.** Note that electronic monitors display pressure in terms of mmHg, rather than cmH_2O. To convert mmHg to cmH_2O, simply multiply the recorded value by 1.40.

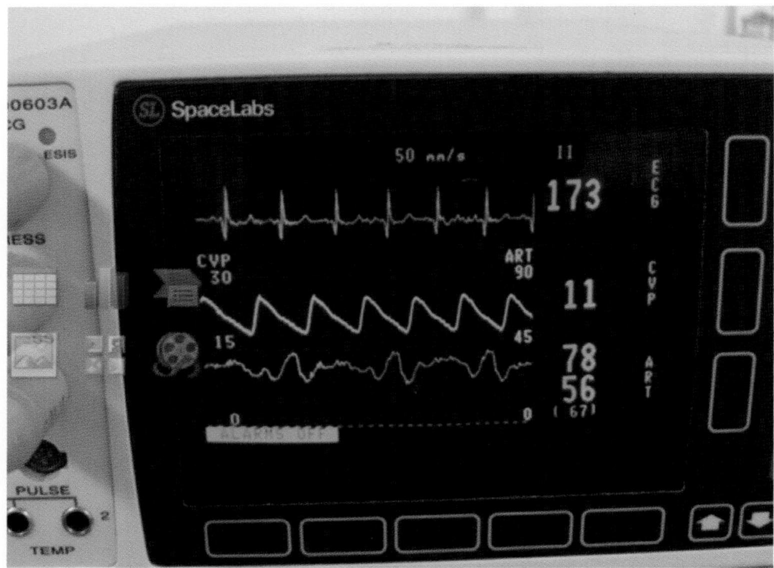

Figure 30-6 Blood pressure monitor. Photo courtesy of S Epstein.

Manometer Technique

Equipment Needed (Fig. 30-7)

- Central venous catheter in place
- A water manometer
- A bag of crystalloid fluids
- A fluid administration set
- A 3-way stopcock
- An extension set

Procedure

Technical Action	Rationale/Amplification
1. Place central venous catheter.	1. See Chapter 4. Jugular catheter is preferred, but long, indwelling saphenous catheters can be used. Tip of catheter should be positioned near the right atrium (confirmed by a lateral radiograph).
2. Connect the stopcock to the manometer.	2. Most manometers are already fitted with one.
3. Attach fluid bag to administration set and connect to the stopcock.	3. A 35 or 60 ml syringe of solution can be used in place of fluid bag (Fig. 30-7).

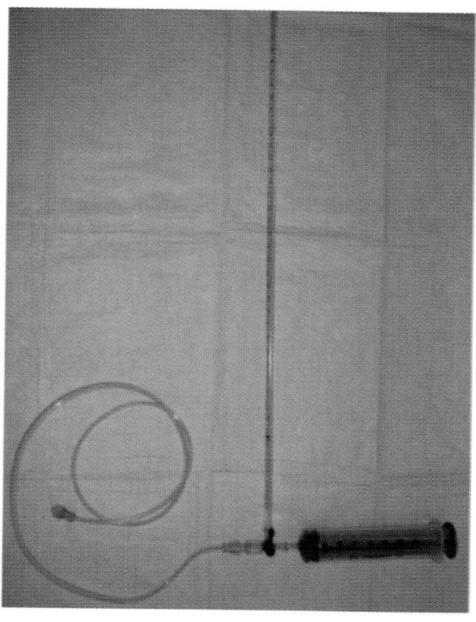

Figure 30-7 Water manometer set up for CVP. Photo courtesy of S Epstein.

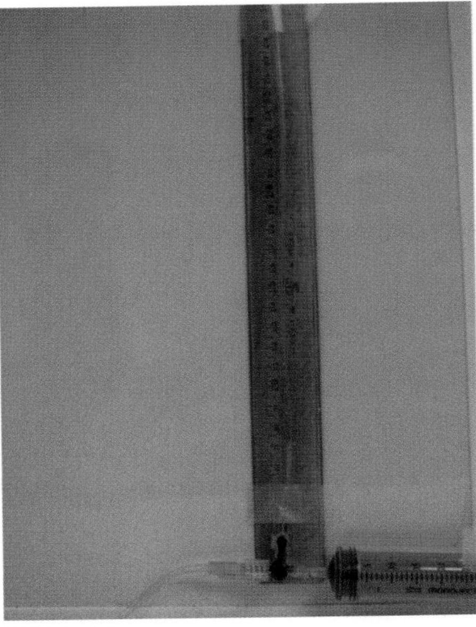

Figure 30-8 Ruler and fluid line extension set up for CVP. Photo courtesy of S Epstein.

Technical Action	Rationale/Amplification
4. Attach extension set to stopcock, turn off to manometer and flush lines.	
5. Attach extension set to patient.	**5.** If using a multi-lumen catheter, be sure that the other port(s) are flushed and closed before opening line to patient.
6. Make sure that the stopcock is level with the right atrium using a level. This serves as the reference point and is the "Zero" mark on the manometer.	**6.** When dealing with CVP measurements, trends are very important so the patient should be in the same position every time.
7. With the stopcock closed towards the patient, open the fluid bag line and fill the manometer to about 25–30 cmH_2O.	**7.** If using syringe, push fluid into the manometer to about 25–30 cmH_2O.
8. Open the stopcock towards the patient (turn it off towards the fluid bag).	**8.** The hydrostatic pressure in the manometer forces fluid through the catheter. The fluid continues to fall until the hydrostatic pressure of the manometer reaches equilibrium with the hydrostatic pressure of the blood.
9. At some point the fluid will begin to oscillate with the patient's heart beat and will stop falling as it equilibrates with the pressure in the vena cava.	**9.** This usually takes about 30 seconds.

Technical Action

10. Once the fluid stops falling, note the number. This is your CVP reading.

Rationale/Amplification

10. If the fluid runs out of the manometer and into the fluid tubing, the patient has a "negative" CVP. This can occur if the manometer/stopcock are considerably higher than the right atrium, or if the patient has hypovolemia.

NOTE: *CVP can be measured without a transducer or manometer by replacing the water manometer with an extension set taped to a ruler and open at the top (Fig. 30-8) and following the manometer procedure.*

Bibliography

Belew AM, Barlett T, Brown SA: Evaluation of the white-coat effect in cats. J Vet Intern Med. Mar–Apr; 13(2): 134–42, 1999

Burkitt J and Davis H: Advanced Monitoring and Procedures for Small Animal Emergency and Critical Care. Oxford, Wiley-Blackwell, 2012

Garofalo NA, Teixeira Neto FJ, Alvaides RK, de Oliveira FA; Pignaton W, Pinheiro RT: Agreement between direct, oscillometric and Doppler ultrasound blood pressures using three different cuff positions in anesthetized dogs. Vet Anaesth Analg 39(4): 324–34, July 2012

Hansen B: Use of CVP for Monitoring and as a Diagnostic Tool, International Veterinary Emergency and Critical Care Symposium, 2006

Holowaychuk M: Central Venous Pressure: Underused or Obsolete? International Veterinary Emergency and Critical Care Symposium, 2013

Raffe MR: Direct Blood Pressure Monitorig. IVECCS, 2005

Robben J H: How to Place a Central Line and Measure CVP, WSAVA/FECAVA/BSAVA World Congress, 2012

Rondeau DA, Mackalonis ME, Hess RS: Effect of body position on indirect measurement of systolic arterial blood pressure in dogs. J Am Vet Med Assoc 242(11): 1523–7, June 2013

Steele A M: Under Pressure, ABP, CVP: What Are the Numbers Really Telling Us? British Small Animal Veterinary Congress, 2010

Waddell LS: Blood Pressure Monitoring for the Critically Ill. Western Veterinary Conference 2004

Chapter 31

Transfusion of Blood and Plasma

Fortune favors the prepared mind.
LOUIS PASTEUR

Purposes

1. Supply red blood cells (RBCs) to patients with anemia
2. Provide clotting factors to patients with clotting disorders
3. Correct massive acute hemorrhage

Complications

1. Sepsis
2. Vascular overload
3. Coagulopathy
4. Hemolysis
5. Pulmonary microembolism

Equipment needed:

- IV catheter with T-connection
- 3 mL of heparinized saline
- Y-type blood administration set
- Extension sets
- One 250-mL bag of 0.9% NaCl
- Hemo-Nate filter (if administering blood or plasma from a syringe)
- Temperature probe
- Blood rocker (if administering fresh whole blood)
- 250 mL 0.9% saline

Crow and Walshaw's Manual of Clinical Procedures in Dogs, Cats, Rabbits, and Rodents, Fourth Edition. Edited by Jennifer E. Boyle. Published 2016 by John Wiley & Sons, Inc.
Companion Website: www.wiley.com/go/boyle/manual4e

Pretransfusion Setup

Technical Action	Rationale/Amplification
1. Place intravenous or intraosseous catheter or, if catheter is already in place, check for patency (see Chapter 4 or Chapter 32).	1. Large lumen catheters are less likely to damage or lyse RBCs. Do not give blood through a catheter smaller than 22 gauge.
2. Perform a blood typing procedure and record results.	2. Due to the risk of severe incompatibility reactions, cats must always be typed before transfusion.
3. If patient has received a prior transfusion, perform a donor-recipient cross-match procedure and record results.	3. Cross matches should be done on any animal that has had a transfusion reaction to a prior blood transfusion or that has received a blood transfusion previously, even if it was several years ago.
4. If using stored blood or plasma, warm products prior to administration: a) Thaw fresh frozen plasma (FFP) at room temperature for 20 minutes, then defrost in lukewarm water. b) Warm refrigerated whole blood and packed RBCs in lukewarm water.	4. FFP can be defrosted without thawing first in emergent circumstances. If denaturing occurs, you will note an area of white congealed proteins in the plasma. Blood can be given cold in emergent situations, but the oxygen-carrying capacity will not occur until the RBCs reach body temperature.
5. Insert an indwelling temperature probe in rectum, if available.	5. Make sure to give warm fluids and heat externally if the patient is hypothermic.
6. Record baseline vital signs (rectal temperature, pulse rate, respiratory rate).	6. It is essential to monitor the animal's vital signs and respiratory pattern throughout the entire transfusion.
7. Attach 1 or 2 extension sets to outlet of Y-type administration set.	7. Aseptic technique should be used while connecting tubes, bags, and filters to avoid contamination of the products to be transfused.
8. Attach blood component or plasma bag to one input port and 0.9% NaCl bag to other input port (Fig. 31-1). 9. Open roll clamp and fill filter halfway, then invert hand pump. 10. Fill hand pump with plasma or blood product; when full, return hand pump to normal position. 11. Fill remaining line and extension sets with plasma or blood product.	8–11. These steps "prime" the line, making it ready for administration. Expel any large air bubbles from the line before proceeding. Do not use the Y-type blood administration set in standard fluid pumps. The pump will compress the line, causing damage to the cells. If available, fluid pumps that are labeled to give RBC can be used. Blood is incompatible with D5W and LRS. Use 0.9% saline.

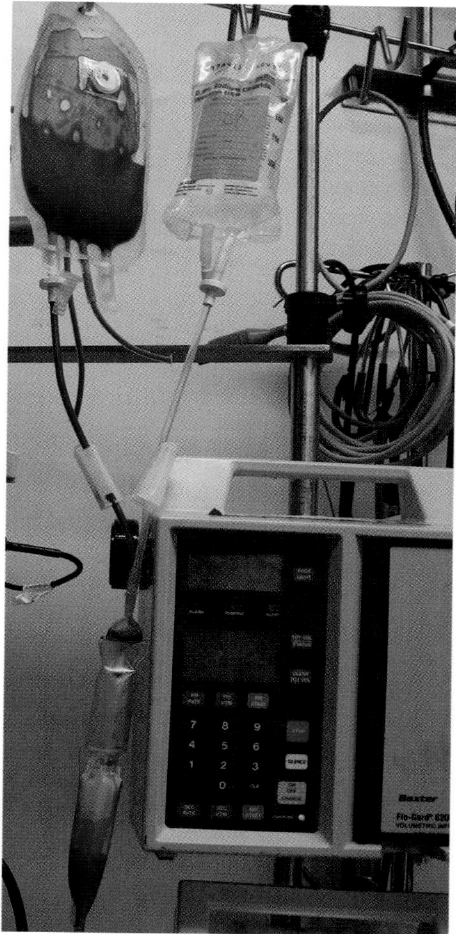

Figure 31-1 Blood and plasma connected to Y-type administration set. Photo courtesy of C Knightly.

NOTE: *If fluid volume overload is a concern, administering blood via syringe (Fig. 31-2) is indicated because it takes less saline to flush line and blood can be given at a more controlled rate. If administering blood products or plasma via syringe, do the following in place of Nos. 7 through 11 above.*

- Insert an injection port (e.g. Baxter sampling site coupler) into plasma or blood product bag
- Draw blood product into syringe
- Attach Hemo-Nate filter between syringe and an extension set

Transfusion Procedure

Technical Action	Rationale/Amplification
1. If animal is actively bleeding and there is not time to give a controlled	1. Patients with hemorrhagic shock can receive up to 22 mL/kg/hr.

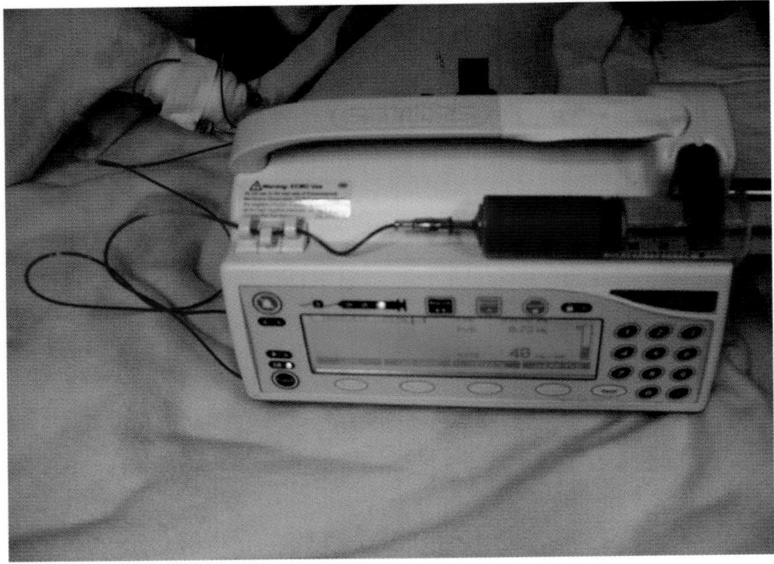

Figure 31-2 Blood administered through syringe pump. Photo courtesy of C Knightly.

Technical Action	Rationale/Amplification
transfusion, blood can be given at a rapid rate.	
2. If animal is relatively stable, begin infusing plasma or blood product at 2.5 mL/kg/hr.	**2.** Watch for signs of transfusion reactions. Most reactions occur because blood is being administered too rapidly. If only a mild temperature increase is noted, decrease the rate of infusion.
3. Vital signs should be monitored every 15 minutes for first 45 minutes, and then every hour until transfusion is completed.	**3.** Discontinue the transfusion if any of the following reactions are observed: **a)** Evidence of vascular overload such as pulmonary edema or dyspnea. **b)** Evidence of an immune-mediated reaction such as restlessness, nausea, vomiting, tachypnea, tachycardia, urticaria, facial edema, swelling, or pruritus (in cats, especially noted by face rubbing).
4. Increase rate of infusion, if indicated.	**4.** If after 20 minutes no signs of adverse reaction are noted, rate of infusion may be increased to 5–10 mL/kg/hr. Heart failure patients should receive no more than 1–2 mL/kg/hr.

Technical Action

5. When transfusion is completed, administration set should be flushed with 0.9%NaCl at same rate until fluid line is mostly clear.

Rationale/Amplification

5. Blood is not compatible with 5% dextrose in water (D5W) or lactated Ringer's solution (LRS). Saline should be run at the same rate as the blood or plasma to avoid administering the remaining in the line too rapidly.

Bibliography

Kirk RW, Bistner SI: Handbook of Veterinary Procedures and Emergency Treatment, 7th edition. Philadelphia, WB Saunders, 2000

Macintire DK, Drobratz KJ, Haskins SC, Saxon WD: Manual of Small Animal Emergency and Critical Care Medicine. Philadelphia, Lippincott, 2005

WSAVA 2003 Congress: Blood Transfusion Guidelines; Bernard F. Feldman, DVM, PhD

Chapter 32

Placement of Intraosseous Catheters

Small things, done in love, bring joy and peace.
MOTHER TERESA

Intraosseous catheterization is the placement of a hollow device, a catheter or needle, through the bone's hard cortex and into the soft marrow interior. * **The following procedure is considered invasive and is typically performed exclusively by veterinarians.**

Indications

Intraosseous catheterization can be used for animals with inaccessible peripheral vessels (i.e. neonates, hypovolemic, hypotensive). This route of fluid and medication administration is an alternate one to the preferred IV route when the latter cannot be established in a timely manner, especially during cardiac arrest. NOTE: *Almost anything that can be given IV can be given IO and at similar rates.*

Purposes

1. To administer fluids, medication, and blood to neonates or very small animals
2. To provide ready access to the circulatory system for anticipated metabolic emergencies (e.g. seizures, hypoglycemia, shock)

Complications

1. Sepsis
2. Osteomyelitis
3. Contraindicated in fractured bones

Crow and Walshaw's Manual of Clinical Procedures in Dogs, Cats, Rabbits, and Rodents, Fourth Edition. Edited by Jennifer E. Boyle. © 2016 John Wiley & Sons, Inc. Published 2016 by John Wiley & Sons, Inc.
Companion Website: www.wiley.com/go/boyle/manual4e

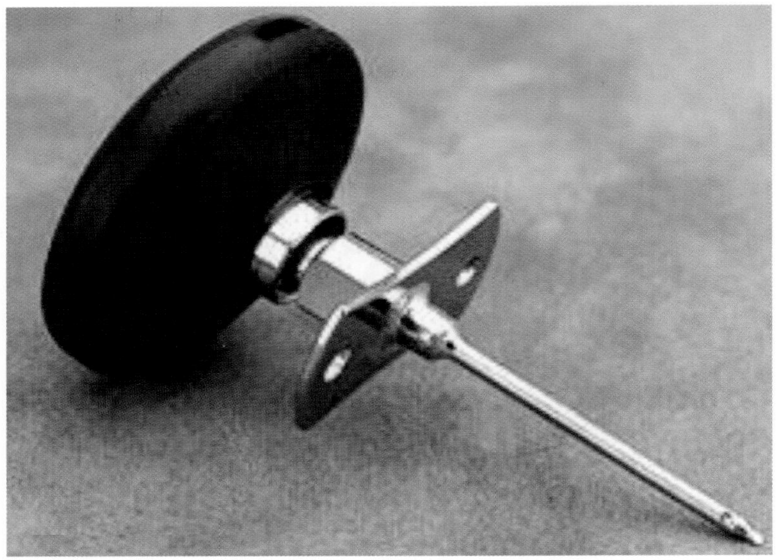

Figure 32-1 Commercial intraosseous catheter.

Equipment Needed (Fig. 32-1)

- 18–20-gauge needle or commercial intraosseous catheter
- Clipper with No. 40 blade
- Skin preparation materials:
  - 2% chlorhexidine scrub
  - 70% alcohol
  - Sterile gauze sponges (2 inch × 2 inch)
- Scissors, needle holder, thumb forceps
- Suture material
- Bandaging material:
  - Sterile gauze sponges
  - Gauze bandage
  - Adhesive tape (½ inch and 1 inch)
- Syringe containing 1 mL of heparinized saline
- Fluid administration set (if necessary)

RESTRAINT AND POSITIONING

The best sites for intraosseous catheterization are the trochanteric fossa of the proximal femur, the iliac crest, and the medial side of the proximal tibia (distal to the tibial tuberosity). When the trochanteric fossa is cannulated, the animal is positioned in lateral recumbency, with the femur to be catheterized facing up. If the medial tibia is selected, the animal should be placed in lateral recumbency with the tibia to be catheterized touching the table.

Procedure

Technical Action	Rationale/Amplification
1. Clip and surgically prepare area over coxofemoral joint.	**1.** Every precaution must be taken to reduce the chance of causing iatrogenic infection.
2. Apply local anesthetic (2% lidocaine) to skin and subcutis at insertion point, then down onto periosteum of trochanteric fossa.	**2.** Feel for the depression between the greater trochanter and the head of the femur. The needle should be introduced on the medial side of the greater trochanter and "walked" down the bone into the fossa, injecting small amounts of the local anesthetic as the needle is advanced.
3. While stabilizing leg with other hand, make a small stab incision through skin to allow insertion of hypodermic or spinal needle.	**3.** A needle with stylet is preferable to avoid occlusion with cortical bone or marrow during insertion.
4. Locate depression between greater trochanter and femoral head. Point needle slightly distal and advance it down medial side of greater trochanter into trochanteric fossa (Fig. 32-2).	**4.** By introducing the needle in this fashion, the sciatic nerve is avoided.

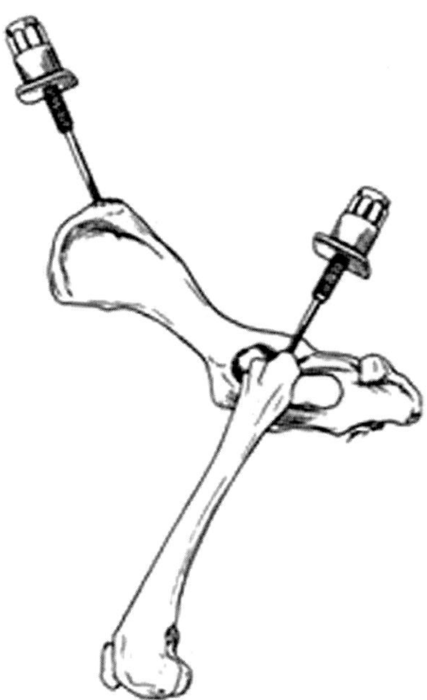

Figure 32-2 Possible sites (proximal femur, iliac crest) for introduction of intraosseous catheter.

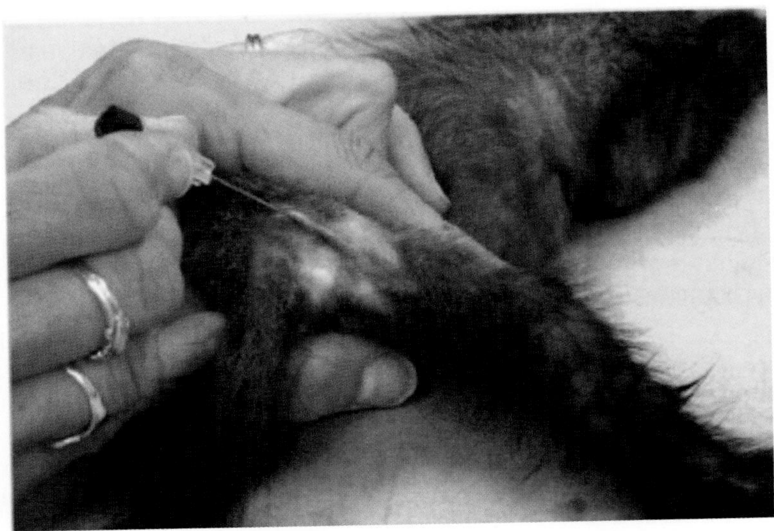

Figure 32-3 Placing 20-gauge needle into the femur of a kitten. With permission from: Advanced Monitoring and Procedures for Small Animal Emergency and Critical Care, Burkitt Creedon J and Davis H. Catheterization of Venous Compartment. p. 66, Copyright Wiley-Blackwell (2012).

Technical Action	Rationale/Amplification
5. Once in position, push needle through cortex into medullary cavity by downward pressure and rotation (about a quarter turn at a time) (Fig. 32-3).	**5.** Upon entering the marrow cavity, resistance will diminish. A properly seated needle will feel solidly in place.
6. Check needle for proper position by manipulation of femur; then flush needle with heparinized saline (Fig. 32-4).	**6.** When manipulating the femur, the needle should move in the same direction easily and you should not be able to see or feel the shaft of the needle. The saline should infuse easily through the needle.
7. Secure needle with butterfly tape and suture in place.	**7.** Patency is maintained by flushing every 6 hours with heparinized saline. The same bone cannot be reused as fluids infused may leak out from original hole in cortex.
8. Apply a bandage to protect needle and insertion site.	**8.** Intraosseous catheters can remain in place for up to 72 hours.

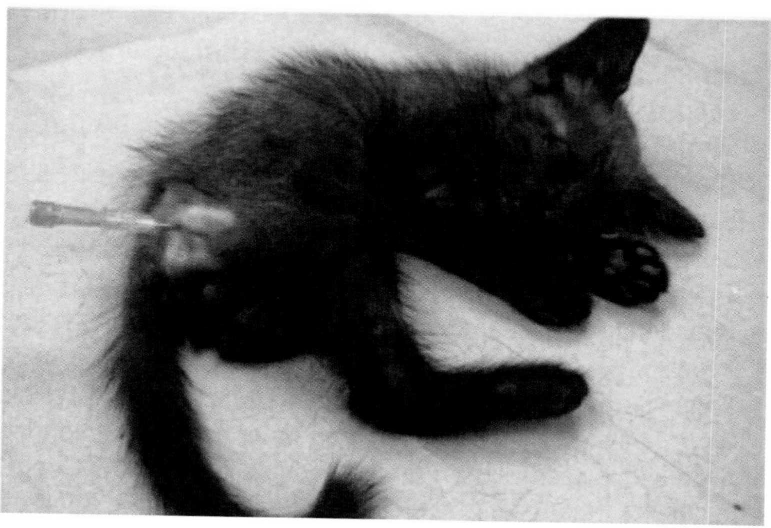

Figure 32-4 Successful placement of intraosseous catheter. With permission from: Advanced Monitoring and Procedures for Small Animal Emergency and Critical Care, Burkitt Creedon J and Davis H. Catheterization of Venous Compartment. p. 66, Copyright Wiley-Blackwell (2012).

Bibliography

Burkitt J and Davis H: Advanced Monitoring and Procedures for Small Animal Emergency and Critical Care, Oxford, Wiley-Blackwell, 2012

Hackett TB, Lehman TL: Practical considerations in emergency drug therapy. Vet Clin N Amer: Small Animal Practice 35: 517–525, 2005

Kirk RW, Bistner SI: Handbook of Veterinary Procedures and Emergency Treatment, 7th edition. Philadelphia, WB Saunders, 2000

Chapter 33

Arterial Blood Collection

Luck is what happens when preparation meets opportunity.
SENECA

ARTERIAL PUNCTURE

Purposes

To obtain a sample of arterial blood for determination of blood gas concentrations and acid-base status.

Complications

1. Arterial spasm
2. Iatrogenic hemorrhage
3. Subcutaneous hematoma formation
4. Arterial thrombosis
5. Hemolysis
6. Sample dilution

Equipment Needed

- Cotton
- Clipper with No. 40 blade
- Skin preparation material
  - 2% chlorhexidine scrub
  - 70% alcohol
  - Sterile gauze sponges (2 inch × 2 inch)

Crow and Walshaw's Manual of Clinical Procedures in Dogs, Cats, Rabbits, and Rodents, Fourth Edition. Edited by Jennifer E. Boyle. Published 2016 by John Wiley & Sons, Inc.
Companion Website: www.wiley.com/go/boyle/manual4e

- 3-mL syringe with a 25- or 22-gauge needle coated with sodium heparin
  OR
- A vented arterial blood gas syringe
- Rubber stopper
- Container of ice large enough to hold syringe
- Adhesive tape, 1 inch wide

NOTE: *Make sure the blood gas analyzer and any associated cartridges are available for immediate use.*

Restraint and Positioning

The femoral or pedal artery may be used in the dog or cat for routine arterial blood collection. The femoral is the larger of the two arteries; however, it is also more difficult to apply adequate pressure after blood collection and therefore holds a higher risk of hemorrhage. For femoral artery blood collection, the animal is placed in lateral recumbency with its uppermost pelvic limb abducted so that the femoral artery can be palpated on the proximal, medial aspect of the opposite leg. For pedal artery puncture, the animal is placed in lateral recumbency as well, with the down side extended to access the medial aspect of the pedal artery.

Procedure

Technical Action	Rationale/Amplification
1. Clip hair from area.	
2. Palpate the pulse in the desired artery.	**2.** Appendage can be mechanically restrained by securing the animal's foot to the table using adhesive tape.
3. Prepare skin over artery, using 2% chlorhexidine and alcohol.	**3.** To minimize the possibility of iatrogenic infection, it is advisable to prepare the skin over the artery as for surgery.
4. Stabilize artery.	**4.** The artery will move; a single digit may be placed directly over the artery to stabilize or a digit on each side of artery. Avoid contaminating exact site where arterial puncture will be performed.
5. Insert the needle through the skin only, allowing the animal time to react to any skin discomfort.	
6. Hold barrel of syringe so that needle bevel is up. Insert needle through skin at approximately 45–60-degree angle with skin.	**6.** If using 1-digit stabilizing technique, advance the needle of heparinized syringe into the vessel at a 45-degree angle, directly below the finger (Fig. 33-1). If using the 2-digit stabilizing technique, insert the needle between the 2 fingers and advance into the vessel at a 90-degree angle (Fig. 33-2).

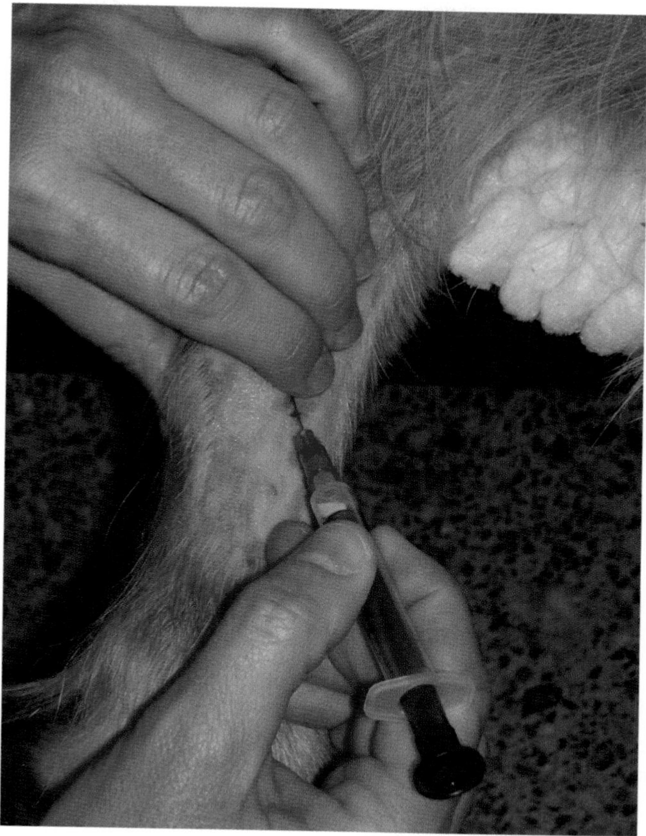

Figure 33-1 Advancing needle using 1-digit stabilizing technique. Photo courtesy of C Knightly.

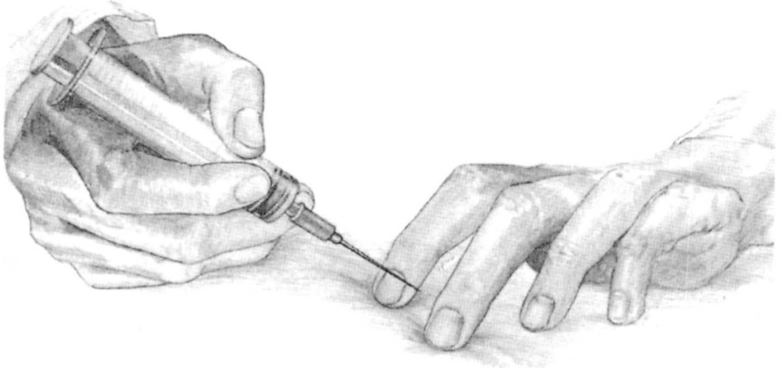

Figure 33-2 Advancing needle using 2-digit stabilizing technique.

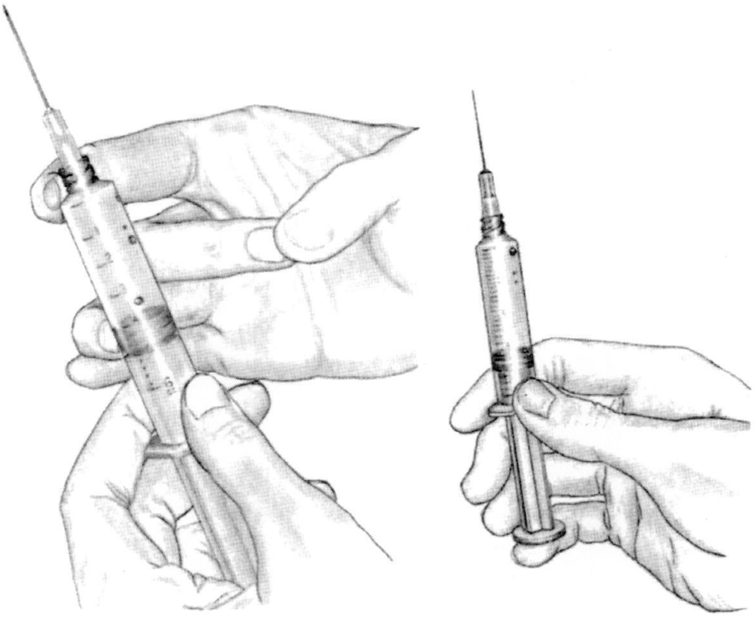

Figure 33-3 Removing air bubbles from syringe (A and B).

Technical Action	Rationale/Amplification
7. Arterial puncture should result in a flash in the hub of the needle or filling of the syringe with arterial blood.	**7.** The syringe may need to be aspirated to obtain a full sample. If using a vented syringe, the syringe is made to fill with blood until it reaches the volume preset by the plunger.
8. Hold syringe upright, tap on syringe to cause air bubbles to rise (Fig. 33-3A), eject air bubbles from syringe (Fig. 33-3B), and insert needle into rubber stopper.	**8.** Evacuation of air from the syringe and insertion of needle into rubber stopper prevent inaccurate results.
9. Following arterial puncture, apply direct pressure to the puncture site for at least 5 minutes to ensure there is no bleeding.	**9.** Firm pressure on the arterial puncture site decreases the possibility of hemorrhage and subcutaneous hematoma formation. Hold pressure on arterial puncture site for 3–5 minutes. Hold pressure for 15 minutes or until bleeding has stopped if animal has a bleeding problem.
10. It is recommended that samples be analyzed immediately.	**10.** If the analysis will not be performed within 5 minutes, place the blood-filled syringe in a container with ice to preserve the condition of the blood for up to 1 hour.

ARTERIAL CATHETER PLACEMENT

Purposes

1. Sampling arterial blood for blood gas and acid base status
2. Direct (invasive) blood pressure measurement

Complications

1. Arterial spasm
2. Vascular injury
3. Iatrogenic hemorrhage possibly leading to exsanguination
4. Subcutaneous hematoma formation
5. Arterial thrombosis
6. Infection
7. Iatrogenic coagulation abnormalities secondary to frequent heparin administration in some small patients

NOTE: *Accidental removal or dislodgment of catheter can produce rapid exsanguination, with the risk of hypotension, shock and death if not immediately identified. Constant monitoring of the animal is important to avoid this complication.*

Equipment Needed

- Clipper with No. 40 blade
- Skin preparation material
  - 2% chlorhexidine scrub
  - 70% alcohol
  - Sterile gauze sponges (2 inch × 2 inch)
- 20–24 gauge catheter depending on size of patient
- No. 11 blade or 18-gauge needle
- Bandaging material
  - Sterile gauze sponges (and/or sterile Band-aid®)
  - Gauze bandage
  - Adhesive tape (½ inch, 1 inch, and 2 inch)
- Injection cap
- T-port (if necessary)
- Heparinized saline flush

Restraint and Positioning

The femoral or pedal arteries are the most commonly used for catheterization. Additional sites include the auricular, radial, and coccygeal arteries. Again, the femoral is a larger artery allowing for potentially easier catheter placement, but at the same time holds a greater risk of hemorrhage. The animal is placed in lateral recumbency for both femoral and pedal arterial catheterization. Animals with arterial catheters must be strictly supervised at all times to prevent dislodgement or removal of catheter.

Procedure

Technical Action	Rationale/Amplification
1. Clip hair from area.	
2. Palpate the pulse in the desired artery	2. Appendage can be mechanically restrained by securing the animal's foot to the table using adhesive tape.
3. Perform surgery scrub over clipped area.	3. To minimize the possibility of iatrogenic infection, it is advisable to prepare the skin over the artery as for surgery.
4. Insert the needle through the skin only, allowing the animal time to react to any skin discomfort. NOTE: *A local anesthetic block can be performed using 2% lidocaine.*	4. To avoid catheter drag, a small nick incision should first be made using an 18-gauge needle or No. 11 blade.
5. The catheter should then be advanced in small, steady increments at a 10–20-degree angle toward the arterial pulse (Fig. 33-4).	5. Use a gloved finger to palpate the pedal pulse within the surgical field.

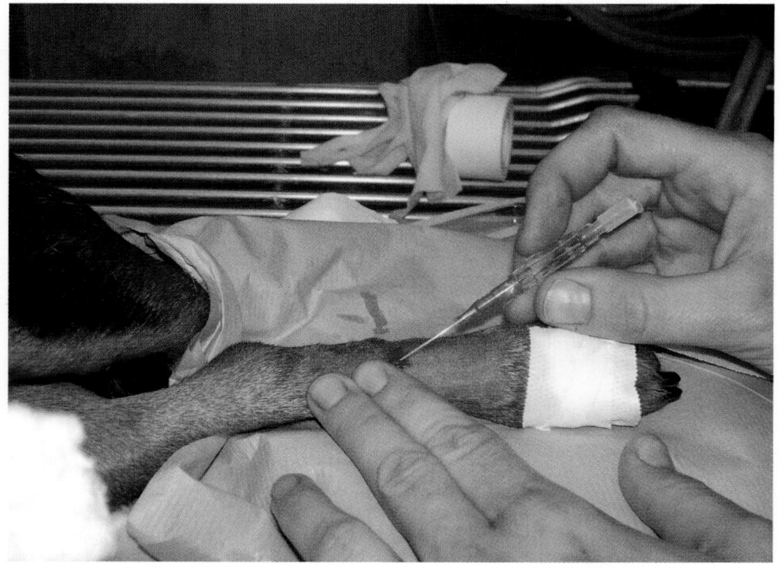

Figure 33-4 Arterial catheter placement. Photo courtesy of C Knightly.

Technical Action	Rationale/Amplification
6. Once a flash of blood is noted in the catheter hub, the catheter should be advanced slightly to ensure the catheter tip is fully through the arterial wall.	6. If a flash is not seen once catheter is at an adequate depth for arterial puncture, the catheter should be withdrawn in small increments, as it is possible to puncture through the arterial wall on initial insertion and a flash may be achieved while withdrawing the catheter.
7. Advance the catheter off of the stylet into the artery, careful not to back the stylet out.	
8. If the catheter will not feed, but an arterial pulse is still palpable, the catheter can be withdrawn slightly and redirected adjacent to the first site without fully removing the catheter.	8. This may help avoid formation of a hematoma that can prevent further attempts at catheterizing the same vessel. If arterial spasm occurs, catheterization will be futile until the spasm resolves. NOTE: *DO NOT attempt to feed catheter back on to stylet if it only partially feeds as this could cause the tip of the catheter to shear off into the artery.*
9. Remove the stylet, place a male adapter or T-port into the catheter hub and flush with heparinized saline.	9. Heparinized saline will keep the catheter patent while the bandage is placed on the leg.
10. Wrap adhesive tape strip around catheter hub and then around animal's leg. Secure an additional strip of tape around the T-port or male adapter plug.	10. This tape anchors the catheter to the leg. Firm anchoring of the catheter prevents the catheter from backing out of the artery. This tape can be further secured by suturing or gluing it to the animal's skin.
11. Cleanse puncture site of any blood.	11. Blood is a good culture medium for bacterial growth. Removal of any blood extravasated during the procedure will help to decrease the possibility of infection.
12. Place sterile gauze sponge or Band-aid® over insertion site.	12. The CDC has determined that the most effective way to prevent catheter-related infections is to avoid multiuse antimicrobial ointment. A sterile gauze sponge or sterile Band-aid® should be aseptically placed over the catheter insertion site.
13. Bandage area above and below the catheter using gauze bandaging material and adhesive tape, leaving only the T-port and injection cap exposed.	13. Bandaging of the leg with gauze helps to prevent contamination of the catheter insertion site and resulting infection.

Technical Action	Rationale/Amplification
14. Flush catheter with heparinized saline every 2–4 hours when not in continuous use.	**14.** Arterial catheters should be flushed every 2–4 hours with small amounts of heparinized saline to maintain patency. Care should be taken to avoid over heparinizing or volume overloading small patients.
15. Remove bandage and evaluate catheter site 24 hours.	**15.** The bandage should be changed immediately if it becomes wet or soiled. The bandage should be changed and the leg inspected for swelling, pain, redness, or discharge every 24 hours. If any of these signs are present, the catheter should be removed and the catheter tip should be submitted for bacteriologic culture.
16. When catheter is removed, immediately apply pressure to catheterization site with dry cotton ball for 5 minutes or more. Then apply previously prepared bandage.	**16.** Pressure on the catheterization site and bandaging of the site following catheter removal will decrease the possibility of hemorrhage and subcutaneous hematoma formation.

NOTE: *The tape and T-connector should be clearly labeled to indicate that this is an arterial catheter. Arterial catheters should never be used for drug or fluid administration* (Fig. 33-5).

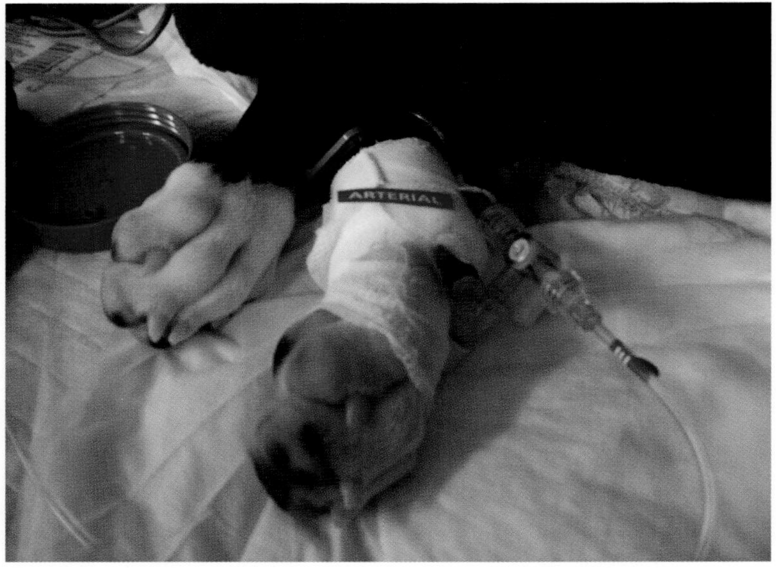

Figure 33-5 Clearly labeled arterial catheter. Photo courtesy of C Knightly.

BLOOD SAMPLING FROM ARTERIAL CATHETER

Equipment Needed

- 70% alcohol
- Sterile gauze sponges (2 inch × 2 inch)
- 3-mL syringe with 0.5 mL heparinized saline
- 3-mL syringe with a 25- or 22-gauge needle coated with sodium heparin
  OR
- A vented arterial blood gas syringe
- Rubber stopper
- Container of ice large enough to hold syringe
- Heparinized saline flush

Procedure

Technical Action	Rationale/Amplification
1. Clean male adapter plug with alcohol.	1. Injection cap should be clean and free of any biological material before insertion of needle to minimize the possibility of iatrogenic infection.
2. Draw 2.5 mL of blood into a syringe contains 0.5 mL of heparinized saline.	2. If using a T-port, draw from the length T-port rather than the base to be sure to clear the line of heparinized saline.
3. Draw arterial sample using 3-mL syringe with a 25- or 22-gauge needle coated with sodium heparin OR a vented arterial blood gas syringe.	3. Hold syringe upright, tap on syringe to cause air bubbles to rise (Fig. 33-3A), eject air bubbles from syringe (Fig. 33-3B), and insert needle into rubber stopper.
4. Flush the catheter with heparinized saline.	4. The heparinized saline will keep the catheter patent.
5. The blood that was obtained first should be administered back to the patient via a peripheral venous catheter.	5. No drugs or intravenous fluids should ever be administered through an arterial catheter.

Bibliography

Burkitt Creedon JM, Davis H: Advanced Monitoring and Procedures for Small Animal Emergency and Critical Care. Oxford, Wiley Blackwell, 2012

Ettinger SJ, Feldman EC: Textbook of veterinary internal medicine. 6th edition. St. Louis, Mo, Elsevier Saunders, 2005

Macintire DK, Drobatz KJ, Haskins SC (eds.): Manual of Small Animal Emergency & Critical Care Medicine. Philadelphia, Lippincott Williams & Wilkins, 2005
Mazzaferro EM: Arterial Catheterization. International Veterinary Emergency and Critical Care Symposium, 2004
McMillan S: Collect an Arterial Blood Gas Sample. British Small Animal Veterinary Congress, 2010

Chapter 34

Tracheostomy

Act as if it were impossible to fail.
DOROTHEA BRANDE

Tracheostomy is the surgical formation of an opening into the cervical trachea to allow for passage of air. * **The following procedure is considered surgical and is performed exclusively by veterinarians.**

Purposes

1. To circumvent upper respiratory obstructions and establish adequate ventilation
2. To reduce resistance to respiration
3. To facilitate artificial respiration

Complications

1. Obstruction of the airway with secretions
2. Tracheal inflammation or necrosis
3. Infection at insertion site
4. Subcutaneous emphysema secondary to tracheal trauma
5. Pneumomediastinum and/or pneumothorax

Equipment Needed

- Sterile tracheostomy tube of appropriate size and type
- Clipper with No. 40 blade
- Skin preparation material (see Chapter 16)
- Scissors, needle holder, thumb forceps
- Scalpel blade/handle
- Suture material
- Umbilical tape or gauze

Crow and Walshaw's Manual of Clinical Procedures in Dogs, Cats, Rabbits, and Rodents, Fourth Edition. Edited by Jennifer E. Boyle. Published 2016 by John Wiley & Sons, Inc.
Companion Website: www.wiley.com/go/boyle/manual4e

- Bandaging material:
  - Sterile gauze sponge
  - Gauze bandage
  - Adhesive tape
- Additional equipment depending on circumstances:
  - Ambu bag
  - Emergency drugs

Procedure

Technical Action	Rationale/Amplification
1. Select tracheostomy tube of appropriate diameter.	**1.** Attempting to use a tube that is too large can cause trauma to the trachea. A tube that is too small will not provide an adequate airway.
2. Clip and surgically prepare ventral cervical area (see Chapter 16).	**2.** Ideally, sterile technique is preferred, but in an emergency situation that may not be possible. Care should be taken to clip and clean the area once the patient is stabilized.
3. Make a longitudinal ventral midline skin incision from cricoid cartilage to sixth tracheal ring (Fig. 34-1).	**3.** This incision should be 2–3 times the diameter of the tube to be inserted.
4. Using forceps, separate muscles overlying trachea to visualize tracheal rings.	**4.** The fascia should be completely cleared away over a length of three to four tracheal rings.
5. Grasp trachea by a tracheal ring with forceps or secure a stay suture around ring to lift and stabilize trachea.	
6. Make a tranverse incision with scalpel blade through ligament between third and fourth cartilage rings (Fig. 34-2).	**6.** This incision should be just long enough to accommodate the tube comfortably.
7. *Alternative technique:* Make a midline, longitudinal incision starting from second or third tracheal ring and extending caudally so that tube rests comfortably within lumen of trachea (Fig. 34-3).	**7.** Small, transverse incisions can be made at either end of the incision to assist with tube insertion.
8. If an orotracheal tube is in place, remove it; then insert tracheostomy tube through incision and into trachea, with curve of tube directed aborally (toward thorax) (Fig. 34-4).	**8.** The tracheostomy tube is inserted while stabilizing the trachea with forceps or suture.

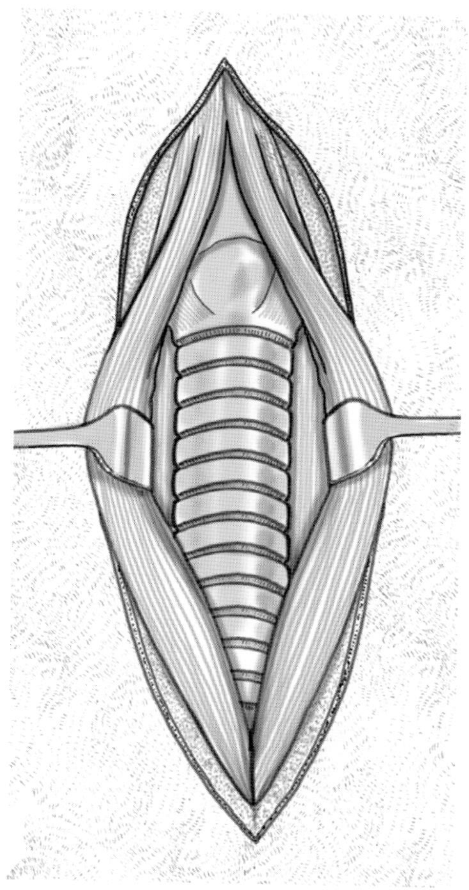

Figure 34-1 Midline ventral cervical skin incision from cricoid cartilage to fifth or sixth tracheal ring.

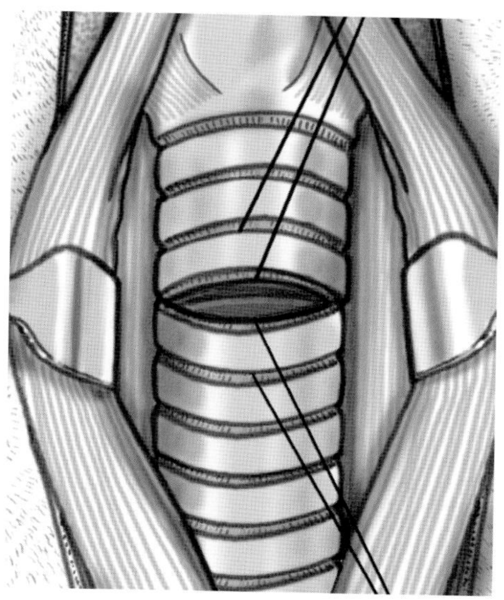

Figure 34-2 Transverse incision in trachea. Stay sutures are placed around rings cranial and caudal to incision.

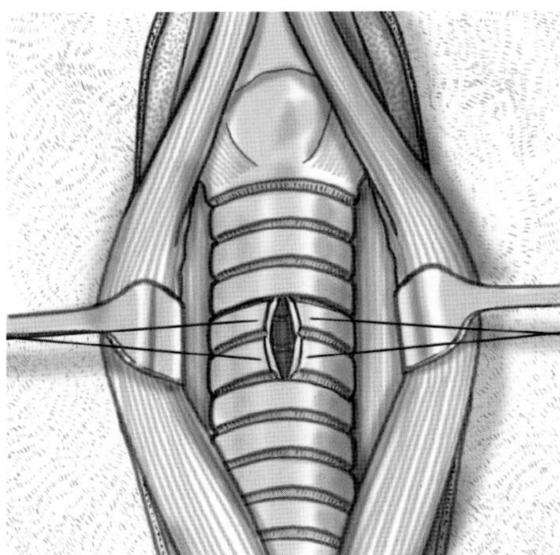

Figure 34-3 Longitudinal incision in trachea. Stay sutures are placed around third tracheal ring lateral to the center of the incision.

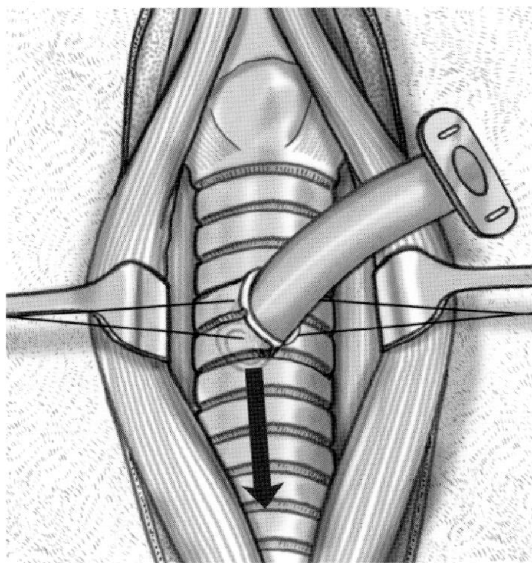

Figure 34-4 Inserting tracheostomy tube through tracheal stoma with curve directed aborally.

Technical Action	Rationale/Amplification
9. Place stay suture loops around tracheal rings cranial and caudal to tracheal incision, and leave long enough to be reached from outside of animal.	**9.** These stay sutures are left in the trachea to facilitate removal and cleaning of the tube and to allow easy access to the airway in an emergency.
10. Administer 100% oxygen and assist with ventilation if needed.	**10.** Oxygenate immediately after placing tube.

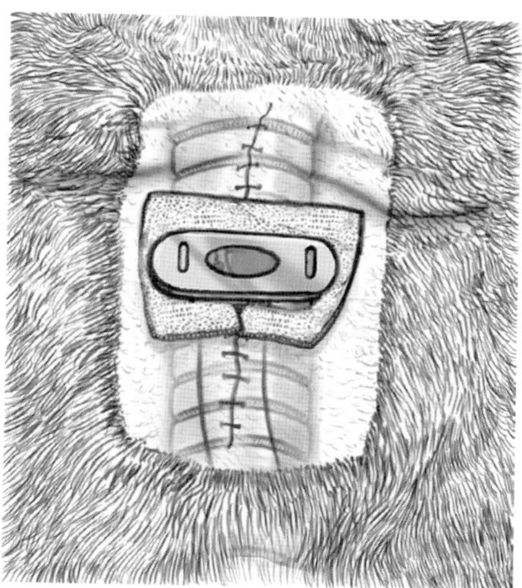

Figure 34-5 Sterile gauze placed around base of tracheostomy tube after skin closure.

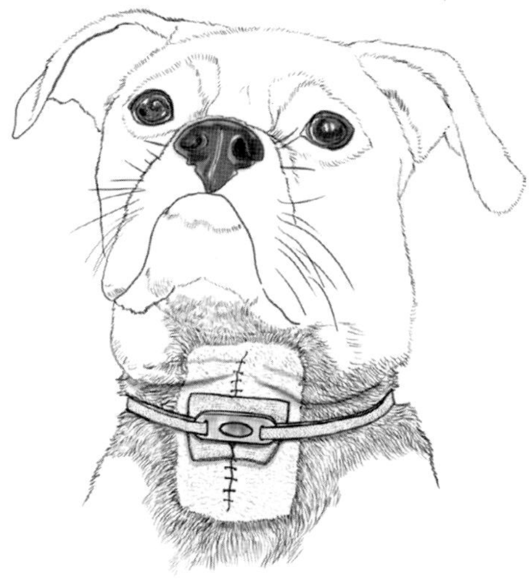

Figure 34-6 Tracheostomy tube secured to neck with umbilical tape.

Technical Action

11. Close majority of incision with simple interrupted sutures, but avoid an airtight seal around tube to allow venting of air from insertion site.

Rationale/Amplification

11. Air will often escape from the tracheal incision and must be allowed to vent to the outside of the patient. Otherwise, the air will accumulate subcutaneously, as well as into the mediastinum.

Technical Action	Rationale/Amplification
12. Cover skin incision with sterile gauze that has been cut to fit around tube (Fig. 34-5) and cover loosely with roll gauze.	**12.** Applying a light bandage will allow the necessary air leakage into the environment.
13. Secure tracheostomy tube to neck using umbilical tape or roll gauze (Fig. 34-6).	**13.** The tube should be double-tied around the neck.
14. If using a cuffed tube, inflate only if mechanical ventilation is required or to prevent aspiration in first 24 hours.	**14.** High pressure inflation of the cuff should be avoided to prevent tracheal necrosis.

Bibliography

Aron DN, Crowe DT: Upper airway obstruction. Vet Clin North Am Small Anim Pract 15: 897, 1985

Hedlund CS: Tracheostomies in the management of canine and feline upper respiratory disease. Vet Clin North Am Small Anim Pract 24: 873–886, 1994

Hedlund CS, Tangner CH, Montgomery DL, Hobson HP: A procedure for permanent tracheostomy and its effects on tracheal mucosa. Vet Surg 11: 13, 1982

Jandrey K: Tracheostomies; UCD SVECCS Respiratory Watch, 2003

Kirk RW, Bistner SI: Handbook of Veterinary Procedures and Emergency Treatment, 7th edition. Philadelphia, WB Saunders, 2000

MacIntire DK, Drobratz KJ, Haskins SC, Saxon WD: Manual of Small Animal Emergency and Critical Care Medicine. Philadelphia, Lippincott, 2005

MacIntire DK, Henderson RA, Wilson ER, Huber ML: Transverse flap tracheostomy: A technique for temporary tracheostomy of intermediate duration. J Veterinary Emergency & Critical Care 5: 25–31, 1995

Chapter 35

Cardiopulmonary Resuscitation

Each morning we are born again. What we do today is what matters most.

BUDDHA

Cardiopulmonary resuscitation (CPR) is the treatment used to establish effective perfusion to the heart and brain post-CPA (cardiopulmonary arrest).

New guidelines for veterinary CPR were established in 2012 by the RECOVER initiative (http://acvecc-recover.org), which discourages the use of the term CPCR (cardiopulmonary-cerebral resuscitation). CPR is an easily recognizable term that is used by both veterinary and medical professionals, thereby lessening the likelihood of confusion.

Purposes

1. Provide pulmonary blood flow for oxygen uptake and CO_2 elimination during CPA
2. Provide tissue perfusion for oxygen delivery to restore cellular metabolic activity during CPA

Complications

1. Tracheal laceration/rupture from ET tube placement
2. Internal hemorrhage due to chest/abdominal compressions
3. Other complications directly relating to CPA
4. Death

Equipment Needed (Figures 35-1 and 35-2)

Crash cart or crash box containing:
- Tracheal intubation supplies

Crow and Walshaw's Manual of Clinical Procedures in Dogs, Cats, Rabbits, and Rodents, Fourth Edition. Edited by Jennifer E. Boyle. Published 2016 by John Wiley & Sons, Inc.
Companion Website: www.wiley.com/go/boyle/manual4e

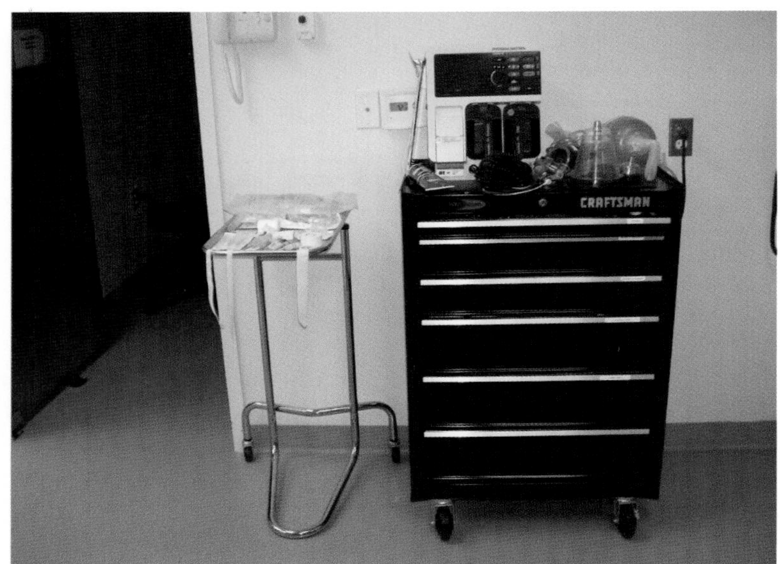

Figure 35-1 Crash cart.

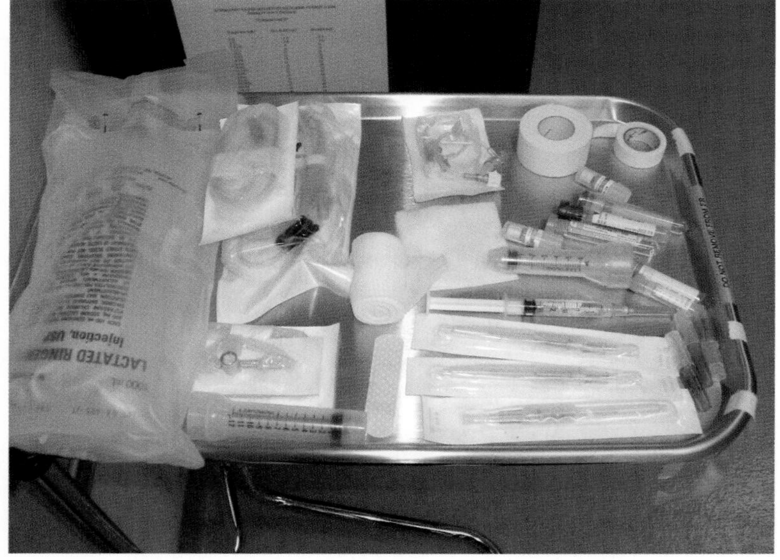

Figure 35-2 Tray prepared with CPR supplies.

- IV catheter supplies
- Stethoscope
- ECG
- Resuscitation drugs:
  - Epinephrine
  - Vasopressin

  - Atropine
  - Reversal agents
  - Sodium bicarbonate
- Defibrillator*
- Doppler*
- ETCO2 monitor*

* *If available.*

Restraint and Positioning

Patients should be positioned in right lateral recumbency. Dorsal recumbency can be used in barrel-chested dogs.

Note: *The ideal number of participants in a resuscitation attempt is 3–5. In a small practice, when staffing is limited, it may be helpful to train the receptionists and kennel help to be a part of the CPR team. Each person can be taught to carry out a specific task.*

SMALL DOGS AND CATS

Procedure (Fig. 35-3)

Technical Action	Rationale/Amplification
1. Intubate using appropriate sized endotracheal tube.	1. See Chapter 17 Endotracheal intubation. Human studies show that chest compressions should be initiated first, but unlike humans, most animal arrests are non-cardiac in nature. Ideally, ventilation and chest compressions should happen simultaneously, but chest compressions can be started while preparing to intubate.
2. Start ventilation at a rate of 10 breaths per minute with a tidal volume of 10 mL/kg and an inspiratory time of 1 second.	2. In non-intubated dogs and cats or if there is only one participant, a compression to ventilation ratio of 30:2 is recommended. In intubated patents with multiple participants, continuous chest compressions with simultaneous ventilation are recommended. NOTE: *Non-intubated patients can be ventilated using mouth to snout technique: however, as they cannot be performed simultaneously, 2 breaths would be followed by 30 chest compressions.*

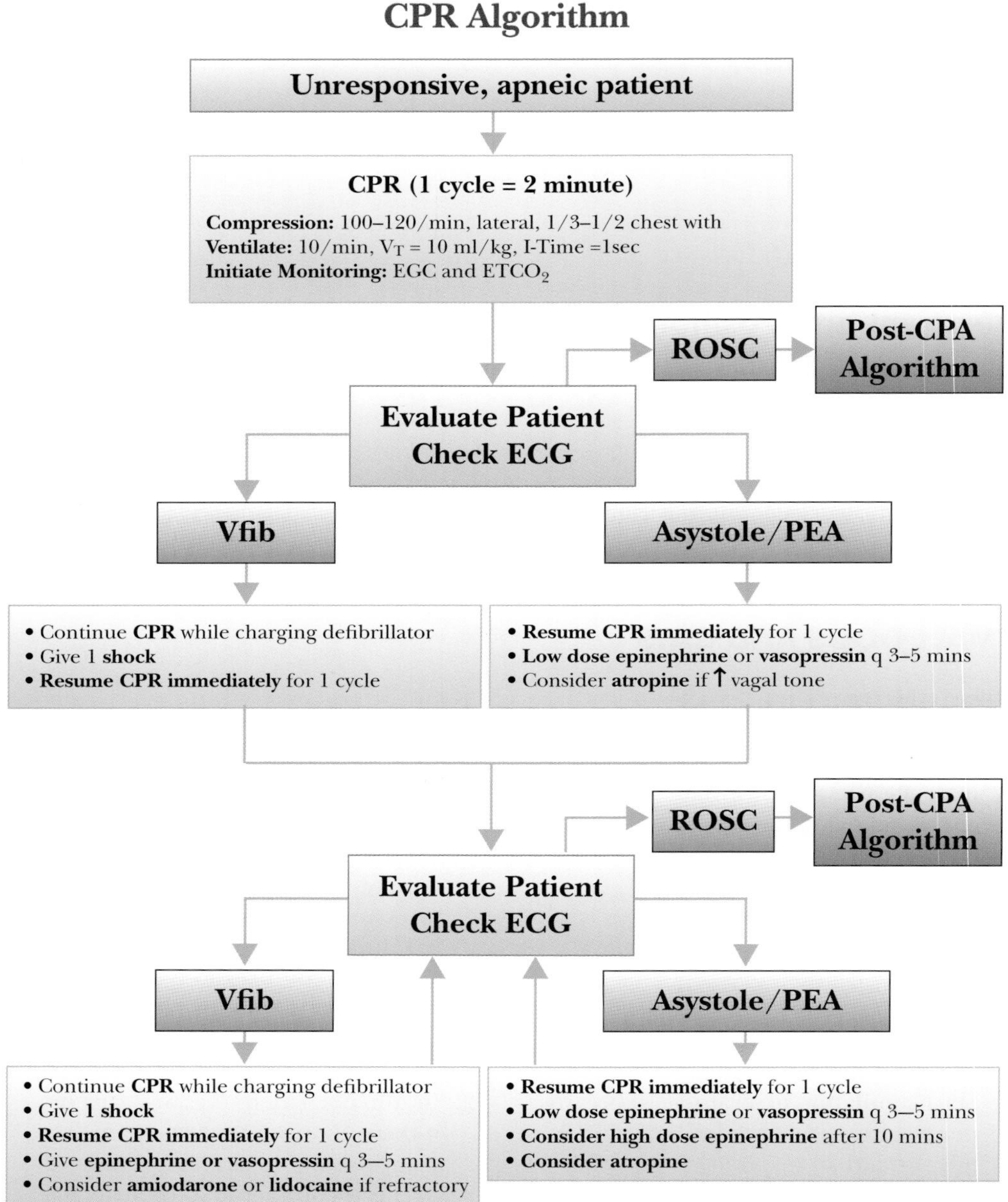

Figure 35-3 RECOVER CPR Algorithm. This figure is duplicated with permission from: J Vet Emerg Crit Care, Fletcher DJ, Boller M, Brainard BM, Haskins SC, Hopper K, McMichael MA, Rozanski EA, Rush JE, Smarick SD. RECOVER evidence and knowledge gap analysis on veterinary CPR. Part 7: Clinical guidelines 22(S1): p. S104, 2012.

Technical Action	Rationale/Amplification
3. Start chest compressions at a rate of 100–120 compressions/minute.	3. Chest compressions should be done in lateral recumbency with a compression depth of between 1/3 and 1/2 the width of the chest. In cats and small dogs, circumferential compressions rather than lateral compressions may be considered.
4. Allow the chest wall to fully recoil between compressions.	4. Based on the thoracic pump theory, the compression of the chest results in an increase of overall intrathoracic pressure causing forward blood flow. During recoil of the chest, intrathoracic pressure facilitates blood flow from the periphery into the thorax and lungs.
5. CPR should be performed in 2-minute cycles without interruption, and duration of pauses between cycles minimized.	5. Human studies have shown increased mortality associated with interruptions in chest compressions for defibrillation attempts, obtaining venous access and checking ECG.
6. Rotate chest compressors every 2 minutes to avoid fatigue and ensure that compressions maintain efficacy.	6. A Doppler probe can be used on the eye to assess effectiveness of the compressions.
7. Place ECG and evaluate during intercycle pauses to determine if there is a rhythm. The ECG evaluation should be done rapidly, and should not delay recommencement of compressions.	
8. Place IV catheter (see Chapter 4).	8. An alternative to intravenous is intraosseous (see chapter 33). Intravenous fluid administration is not recommended unless the patient is hypovolemic; however, any drugs given through catheter should be followed by a bolus of fluids to be sure drugs reach the central bloodstream.
9. If catheter placement is unsuccessful, drugs can go intratracheally.	9. The drugs that may be administered by this route include epinephrine, atropine, and vasopressin. If this route used, then the drug dosage is doubled and added to sterile saline or water for volume. The drugs are then injected down the trach tube through a long

Technical Action

Rationale/Amplification

catheter that extends beyond the endotracheal tube.
NOTE: *Intracardiac injections are no longer recommended due to the potential problems that can occur with this route.*

10. Administer epinephrine at an initial dose of 0.01 mg/kg. Dosage can be increased to 0.1 mg/kg in the cases of prolonged arrest. Epinephrine should be redosed every 3–5 minutes (Fig. 35-4).

10. Epinephrine should be administered during every other 2-minute cycle. Vasopressin may be used as a substitute or in combination with epinephrine at a dose of 0.08 U/kg IV.

11. Atropine can be given once at a dose of 0.04 mg/kg if the patient is in asystole.

12. Reversal agents such as naloxone, flumazenil, and atipamezole may be given if an opioid, benzodiazepine or alpha-2-agonist was administered prior to the cardiac arrest.

13. Sodium bicarbonate (NaHCO3) can be given at a dose of 1 mEq/kg to correct metabolic acidosis, if the cardiac arrest is greater than 10–15 minutes.

13. While not recommended in the routine treatment of cardiac arrest, calcium may be indicated when hyperkalemia or hypocalcemia is present. The dose of calcium is 0.1 ml/kg of 10% calcium chloride or 0.4 ml/kg of 10% calcium gluconate.

14. A patient in ventricular fibrillation or pulseless ventricular tachycardia should be defibrillated. If a defibrillator is not available, the patient can be mechanically defibrillated with a precordial thump. After defibrillation, another 2-minute cycle of CPR should be started immediately.

14. Following the application of a contact gel and the defibrillator charged to the desired energy level, chest compressions and ventilation are halted and the patient placed in dorsal recumbency. Place the defibrillator paddles firmly over the heart on each side of the chest. For external defibrillation the joules should be set at 4–6 joules/kg for monophasic and 2–4 joules/kg for biphasic defibrillation. Internal defibrillation is 0.2–0.5 joules/kg. All participants must be clear of the area/patient before the defibrillator is discharged.
NOTE: *In the past, it was suggested to rapidly repeat defibrillation up to three times if the patient had a refractory VF or*

Technical Action	Rationale/Amplification
	PVT. It is now suggested that a full 2-minute cycle of CPR be performed before reevaluating the ECG and defibrillating again.
15. CPR should be continued until resuscitative efforts are successful, or up to 20–30 minutes.	**15.** Success rate is approximately 6%, dependent on the cause of arrest. Anesthetic arrests have a relatively high success rate. Patients surviving arrest are typically resuscitated within 20 minutes, with the majority resuscitated in less than 10 minutes.
16. After the arrest the patient should be monitored closely.	**16.** Up to 68% of dogs and 38% of cats that are successfully resuscitated re-arrest, most within 4 hours of the initial arrest. Continuous monitoring and reassessment is necessary to prevent re-arrest.

LARGE DOGS

Procedure (Fig. 35-3)

Technical Action	Rationale/Amplification
1. Intubate using appropriate sized endotracheal tube.	**1.** See Chapter 17 Endotracheal intubation. Human studies show that chest compressions should be initiated first, but unlike humans, most animal arrests are non-cardiac in nature. Ideally, ventilation and chest compressions should happen simultaneously, but chest compressions can be started while preparing to intubate.
2. Start ventilation at a rate of 10 breaths per minute with a tidal volume of 10 mL/kg and an inspiratory time of 1 second.	**2.** In non-intubated dogs and cats or if there is only one participant, a compression to ventilation ratio of 30:2 is recommended. In intubated patents with multiple participants, continuous chest compressions with simultaneous ventilation are recommended. NOTE: *Non-intubated patients can be ventilated using mouth to snout technique; however, as they*

Technical Action	Rationale/Amplification
	cannot be performed simultaneously, 2 breaths would be followed by 30 chest compressions.
3. Start chest compressions at a rate of 100–120 compressions/minute.	**3.** Chest compressions should be done with a compression depth of between one-third and half the width of the chest. In large and giant breed dogs, chest compressions may prove more effective with the hands placed over the widest portion of the chest. In barrel-chested dogs, chest compressions can be done with the dog in dorsal recumbency and the hands directly over the heart.
4. Allow the chest wall to fully recoil between compressions.	**4.** Based on the thoracic pump theory, the compression of the chest results in an increase of overall intrathoracic pressure causing forward blood flow. During recoil of the chest, intrathoracic pressure facilitates blood flow from the periphery into the thorax and lungs.
5. CPR should be performed in 2-minute cycles without interruption, and duration of pauses between cycles minimized.	**5.** Human studies have shown increased mortality associated with interruptions in chest compressions for defibrillation attempts, obtaining venous access, and checking ECG.
6. Rotate chest compressors every 2 minutes to avoid fatigue and ensure that compressions maintain efficacy.	**6.** A Doppler probe can be used on the eye to assess effectiveness of the compressions.
7. Place ECG and evaluate during intercycle pauses to determine if there is a rhythm. The ECG evaluation should be done rapidly, and should not delay recommencement of compressions.	
8. Place IV catheter (see Chapter 4).	**8.** An alternative to intravenous is intraosseous (see Chapter 33). Intravenous fluid administration is not recommended unless the patient is hypovolemic; however, any drugs given through catheter should be followed by a bolus of fluids to be sure drugs reach the central bloodstream.

Technical Action	Rationale/Amplification
9. If catheter placement is unsuccessful, drugs can go intratracheally.	**9.** The drugs that may be administered by this route include epinephrine, atropine, and vasopressin. If this route used, then the drug dosage is doubled and added to sterile saline or water for volume. The drugs are then injected down the trach tube through a long catheter that extends beyond the endotracheal tube. NOTE: *Intracardiac injections are no longer recommended due to the potential problems that can occur with this route.*
10. Administer epinephrine at an initial dose of 0.01 mg/kg. Dosage can be increased to 0.1 mg/kg in the cases of prolonged arrest. Epinephrine should be redosed every 3–5 minutes (Fig. 35-4).	**10.** Epinephrine should be administered during every other 2-minute cycle. Vasopressin may be used as a substitute or in combination with epinephrine at a dose of 0.08 U/kg IV.

CPR Emergency Drugs and Doses

		Weight (kg)	2.5	5	10	15	20	25	30	35	40	45	50
		Weight (lb)	5	10	20	30	40	50	60	70	80	90	100
	DRUG	**DOSE**	**ml**	**ml**	**ml**	**ml**	**ml**	**ml**	**ml**	**ml**	**ml**	**ml**	**ml**
Arrest	**Epi Low** (1:1000)	**0.01 mg/kg**	0.03	0.05	0.1	0.15	0.2	0.25	0.3	0.35	0.4	0.45	0.5
Arrest	**Epi High** (1:1000)	**0.1 mg/kg**	0.25	0.5	1	1.5	2	2.5	3	3.5	4	4.5	5
Arrest	**Vasopressin** (20 U/ml)	**0.8 U/kg**	0.1	0.2	0.4	0.6	0.8	1	1.2	1.4	1.6	1.8	2
Arrest	**Atropine** (0.54 mg/ml)	**0.05 mg/kg**	0.25	0.5	1	1.5	2	2.5	3	3.5	4	4.5	5
Anti-Arrhyth	**Amiodarone** (50 mg/ml)	**5 mg/kg**	0.25	0.5	1	1.5	2	2.5	3	3.5	4	4.5	5
Anti-Arrhyth	**Lidocaine** (20 mg/ml)	**2-8 mg/kg**	0.25	0.5	1	1.5	2	2.5	3	3.5	4	4.5	5
Reversal	**Naloxone** (0.4 mg/ml)	**0.04 mg/kg**	0.25	0.5	1	1.5	2	2.5	3	3.5	4	4.5	5
Reversal	**Flumazenil** (0.1 mg/ml)	**0.01 mg/kg**	0.25	0.5	1	1.5	2	2.5	3	3.5	4	4.5	5
Reversal	**Atipamezole** (5 mg/ml)	**50 ųg/kg**	0.03	0.05	0.1	0.15	0.2	0.25	0.3	0.35	0.4	0.45	0.5
Defib Monophasic	**External Defib** (J)	**2-10 J/kg**	20	30	50	100	200	200	200	300	300	300	360
Defib Monophasic	**Internal Defib** (J)	**0.2-1 J/kg**	2	3	5	10	20	20	20	30	30	30	50

Figure 35-4 RECOVER Drug Dosage Chart. This figure is duplicated with permission from: J Vet Emerg Crit Care, Fletcher DJ, Boller M, Brainard BM, Haskins SC, Hopper K, McMichael MA, Rozanski EA, Rush JE, Smarick SD. RECOVER evidence and knowledge gap analysis on veterinary CPR. Part 7: Clinical guidelines; 22(S1): p. S107, 2012.

Technical Action	Rationale/Amplification
11. Atropine can be given once at a dose of 0.04 mg/kg if the patient is in asystole.	
12. Reversal agents such as naloxone, flumazenil, and atipamezole may be given if an opioid, benzodiazepine or alpha-2-agonist was administered prior to the cardiac arrest.	
13. Sodium bicarbonate ($NaHCO_3$) can be given at a dose of 1 mEq/kg to correct metabolic acidosis, if the cardiac arrest is greater than 10–15 minutes.	**13.** While not recommended in the routine treatment of cardiac arrest, calcium may be indicated when hyperkalemia or hypocalcemia is present. The dose of calcium is 0.1 ml/kg of 10% calcium chloride or 0.4 ml/kg of 10% calcium gluconate.
14. A patient in ventricular fibrillation or pulseless ventricular tachycardia should be defibrillated. If a defibrillator is not available, the patient can be mechanically defibrillated with a precordial thump. After defibrillation, another 2-minute cycle of CPR should be started immediately.	**14.** Following the application of a contact gel and the defibrillator charged to the desired energy level, chest compressions and ventilation are halted and the patient placed in dorsal recumbency. Place the defibrillator paddles firmly over the heart on each side of the chest. For external defibrillation the joules should be set at 4–6 joules/kg for monophasic and 2–4 joules/kg for biphasic defibrillation. Internal defibrillation is 0.2–0.5 joules/kg. All participants must be clear of the area/patient before the defibrillator is discharged. NOTE: *In the past, it was suggested to rapidly repeat defibrillation up to 3 times if the patient had a refractory VF or PVT. It is now suggested that a full 2-minute cycle of CPR be performed before reevaluating the ECG and defibrillating again.*
15. CPR should be continued until resuscitative efforts are successful, or up to 20–30 minutes.	**15.** Success rate is approximately 6%, dependent on the cause of arrest. Anesthetic arrests have a relatively high success rate. Patients surviving arrest are typically resuscitated within 20 minutes, with the majority resuscitated in less than 10 minutes.

Technical Action

16. After the arrest the patient should be monitored closely.

Rationale/Amplification

16. Up to 68% of dogs and 38% of cats that are successfully resuscitated re-arrest, most within 4 hours of the initial arrest. Continuous monitoring and reassessment is necessary to prevent re-arrest.

Bibliography

Burkitt J and Davis H: Advanced Monitoring and Procedures for Small Animal Emergency and Critical Care. Oxford, Wiley-Blackwell, 2012

Davis H: Cardiopulmonary Resuscitation (CPR) Update. Atlantic Coast Veterinary Conference, 2012

Fletcher DJ: CPR: Basic and Advanced Life Support. International Veterinary Emergency and Critical Care Symposium, 2013

Fletcher DJ, Boller M, Brainard BM, Haskins SC, Hopper K, McMichael MA, Rozanski EA, Rush JE, Smarick SD: RECOVER evidence and knowledge gap analysis on veterinary CPR. Part 7: Clinical guidelines. J Vet Emerg Crit Care22(S1): S102–S131, 2012

Hackett, T: Cardiopulmonary Resuscitation. Central Veterinary Conference, 2013, Kansas City

Wells RJ: CPCR: Overview and Update. International Veterinary Emergency and Critical Care Symposium, 2008

Part IV

Routine Clinical Procedures in Small Mammals

In the last two decades, many people have discovered the joys of owning a house rabbit. Rabbits are curious, affectionate, and playful. They are easily trained to use a litter pan. Spaying or castrating eliminates the few negative behavioral traits these animals have. A rabbit normally naps during the morning and afternoon and is quite lively in the early evening. Thus, the rabbit is quite content to rest in an indoor cage during the day and interact with its owner(s) in the evening.

American and British house rabbit associations advise owners to have their pet rabbits neutered. Veterinarians, therefore, can expect to see young rabbits for surgery and older rabbits for diagnostic and therapeutic procedures.

A rabbit's size approximates that of a cat or small dog. Many clinical procedures that are routinely performed on dogs or cats can be utilized in rabbits. The rabbit section focuses on key differences in restraint and handling as well as modification of some procedures for the rabbit. We encourage our readers to consult with laboratory animal veterinarians and veterinarians in exotic animal practice when dealing with complex medical cases. Rabbits are great patients, so hop to it!

One of the authors has spent more than two decades looking after the special needs of laboratory animals at two universities.The unique nature of each of these rodents makes them interesting and fun to handle and study. Even though their lives are relatively short, they deserve the same respect and gentle, humane treatment that we prescribe for the dog, cat, and rabbit.

Do all the good you can,
In all the ways you can,
In all the places you can,
At all the times you can,
To all the [creatures] you can,
As long as ever you can.

Adapted from JOHN WESLEY

What's up, doc?

BUGS BUNNY

Chapter 36

Restraint of Rabbits

Once there was a little bunny who wanted to run away. So he said to his mother, "I am running away." "If you run away," said his mother, "I will run after you. For you are my little bunny."

MARGARET WISE BROWN, The Runaway Bunny

Restraint is the restriction of an animal's activity by verbal, physical, or pharmacologic means so that the animal is prevented from injuring itself or others.

Purposes

1. To facilitate physical examination, including ophthalmic examinations
2. To administer oral, injectable, and topical materials
3. To apply bandages
4. To perform certain procedures (e.g. intravenous catheterization, pedicure)

Complications

1. Dyspnea
2. Hyperthermia
3. Hind limb paralysis due to fractured back (especially the seventh lumbar vertebra)

Equipment Needed

- Large bath towel
- Cat bag

Crow and Walshaw's Manual of Clinical Procedures in Dogs, Cats, Rabbits, and Rodents, Fourth Edition. Edited by Jennifer E. Boyle. Published 2016 by John Wiley & Sons, Inc.
Companion Website: www.wiley.com/go/boyle/manual4e

MOVING OR CARRYING A RABBIT

Procedure

Technical Action	Rationale/Amplification
1. Observe the rabbit briefly in its cage or pen before attempting to handle it, noting its attitude.	1. If the rabbit seems aggressive, it may be necessary to throw a towel over the rabbit to remove it from the cage or pen. An aggressive rabbit or a nursing doe may quickly inflict painful bites on a hand that is reaching for it.
2. Determine whether the rabbit is breathing effortlessly at the usual rate of 30–60 breaths per minute.	2. Even minimal restraint may cause respiratory arrest in a dyspneic rabbit.
3. Talk quietly to the rabbit.	3. From a rabbit's point of view, a human being is a large potential predator. A calm, quiet approach is always advisable.
4. Try to stroke the rabbit's head, with your hand coming from behind its head.	4. One does not offer a hand for the rabbit to sniff, as with a dog, because a rabbit, with its laterally placed eyes, has relatively poor depth perception and may mistake the person's hand for food.
5. Gently lift the rabbit by grasping skin over its dorsal neck area with one hand while supporting the rabbit's hindquarters with the other hand, with its feet pointing away from you (Fig. 36-1).	5. Keep the rabbit's back curved to prevent dorsiflexion of the spine and possible fracture. The rabbit's feet should be pointed away from you because a rabbit can inflict painful scratches with its sharp toenails.
6. A quiet-natured rabbit can be carried with one hand under its thorax and the other hand supporting the rabbit's hindquarters (Fig. 36-2).	6. This position is more comfortable for large rabbits than being partially supported by the skin of the dorsal neck region.
7. Tuck the rabbit's head and front feet under your upper arm and carry the rabbit a short distance with its body supported by your forearm (Fig. 36-3).	7. When transporting a rabbit in a noisy area or to another room, it is safer to place the rabbit in a box or commercial carrier before moving it.
8. When placing the rabbit back into the cage or pen, it should be placed hind-end first.	8. This can help prevent potential spinal injury from the rabbit from kicking out/moving away from restraint.

NOTE: *It is essential to keep the rabbit's back in its normal curved posture during handling and restraint. The rabbit's relatively fragile skeleton and large lumbar muscles render it susceptible to spinal fracture while struggling.*

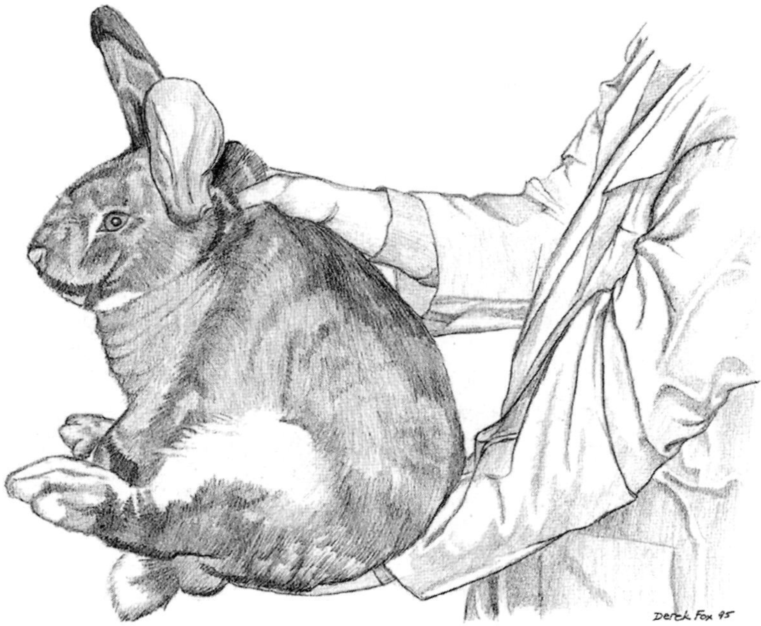

Figure 36-1 Carrying a rabbit by lifting dorsal neck skin while supporting rabbit's hindquarters.

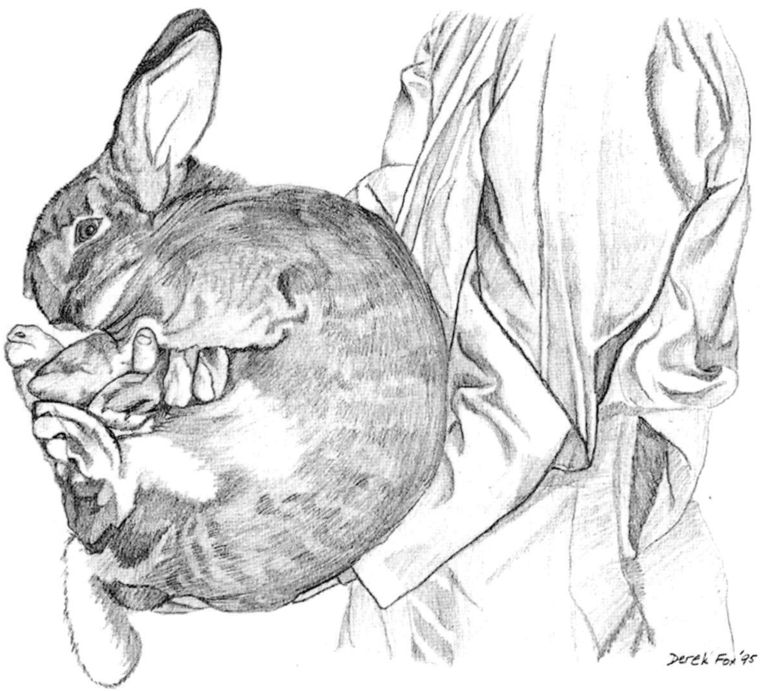

Figure 36-2 Carrying a rabbit by placing one hand under rabbit's thorax while supporting its hindquarters.

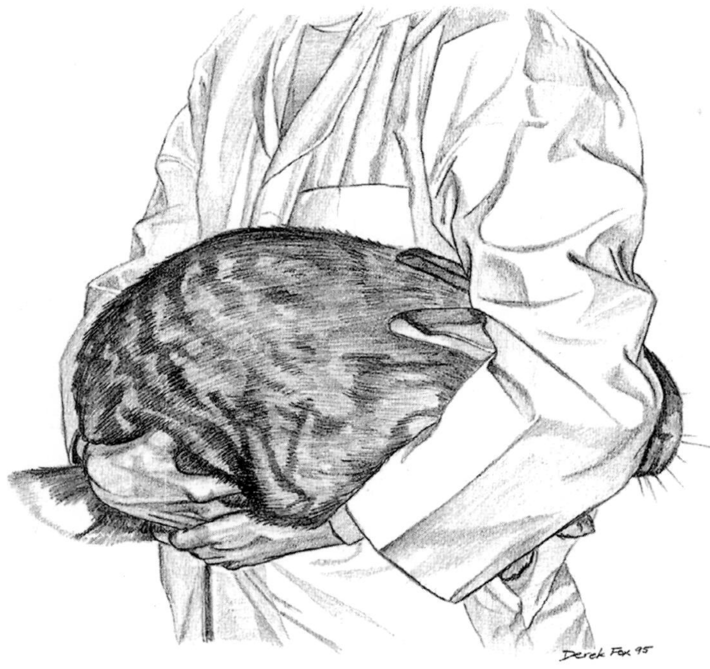

Figure 36-3 Carrying a rabbit by tucking its head under the handler's upper arm and supporting the rabbit's body with a forearm.

TOWEL RESTRAINT OF A RABBIT

Procedure

Technical Action	Rationale/Amplification
1. Place the rabbit in the middle of a large towel (Fig. 36-4).	1. If the rabbit is struggling, do this entire procedure on the floor to prevent injury to the animal and the handler if the rabbit tries to jump off the table.
2. Pull up on one end of the towel while wrapping and tucking the towel securely around the rabbit's neck and covering one front foot (Fig. 36-5).	2. Tension on one end of the towel helps ensure a secure wrap around the rabbit's neck. It is important to completely enclose one front foot in the underneath towel wrap. The rabbit tends to hop with its front feet simultaneously and having a front foot securely restrained by the towel has a calming effect.

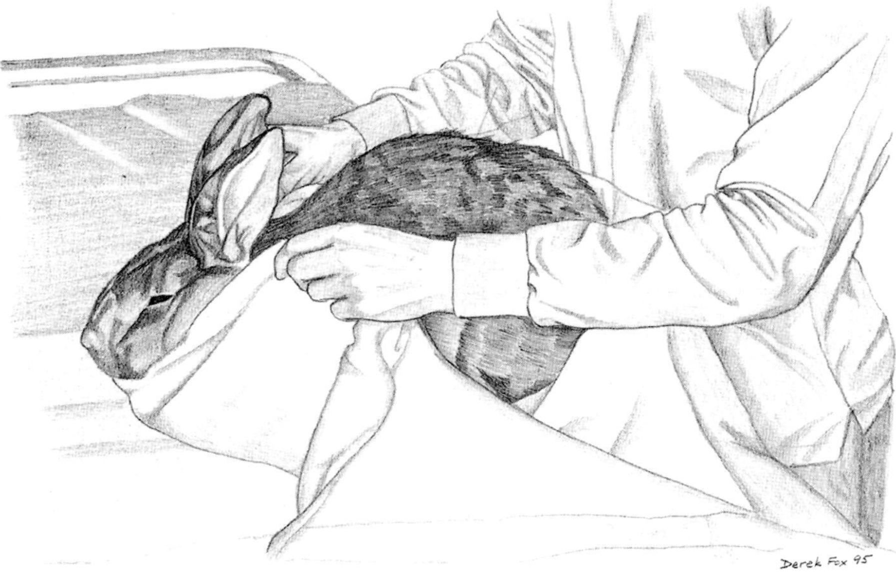

Figure 36-4 Placing rabbit in middle of towel for towel restraint wrap.

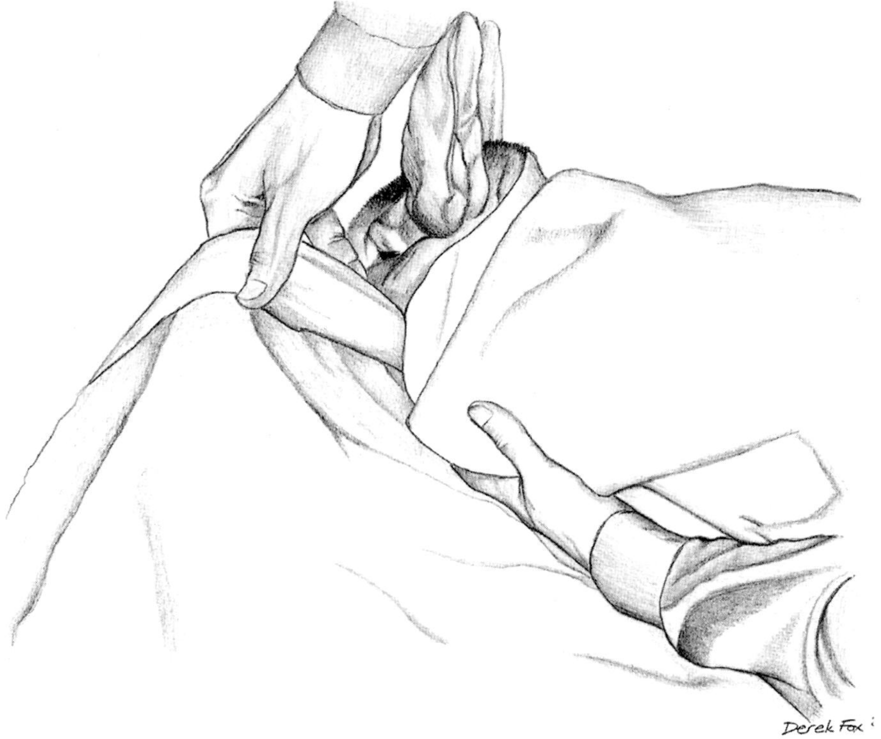

Figure 36-5 Wrapping one end of the towel around the rabbit and under its front foot while keeping upward tension on the other end of the towel.

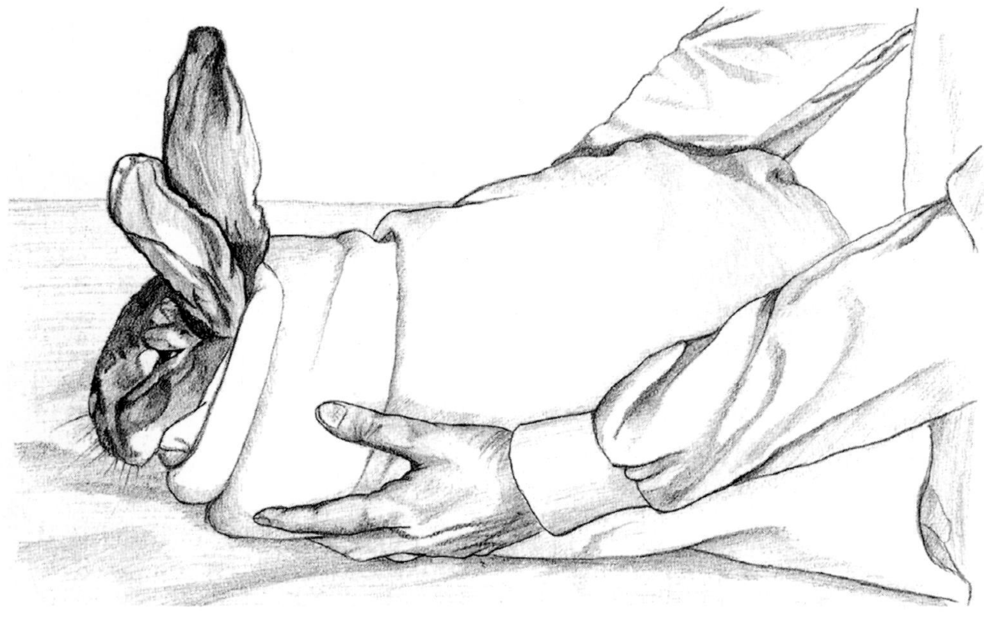

Figure 36-6 Rabbit securely wrapped in a towel.

Technical Action	Rationale/Amplification
3. Wrap the other end of the towel securely around the rabbit, leaving only the head exposed (Fig. 36-6).	3. Covering the rabbit's front feet with the towel prevents the animal from squirming out of the towel.
4. Leave towel in place for such procedures as ophthalmic procedures (Chapter 9), blood collection from ear artery or vein, intravenous catheter placement in ear vein, and oral examination and administration of oral medications.	4. The towel is warm and comfortable, perhaps explaining why rabbits tend to relax and their ear blood vessels dilate when the towel restraint method is used.
5. Unwrap small areas of rabbit for performing procedures such as toenail clipping or injections.	

CAT BAG RESTRAINT OF A RABBIT

Procedure

Technical Action	Rationale/Amplification
1. Place the rabbit in the cat bag by grasping skin over the rabbit's dorsal neck area with one hand and supporting the rabbit's hindquarters with the other hand and slipping the rabbit backwards into the bag.	1. Supporting the rabbit's back will help prevent struggling without using excessive force to restrain.
2. Secure the cat bag as necessary, leaving only the head exposed.	
3. Procedures such as ophthalmic procedures (Chapter 9), blood collection from ear artery or vein, intravenous catheter placement in ear vein, and oral examination and administration of oral medications can be accommodated in this manner.	
4. Sections of the cat bag can be unzipped for performing procedures such as toenail clipping or injections.	
5. Remove rabbit from cat bag by backing the rabbit out of the bag.	5. Rabbits are less likely to jump or kick out, thus fracturing their spine, if they are placed backward into cages and such.

RESTRAINT OF AN AGGRESSIVE RABBIT

Procedure

Technical Action	Rationale/Amplification
1. To remove an aggressive rabbit from a cage or carrier, throw a towel over the animal and quickly bundle it up with its head completely covered.	1. Some rabbits will attack the first towel thrown into the cage. While this is occurring, throw a second towel over the rabbit.
2. Place the "bundle" of aggressive rabbit on the floor, rather than on a table, for rewrapping in a more efficient manner.	2. Once on the floor, the rabbit cannot scratch the handler's face and also may "freeze" in position in the unfamiliar surroundings.

Technical Action	Rationale/Amplification
3. After placing an aggressive rabbit on the floor, try putting pressure over the rabbit's shoulder area, immobilizing the front legs, while also applying pressure over the hip area.	

NOTE: *Female rabbits that have not been spayed may become territorial and aggressive. Ovariohysterectomy often results in dramatic improvement in behavior within a few weeks.*

Bibliography

Ackerman S: Aggressive rabbits. Rabbit Health News 8: 4–5, 1993

Beynon PH, Cooper JE: BSAVA Manual of Exotic Pets. Cheltenham, England, British Small Animal Veterinary Association, 1991

Harkness JE, Wagner JE: The Biology and Medicine of Rabbits and Rodents, 4th edition. Philadelphia, Williams and Wilkins, 1995

Hillyer EV: Pet rabbits. Vet Clin North Am: Small Animal Practice 24(1): 25–65, 1994

Laber-Laird K, Swindle MM, Flecknell P: Handbook of Rodent and Rabbit Medicine. Oxford, England, Pergamon Press, 1996

Manning PJ, Ringler DH, Newcomer CH (eds): The Biology of the Laboratory Rabbit, 2nd edition. San Diego, Academic Press, 1994

Okerman L: Diseases of Domestic Rabbits, 2nd edition. Oxford, England, Blackwell Scientific Publications, 1994

Podberscek AL, Blackshaw JK, Beattie AW: The effects of repeated handling by familiar and unfamiliar people on rabbits in individual cages and group pens. Applied Animal Behaviour Science 28: 365–373, 1991

Chapter 37

Selected Clinical Procedures in Rabbits

Peter was not very well during the evening. His mother put him to bed, and made some camomile tea; and she gave a dose of it to Peter! "One table-spoonful to be taken at bed-time."

BEATRIX POTTER, The Tale of Peter Rabbit

Routine clinical procedures in rabbits include blood collection, injections, placement of intravenous catheters, oral administration of medications, and a variety of diagnostic and therapeutic procedures described in Part I and Part II of this book. This chapter highlights the modifications of some of these routine procedures for ease in performing the procedures on the rabbit. If not otherwise specified, a procedure should be performed on a rabbit using the same technique as for a dog or cat.

INTRAVENOUS CATHETERIZATION OF THE RABBIT

Intravenous catheterization is useful in rabbits for collecting blood as well as for administering intravenous fluids to a rabbit.

Blood Collection from the Blood Vessels of a Rabbit's Ear

NOTE: *The marginal ear vein is a good choice for routine blood collection for any rabbit weighing at least 2 kg. The central artery of the ear is accessible and blood collection is rapid unless the vessel is constricted in a cold or nervous rabbit. Small amounts (1–3 mL) of blood may be collected from a rabbit's cephalic vein or lateral saphenous vein.*

Crow and Walshaw's Manual of Clinical Procedures in Dogs, Cats, Rabbits, and Rodents, Fourth Edition. Edited by Jennifer E. Boyle.

Published 2016 by John Wiley & Sons, Inc.
Companion Website: www.wiley.com/go/boyle/manual4e

Equipment Needed

- Cloth towel
- Gauze sponges
- Warm soapy water
- Syringe
- Blood collection tubes
- Drugs for tranquilization (if necessary), for example, acepromazine
- Petroleum jelly
- 24-gauge, over-the-needle intravenous catheter

NOTE: *Rabbit blood clots in 20–90 seconds, especially when collected using a metal needle. For this reason, Teflon-coated intravenous catheters are preferred for blood collection from ear blood vessels.*

Procedure

Technical Action	Rationale/Amplification
1. Administer tranquilizing agent to excitable rabbit.	**1.** It is difficult to collect blood from a frightened rabbit. Peripheral vessels will constrict in such situations.
2. Wrap rabbit in a cloth towel (See Chapter 35).	**2.** Even a tranquilized rabbit should be wrapped in a towel to provide the comfort and warmth that will enhance relaxation of the rabbit during the procedure.
3. Pluck hair over central artery of ear and/or marginal ear vein along edge of ear (Fig. 37-1).	**3.** Removing the hair with an electric clipper is likely to irritate the delicate skin on the rabbit's ear.
4. Clean ear with warm soapy water, if dirty.	**4.** Surface debris should be removed, but cool substances such as alcohol will cause vasoconstriction of the ear blood vessels.
5. Inspect intravenous catheter for flaws.	**5.** Discard any catheter with a barbed needle or with immobile parts.
6. Cover rabbit's eyes with fold of towel (or ask assistant to cover rabbit's eyes with hand).	**6.** A rabbit may tend to move if it sees someone approaching it with an instrument.
7. If necessary, distend (or ask assistant to distend) vein with blood by applying firm pressure on vein at base of ear near rabbit's head.	**7.** Pressure at the base of the ear should be great enough to keep the vein distended but not so much as to shut off arterial flow. Distention of the artery is not necessary.
8. Insert needle and catheter into blood vessel with bevel up.	**8.** Flow of blood into the hub of the needle indicates entry into the blood vessel.
9. Advance needle into blood vessel until at least one-half of needle is within blood vessel (Fig. 37-2).	**9.** The catheter is slightly shorter than the needle in an over-the-needle catheter. Entry of the catheter into the lumen of the blood vessel is ensured by placing at least one-half of the needle within the lumen of the blood vessel.

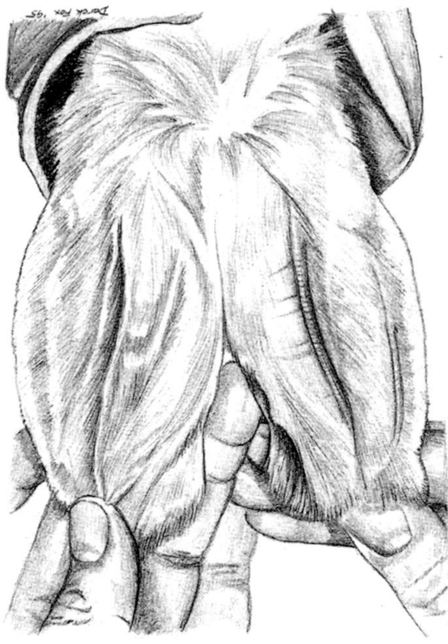

Figure 37-1 Central artery of ear and marginal ear vein of rabbit.

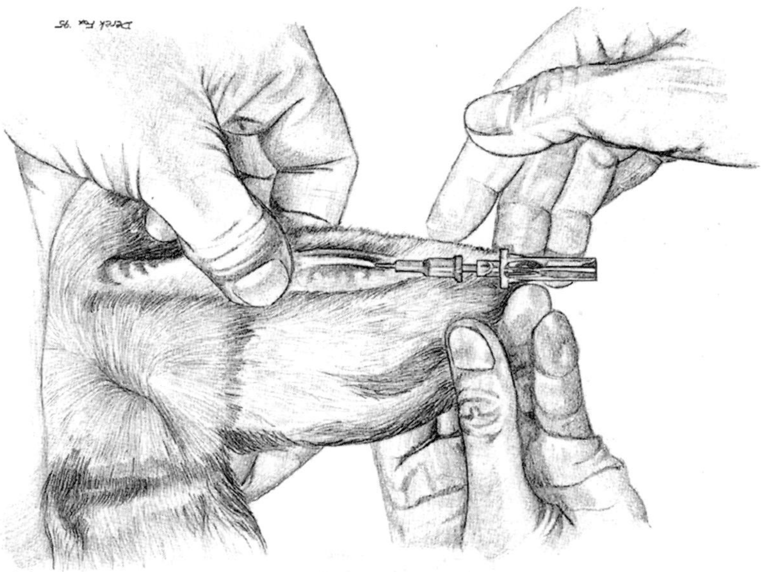

Figure 37-2 Intravenous over-the-needle catheter placed into marginal ear vein of rabbit.

Technical Action	Rationale/Amplification
10. Hold needle in place with fingers of one hand and slowly advance catheter farther into blood vessel with fingers of other hand (Chapter 4).	**10.** Once the advancing of the catheter has begun, the metal needle must not be reinserted through the catheter because the needle could cut the catheter while the catheter is in the vessel.
11. Hold catheter hub and withdraw needle from catheter.	**11.** The catheter can be removed inadvertently if it is not held in place while the needle is withdrawn.
12. Attach syringe to catheter hub and withdraw needle from catheter.	**12.** It may be necessary to hold pressure on the vein at the base of the ear during blood collection.
13. If blood flow stops, rotate catheter within blood vessel or withdraw it slightly.	**13.** The tip of the catheter may be wedged up against the wall of the blood vessel.
14. When catheter is removed, immediately apply pressure to catheterization site with dry gauze sponge.	**14.** Pressure on the catheterization site for 1–3 minutes following catheter removal will decrease the possibility of hemorrhage and subcutaneous hematoma formation.
15. Clean ear thoroughly with warm soapy water. Apply petroleum jelly to area of ear where hair was removed to soothe skin and promote healing.	**15.** Blood is a good culture medium for bacteria and must be removed from the animal's ear or fur at the end of the procedure.

BANDAGING INTRAVENOUS CATHETER FOR ADMINISTERING FLUIDS TO A RABBIT

Procedure

Technical Action	Rationale/Amplification
1. Insert intravenous catheter into marginal ear vein as for blood collection.	**1.** See **Intravenous Catheterization of the Rabbit**.
2. Place injection cap or T-port on catheter (see Chapter 4).	**2.** An injection cap provides a sterile seal to the intravenous catheter. A T-port should be placed on the catheter for continuous fluid administration.
3. Flush catheter with heparinized saline.	**3.** Heparinized saline will keep the catheter patent while the bandage is placed on the ear.
4. Insert small roll of gauze sponges into rabbit's ear.	**4.** The small roll of gauze sponges helps keep the ear cartilage in a natural, comfortable position under the bandage.

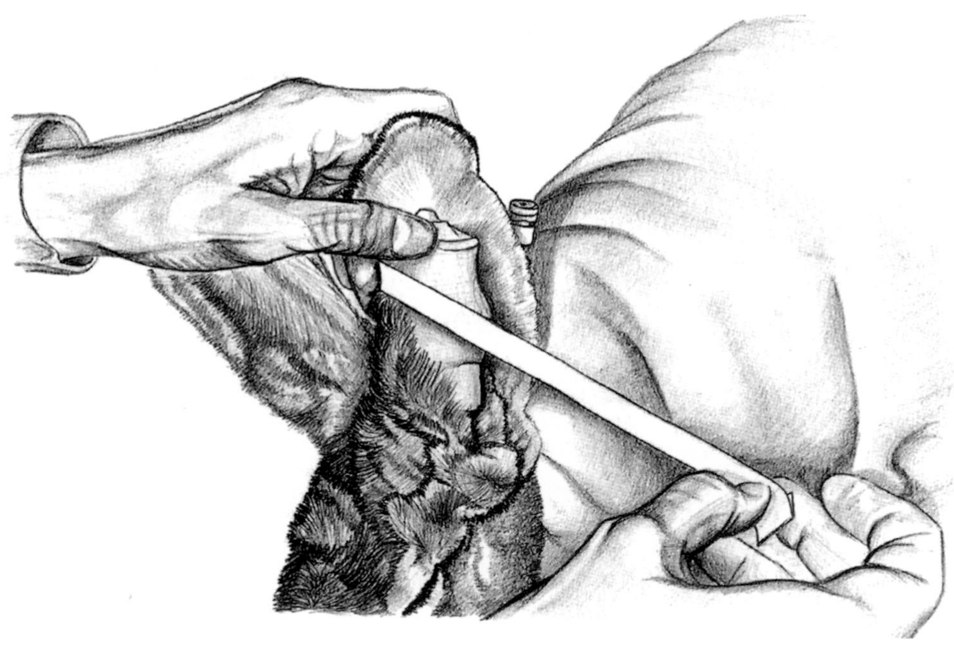

Figure 37-3 Bandaging of intravenous catheter to rabbit's ear.

Technical Action	Rationale/Amplification
5. Wrap adhesive tape strip attached to catheter hub around ear (Fig. 37-3).	**5.** This tape anchors the catheter to the ear. Firm anchoring of the catheter prevents trauma to the vein caused by excessive movement of the catheter.
6. Bandage ear using gauze bandaging material, leaving only injection cap exposed.	**6.** Careful bandaging of the ear over a wide area helps to prevent contamination of the catheter insertion site and resulting infection.
7. Insert small roll of gauze sponges into rabbit's other ear.	**7.** The small roll of gauze sponges will keep the other (noncatheterized) ear in a natural, comfortable position when the two ears are bandaged together.
8. Bandage both ears together and hook up intravenous drip set (Fig. 37-4).	**8.** The rabbit is less likely to scratch at the catheter with front or hind legs if the ears are bandaged together. A single bandaged ear with an intravenous catheter in place will hang down on the side of the rabbit and be a source of annoyance to the animal.

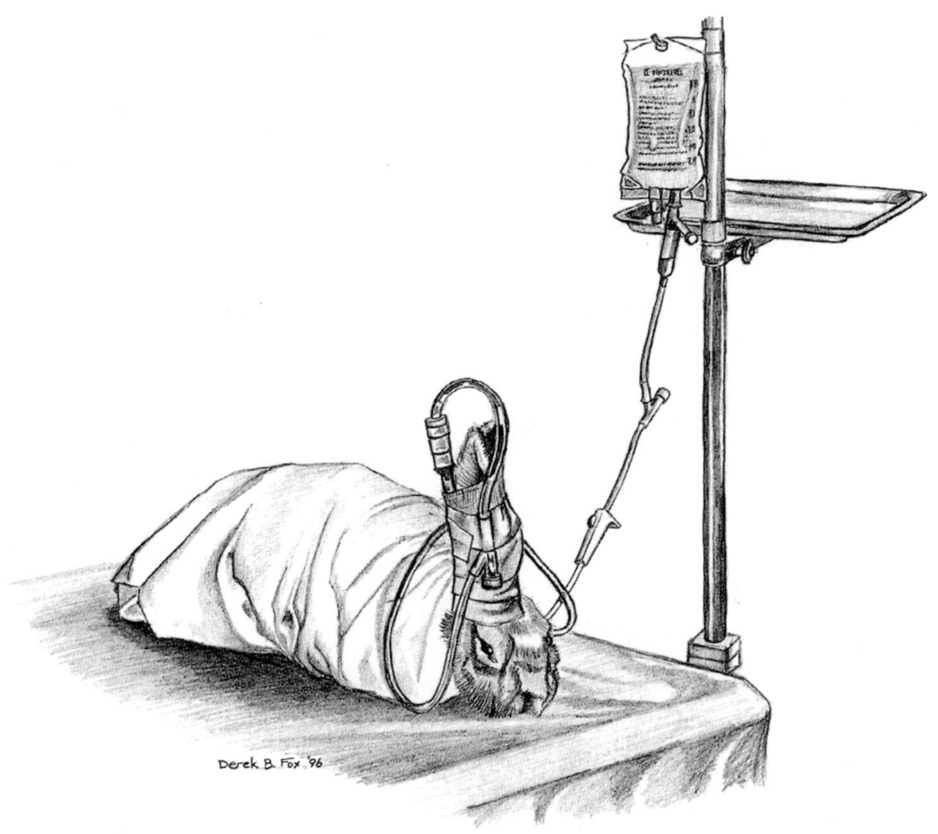

Figure 37-4 Bandaging of ears together for administering intravenous fluids to rabbit via marginal ear vein.

Technical Action	Rationale/Amplification
9. Secure all tubing away from rabbit's mouth.	9. A rabbit will chew through tubes readily, so all tubing must be secured away from the rabbit's mouth. If necessary, an Elizabethan collar can be placed on the rabbit.

BLOOD COLLECTION FROM THE JUGULAR VEIN OF A RABBIT

Procedure

Technical Action	Rationale/Amplification
1. Wrap rabbit in a towel.	1. Tranquilization is advised for this procedure to minimize the possibility of injuring the spine of a struggling rabbit.

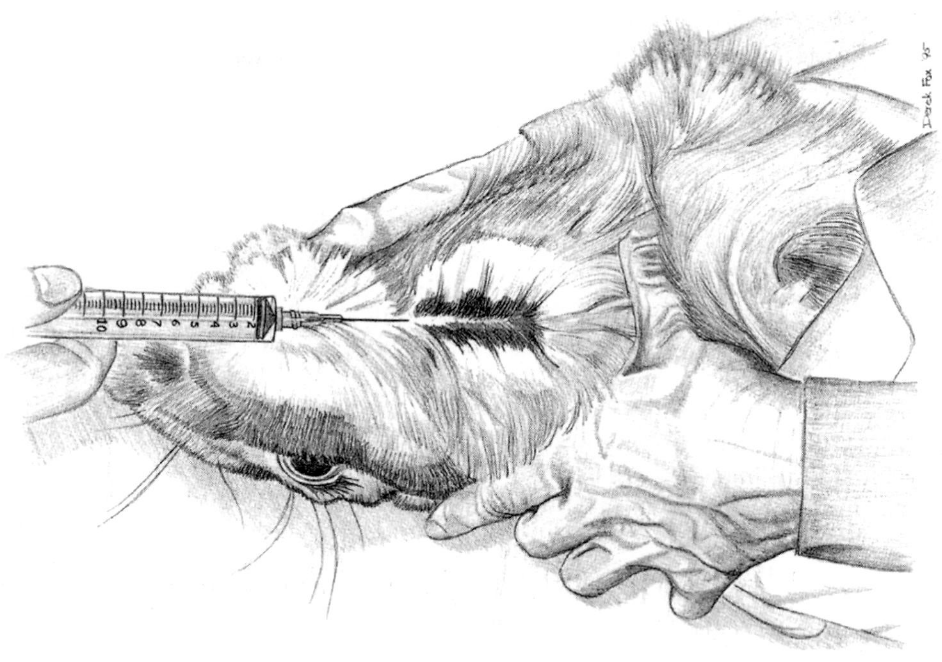

Figure 37-5 Restraint of rabbit for jugular venipuncture.

Technical Action

2. Place towel-wrapped rabbit in dorsal recumbency with its neck extended and its body restrained by an assistant (Fig. 37-5).
3. Collect blood using a needle and syringe.

Rationale/Amplification

2. In a quiet room, some rabbits relax into an almost trancelike state when placed in this position.
3. Hold firm pressure over jugular vein for 1–3 minutes after the needle is removed.

BLOOD COLLECTION FROM THE LATERAL SAPHENOUS VEIN OF A RABBIT

Procedure

Technical Action

1. Wrap rabbit in a towel.

Rationale/Amplification

1. Tranquilization is advised for this procedure to minimize the possibility of back injury to a struggling rabbit.

Technical Action

2. Gently restrain rabbit with the hind leg extended by an assistant.

Rationale/Amplification

2. The ideal site for venipuncture is the lateral saphenous vein. The rabbit is gently restrained with the hind leg extended. The vessel lies across the lateral surface of the tibia, proximal to the hock.

Technical Action

3. Collect blood using a needle and syringe or butterfly catheter.

Rationale/Amplification

3. A butterfly catheter or 25-gauge needle is used with a 1 mL syringe. Hold firm pressure over saphenous vein for 1–2 minutes after the needle is removed.

ORAL ADMINISTRATION OF LIQUID MEDICATION TO RABBITS

Procedure

Technical Action

1. Check medication to be administered, using "The Five Rights": right patient, right drug, right dose, right route, right time and frequency.

Rationale/Amplification

1. It is important to take measures to prevent errors of medication administration.

Technical Action

2. Wash hands.

Rationale/Amplification

2. Washing hands between patients is important in controlling communicable diseases in a hospital. It is advisable to wear examination gloves while administering oral medication to an animal with a communicable disease.

Technical Action

3. Place liquid medication in a small syringe (1-mL syringe for rabbits under 2 kg, 3-mL syringe for rabbits over 2 kg).

Rationale/Amplification

3. The rabbit's mouth does not open widely. Oral dosing may require multiple insertions of a small syringe. A metal ball-tipped feeding needle can also be utilized, but care must be taken to avoid damaging soft tissues in the rabbit's mouth.

Technical Action

4. Place palm of hand on dorsal surface of rabbit's snout and pull back upper lips.

Rationale/Amplification

4. It is important to watch the placement of the syringe in relation to the teeth because a rabbit will generally not swallow liquid placed in the cheek area.

Technical Action

5. With rabbit's nose held parallel with ground, gently insert syringe into rabbit's mouth behind incisor teeth and direct end of syringe back into posterior part of mouth (Fig. 37-6).

Rationale/Amplification

5. Keeping the rabbit's nose parallel to the ground will minimize the possibility of aspiration of the liquid into the respiratory tract.

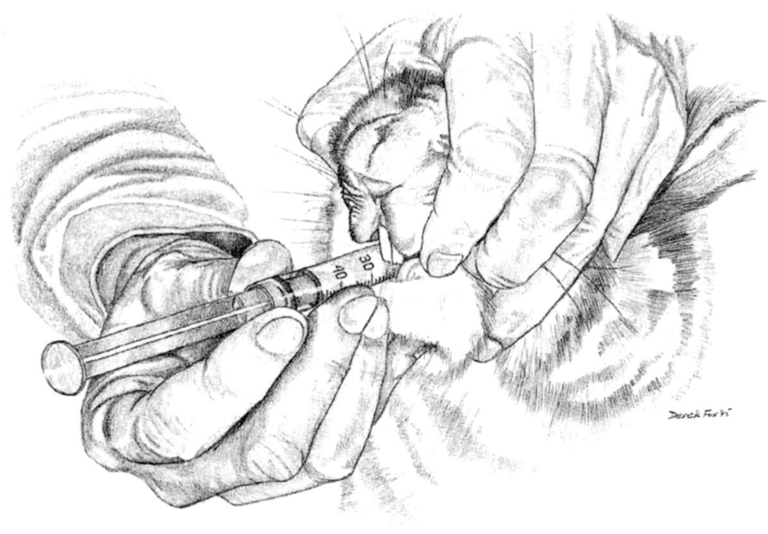

Figure 37-6 Rabbit receiving liquid oral medication.

Technical Action

6. Administer small amount of liquid at a time (3 mL in a 4-kg or larger rabbit) and wait until the rabbit swallows before placing any more liquid into the animal's mouth.
7. Note in rabbit's medical record that medication was given.

Rationale/Amplification

6. A rabbit that refuses to swallow pleasant-flavored liquids may be experiencing abdominal pain.
7. The following information should be noted in the medical record: date, time, medication, dosage, route, initials of individual administering medication, and comments.

NOTE: *A rabbit can be trained to drink from a small-diameter syringe (1–3 mL) if the end of the syringe has been moistened and then dipped into granulated sugar.*

ORAL ADMINISTRATION OF TABLETS TO RABBITS

Some rabbits will eat whole tablets if inserted into a sliced apple or banana. Alternatively, tablets can be crushed and mixed with a variety of treat foods, including bananas, raisins, fruit-flavored yogurt, and fruit jam.

INJECTION TECHNIQUES IN RABBITS

Subcutaneous Injection

The rabbit does not generally object to a subcutaneous injection given in the dorsal neck area. A calm rabbit may be left in its cage and just pushed against one side of the cage while the subcutaneous injection is given. A small-gauge needle (25 or 22 gauge) is suitable.

Intramuscular Injection

The dorsal lumbar muscle group is a large, easily accessible muscle group when a rabbit is partially wrapped in a towel. The quadriceps muscle on the anterior aspect of the femur may also be used.

Intravenous Injection

The marginal ear vein is the most easily accessible vein for intravenous injection in the rabbit. The cephalic and saphenous veins are practical for use only in rabbits that weigh at least 3 kg. Needle size should be 24 gauge or smaller, regardless of the vein used.

URINE COLLECTION

Cystocentesis yields a sterile urine specimen from the rabbit, as for the cat and dog (see Chapter 20). A nonsterile specimen can be obtained by using nonabsorbable veterinary medical litter or aquarium gravel in the rabbit's litter pan.

NOTE: *While cystocentesis is typically performed on conscious animals, sedation may be necessary to limit movement.*

ENDOTRACHEAL INTUBATION IN THE RABBIT

Several factors in the rabbit make endotracheal intubation more challenging than in the dog and cat: a sensitive oropharyngeal area, a long and narrow oral cavity, and a large tongue. There are two techniques commonly used: blind technique and a technique that uses a laryngoscope.

A few drops of local anesthetic placed in the area of the larynx will help minimize laryngospasm. The endotracheal tube should be 2–4 mm internal diameter, depending on the size of the rabbit.

In the blind approach, the sedated rabbit is placed in sternal recumbency with its head held up so that the nostrils point toward the ceiling. An endotracheal tube is lowered gradually into the mouth and observed for misting that would indicate proximity to the larynx. The tube is advanced as the animal takes a breath.

A visual method of endotracheal intubation utilizes a small bladed laryngoscope or an otoscope to locate the vocal folds. A small polypropylene urinary catheter is preplaced in the trachea and the appropriate size endotracheal tube is threaded down into the trachea over the catheter. The catheter is then removed.

Bibliography

Aeschbacher G: Rabbit anesthesia. Comp Contin Educ for Prac Vet 17(8): 1003–1010, 1995

Bradley T: Rabbit care and husbandry. Vet Clin N Amer: Exotic Animal Practice 7(2): 299–313, 2004

Brown C: Diagnostic cystocentesis: technique and considerations, Lab Animal 35, 4, 2006. doi: 10.1038/laban0406-21

Cranney J, Zajac A: A method for jugular blood collection in rabbits. American Association for Laboratory Animal Science: Contemporary Topics 32: 6, 1993

Fick TE, Schalm SW: A simple technique for endotracheal intubation in rabbits. Laboratory Animals 21: 265–266, 1987

Gilroy BA: Endotracheal intubation of rabbits and rodents. Journal of the Amer Vet Med Assoc 179(11): 1295, 1981

Harkness JE, Wagner JE: The Biology and Medicine of Rabbits and Rodents, 4th edition. Philadelphia, Williams and Wilkins, 1995

Hillyer EV: Pet rabbits. Vet Clin North Am: Small Animal Practice 24(1): 25–65, 1994

Kruger J, Zeller W, Schottmann: A simplified procedure for endotracheal intubation in rabbits. Laboratory Animals 28: 176–177, 1994

Laber-Laird K, Swindle MM, Flecknell P: Handbook of Rodent and Rabbit Medicine. Oxford, England, Pergamon Press, 1996

Macrae DJ, Guerreiro D: A simple laryngoscopic technique for the endotracheal intubation of rabbits. Laboratory Animals 23: 59–61, 1989

Okerman L: Diseases of Domestic Rabbits, 2nd edition. Oxford, England, Blackwell Scientific Publications, 1994

Chapter 38

Selected Clinical Procedures in Small Rodents

If you give a mouse a cookie, he's going to ask for a glass of milk.
LAURA JOFFE NUMEROFF, If You Give a Mouse a Cookie

MOVING, CARRYING, AND RESTRAINING SMALL RODENTS

Restraint is the restriction of an animal's activity by verbal, physical, or pharmacologic means so that the animal is prevented from injuring itself or others.

Purposes

1. To facilitate physical examination, including ophthalmic examination
2. To administer oral, injectable, and/or topical materials

Complications

1. Dyspnea
2. Hyperthermia

Equipment Needed

- Handkerchief for mouse, gerbil, or hamster
- Small towel or stockinette for rat, guinea pig, or chinchilla

Crow and Walshaw's Manual of Clinical Procedures in Dogs, Cats, Rabbits, and Rodents, Fourth Edition. Edited by Jennifer E. Boyle. Published 2016 by John Wiley & Sons, Inc.
Companion Website: www.wiley.com/go/boyle/manual4e

Mouse

Technical Action	Rationale/Amplification
1. Lift mouse by base of its tail (Fig. 38-1).	1. If the tail is grasped near the tip, the skin of the tail can be easily torn off.
2. Move mouse quickly to table.	
3. Restrain mouse by grasping skin between its ears and along its back (Fig. 38-2).	3. The mouse can turn around and bite if insufficient skin is held.
4. Hold mouse's tail between fourth and fifth fingers with its back against palm of hand (Fig. 38-3).	4. Supporting the back in this manner is more comfortable for the mouse and prevents it from biting.
5. Observe breathing pattern.	5. The mouse can suffocate if the skin is held too tightly over its neck.

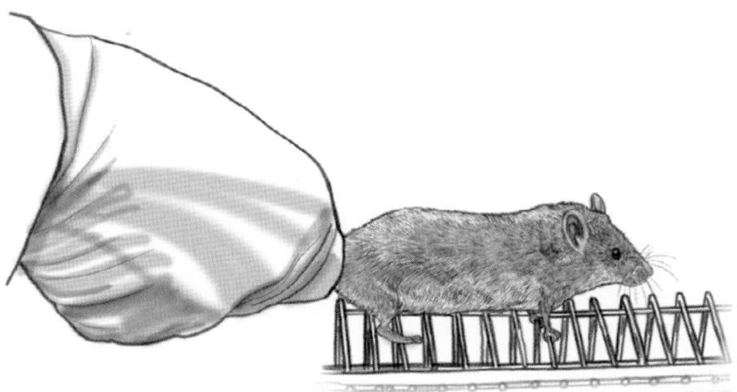

Figure 38-1 Lifting mouse by base of its tail.

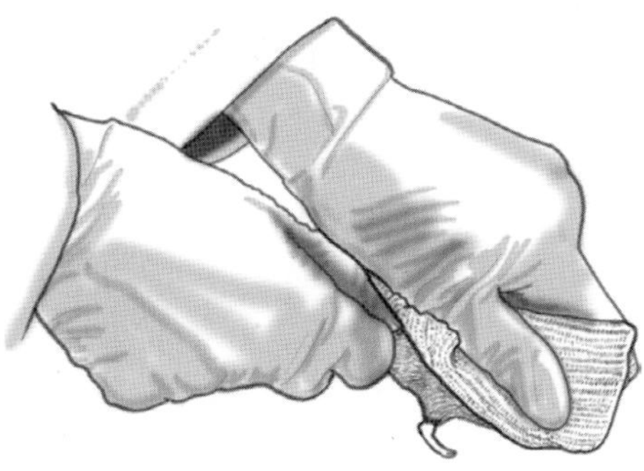

Figure 38-2 Restraining mouse by grasping skin between its ears and along its back.

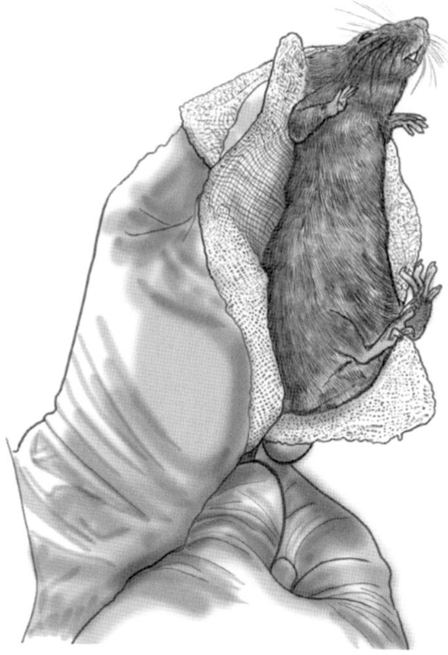

Figure 38-3 Holding tail of mouse between fourth and fifth fingers while resting its back against palm of hand.

Rat

Technical Action

1. Lift rat from cage with tail (Fig. 38-4), then support with two hands and move to table.
2. Support rat on one arm while holding tail with opposite hand (Fig. 38-5).
3. Hold tail, hind legs, and rump with other hand.
4. Place rat in stockinette "sweater" (Fig. 38-6) for minor procedures, including subcutaneous injections and blood collection.

Rationale/Amplification

4. Prepare stockinette "sweater" in advance. Two-inch-wide stockinette is cut to appropriate length. Fold over one end to make collar. One-inch adhesive tape is used to strengthen the collar. The "sweater" must be long enough to cover the whole animal.

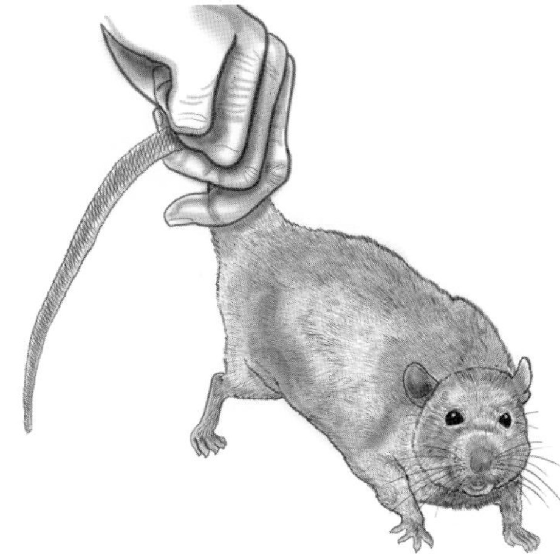

Figure 38-4 Lifting rat from cage with tail.

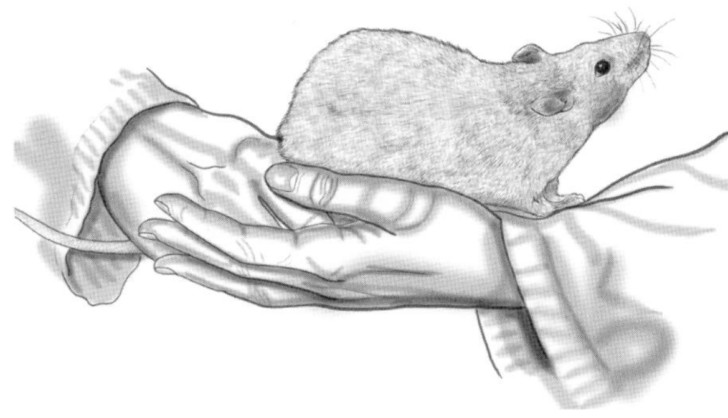

Figure 38-5 Supporting rat on one arm while holding tail with opposite hand.

Guinea Pig, Gerbil, & Chinchilla

Technical Action	Rationale/Amplification
1. Pick up guinea pig by whole body.	1. Guinea pigs are placid animals. Minimal restraint is needed for most simple procedures.
2. Pick up gerbil by whole body.	2. Gerbils have delicate tails. The tail can be "degloved" with aggressive handling.

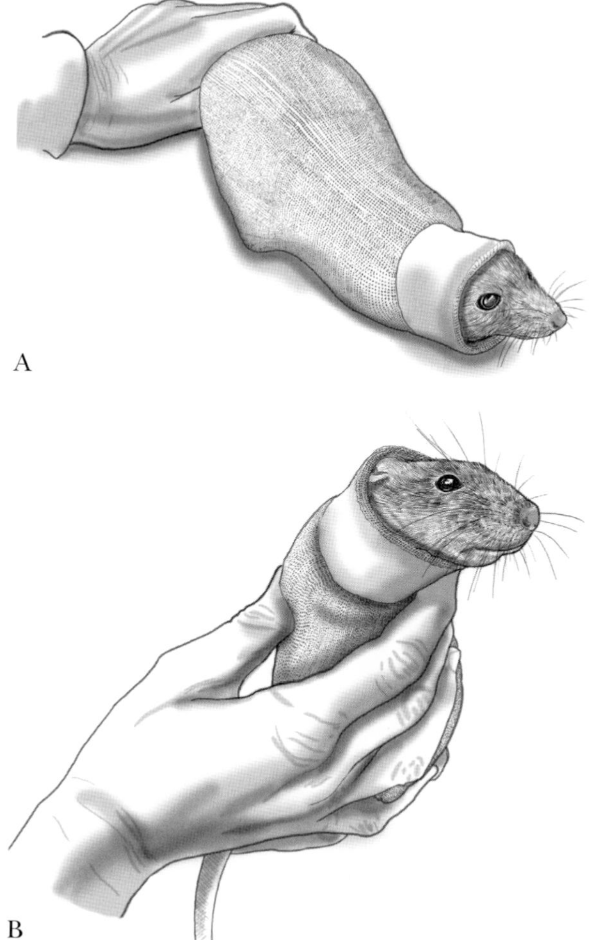

Figure 38-6 Placing rat in stockinette "sweater" for minor procedures.

Technical Action	Rationale/Amplification
3. Pick up chinchilla by whole body.	**3.** Chinchillas are nervous rodents that like to jump and climb. With rough handling, a chinchilla may have "furslip"; however, in most cases, the fur will regrow.
4. Use stockinette "sweater" when working with rats, gerbils, guinea pigs, and chinchillas.	
5. Use small towel for restraint of guinea pigs (Figs. 38-7 and 38-8) and chinchillas.	**5.** It can be used to wrap the animal while administering injections or oral medications (Fig. 38-9).

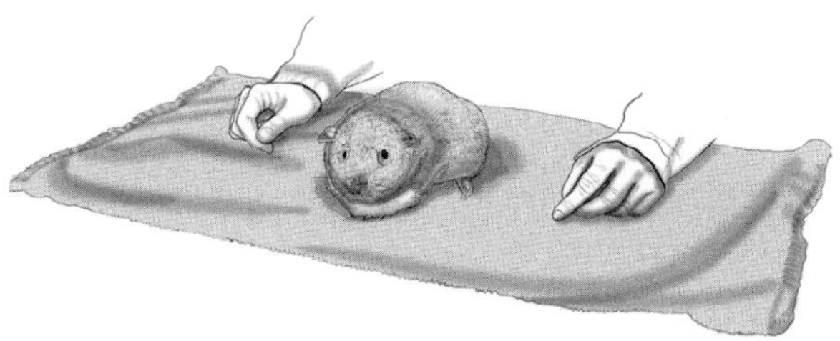

Figure 38-7 Placing guinea pig on small towel for restraint.

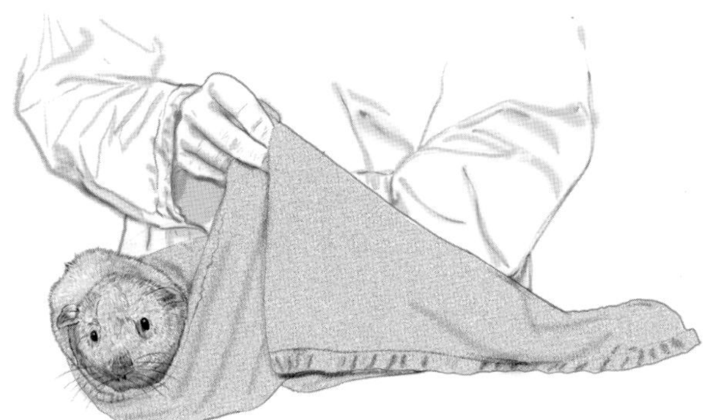

Figure 38-8 Wrapping guinea pig in small towel.

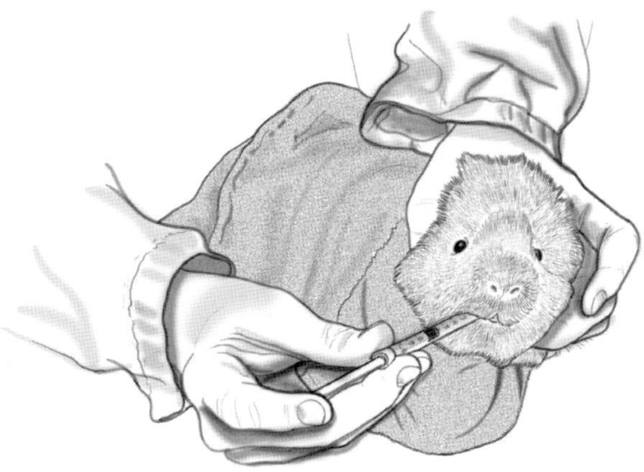

Figure 38-9 Administering oral medications or injections to guinea pig wrapped in towel.

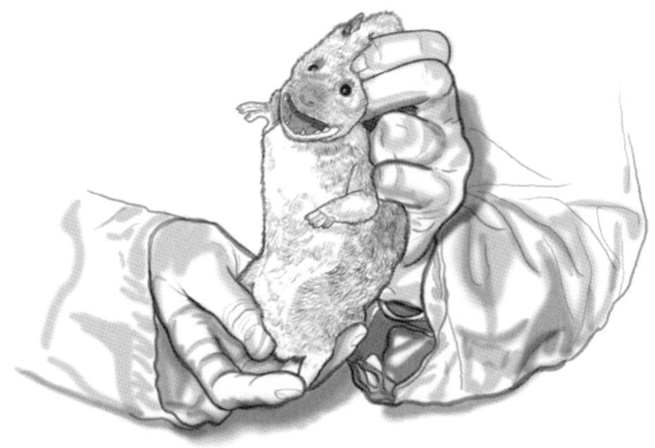

Figure 38-10 Picking up hamster by grasping skin behind shoulders.

Hamster

Technical Action

1. Pick up hamster by grasping skin behind shoulders and supporting body with other hand (Fig. 38-10).
2. Use a full hand grip for restraining a hamster.

Rationale / Amplification

1. Hamsters have tiny tails and deep cheek pouches. When a hamster is sleeping, wake it carefully. Hamsters are nocturnal and like running in an exercise wheel. Adult hamsters are solitary rodents (except for breeding). Hamsters often fill their cheek pouches with food and bedding. Remove any items in the cheek pouches before anesthetizing a hamster.
2. Gripping the dorsal skin in this manner provides control over the animal for technical procedures.

EXAMINING RODENTS

Procedure

Technical Action

1. Observe the animal in cage before attempting to handle it, noting attitude and activity.
2. Determine whether animal is breathing effortlessly and at usual rate.

Rationale/Amplification

1. Place the animal on a small towel or in a small basket.
2. See Table 38-1 for normal respiratory rates of small mammals.

TABLE 38-1 Normal respiratory rates in small mammals.

Species	Respiratory Rate (breaths/minute)
Mouse	100–250
Gerbil	90–140
Hamster	33–127
Rat	70–150
Chinchilla	100–150
Guinea pig	90–150

Technical Action	Rationale/Amplification
3. Observe body condition.	**3.** The condition could be normal, obese, or emaciated.
4. Note hair coat and skin.	**4.** A rough coat may indicate illness or ectoparasites. Crusts, sores, and swellings are examples of abnormal findings.
5. Check nose and eyes.	**5.** A red discharge from nose and/or eyes is abnormal, unless the animal is nervous.
6. Check skin color (foot pads, ears, lips, tongue).	**6.** Pale color may indicate anemia. If the animal is cyanotic, the skin may be gray/blue.
7. Check anal area and feces in the cage.	**7.** Signs of illness include diarrhea and protruding reddened rectal tissue.

Husbandry of Small Rodents

NOTE: *The following statements regarding habits of the rodent species discussed in this chapter are intended to help the reader understand these interesting animals and respond appropriately to their special qualities.*

1. Rats are friendly and confident. They usually enjoy being petted. Most rats enjoy a treat.
2. Guinea pigs have four toes on their front feet and three toes on their back feet. They will squeal for food or after rough handling. When a guinea pig gives birth, the babies' eyes and ears are open and they are able to walk. Dystocia is a common problem in female guinea pigs. Guinea pigs must have vitamin C in their diet (tomatoes, strawberries, or spinach).
3. Chinchillas should have "dust baths" daily or at least several times a week.
4. Male and female gerbils live together naturally, so they should not be housed separately by sex.
5. When a hamster is sleeping, wake it carefully. Hamsters are nocturnal and like running in an exercise wheel. Adult hamsters are solitary rodents (except for breeding). Hamsters often fill their cheek pouches with food and bedding. Remove any items in the cheek pouches before anesthetizing a hamster.

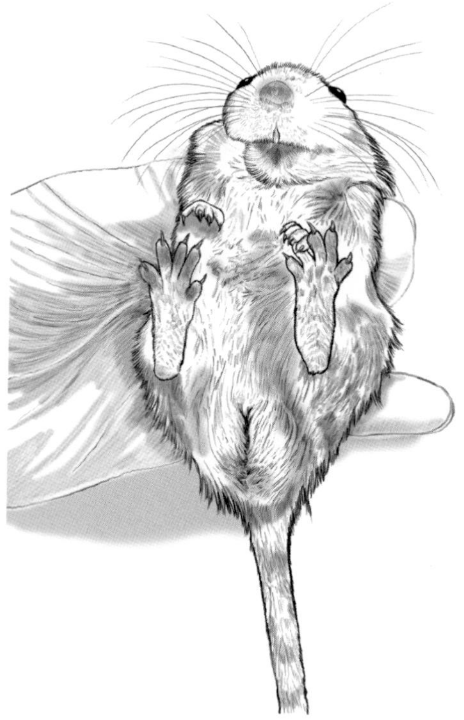

Figure 38-11 A male gerbil.

Determining Gender in Small Rodents

Technical Action	Rationale/Amplification
1. Determine sex by measuring distance between penis or vulva and anus (mouse, rat, gerbil, hamster).	1. A male will have a longer anogenital distance (Fig. 38-11).
2. Determine sex by identifying prominent genitalia in males (guinea pig, chinchilla).	2. In the male guinea pig and chinchilla, the penis can be protruded by pressing gently on either side of the prepuce.

Venipuncture and Fluid Administration in Small Rodents

Technical Action	Rationale/Amplification
1. Give ill rodents fluids subcutaneously (Fig. 38-12) or intraperitoneally (0.03–0.05 mL/gram) (Figs. 38-13 through 38-15).	1. Additional intraperitoneal fluids can be given every 4 hours. Subcutaneous fluids are absorbed more slowly.

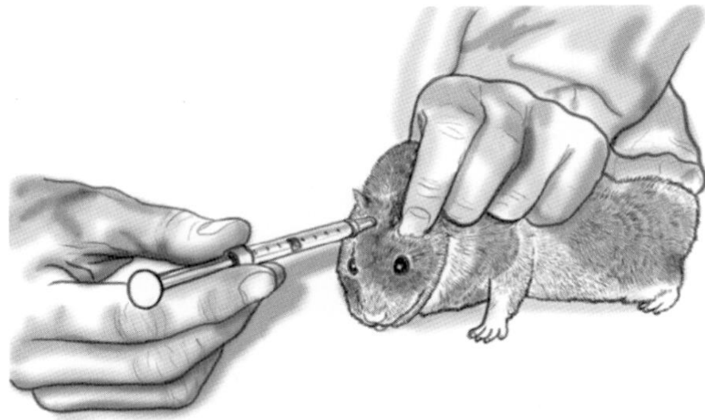

Figure 38-12 Administering a subcutaneous injection to a hamster.

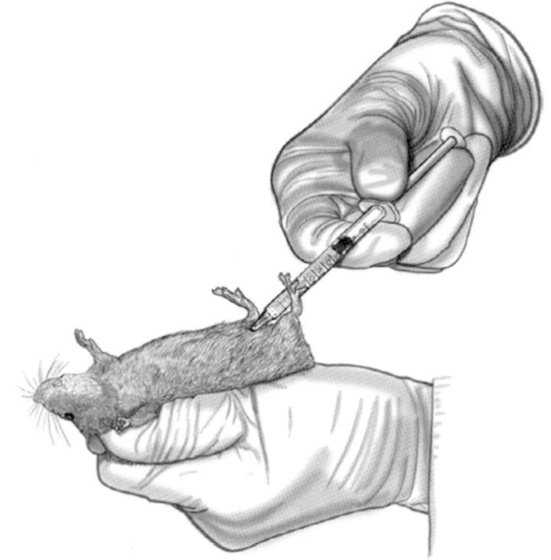

Figure 38-13 Administering an intraperitoneal injection to a mouse.

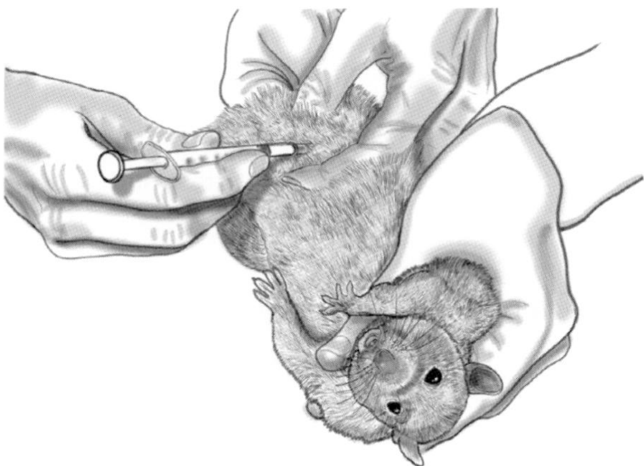

Figure 38-14 Administering an intraperitoneal injection to a rat.

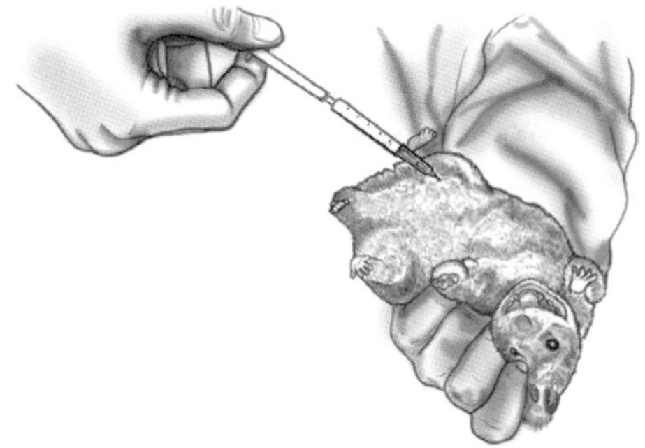

Figure 38-15 Administering an intraperitoneal injection to a hamster.

Technical Action

2. To collect blood from a mouse, gerbil, hamster, guinea pig, rat, or chinchilla, use saphenous vein on pelvic limb (Figs. 38-16 through 38-19).

3. Use syringe case to restrain mouse for venipuncture (Fig. 38-20).

4. Administer oral medication with small syringe (Fig. 38-9 and 38-21).

Rationale/Amplification

2. Apply petrolatum to the site and collect blood using a heparinized tube. The amount of blood to collect from a mouse is 0.3 mL. A larger amount of blood can be collected from the guinea pig, rat, and chinchilla (see Table 38-2).
3. The mouse can be restrained in a plastic tube that is open at both ends. For example, use a syringe case with a hole drilled in the closed end so that air is available for the mouse to breathe.
4. A 1-mL syringe may be sufficient to administer liquid oral medications.

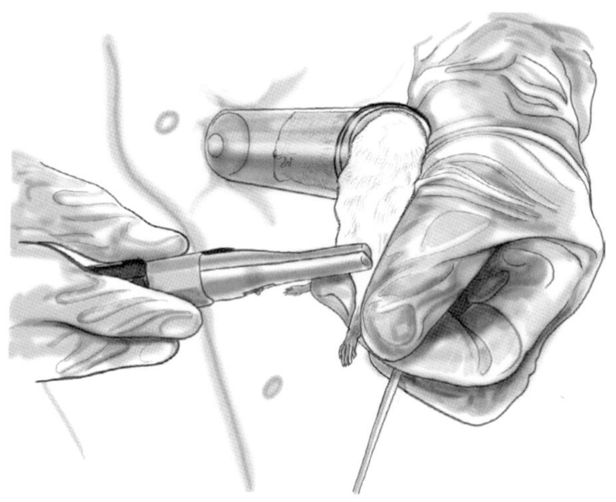

Figure 38-16 Clipping hair of pelvic limb for venipuncture.

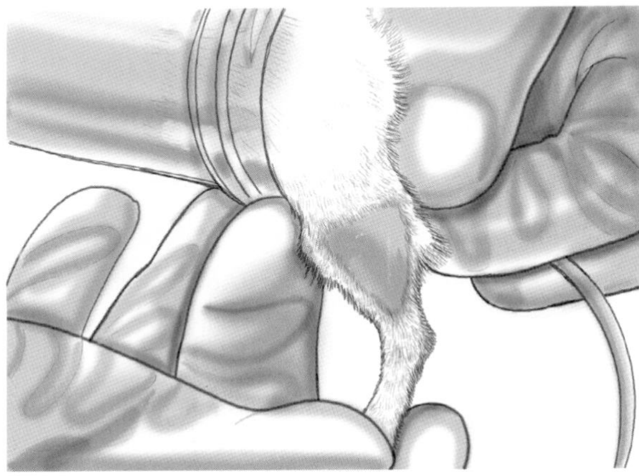

Figure 38-17 Leg prepared for venipuncture.

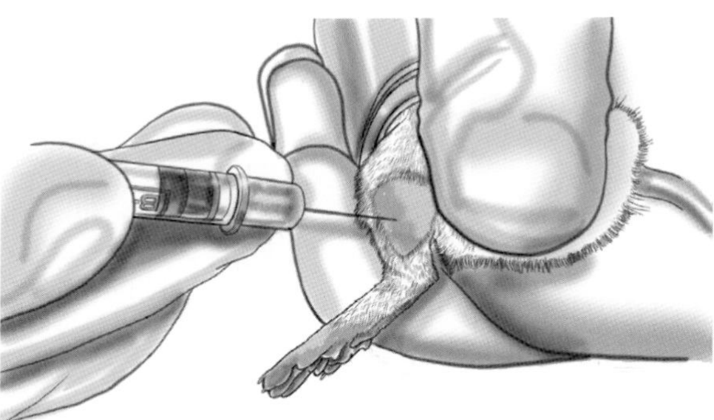

Figure 38-18 Puncturing vein on medial aspect of tibial segment of pelvic limb.

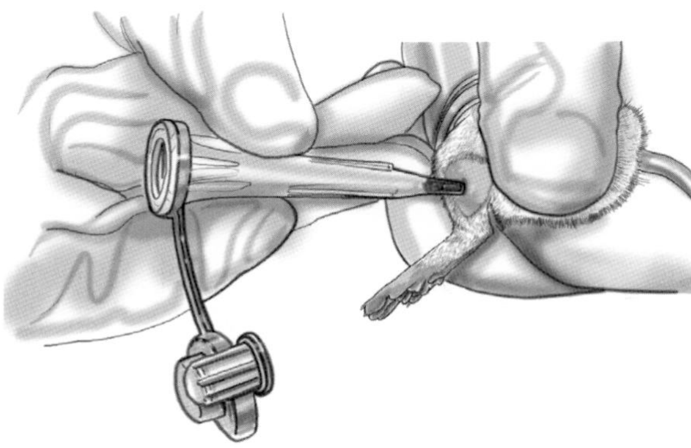

Figure 38-19 Collecting blood into tube using capillary action.

TABLE 38-2 Weight and blood volume of small mammals.

Species	Weight (g)	Total Blood Volume (mL)	Maximum Blood Draw Volume (mL)
Mouse	30	2.2–2.5	0.3–0.4
Gerbil	90	7.0–8.0	0.9–1.0
Hamster	100	7.5–8.5	1.0–1.2
Rat	400	30–35	4.0–4.8
Chinchilla	500	38–42	6.0–7.0
Guinea pig	800	60–70	8.0–9.6

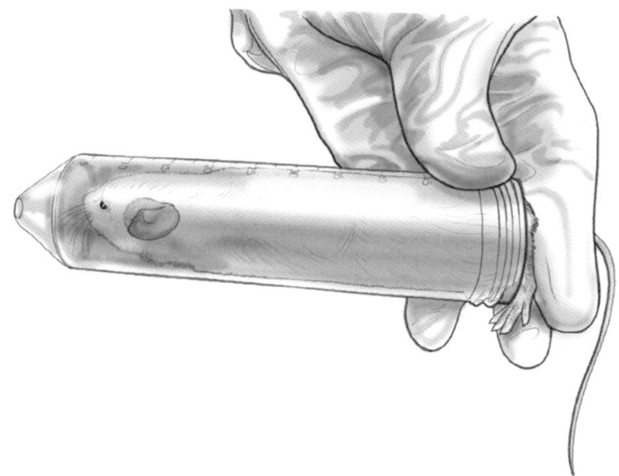

Figure 38-20 Restraining mouse for venipuncture in clear tube.

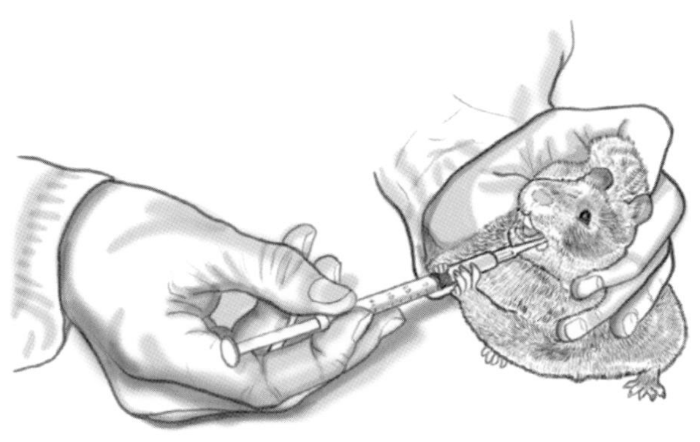

Figure 38-21 Administering oral medication to a hamster.

Suggested websites

http://web.jhu.edu/animalcare/procedures/restraint.html
http://vetmed.duhs.duke.edu/GuidelinesforRodentTechniques.html
http://www.research.psu.edu/arp/training/videos/handling-and-restraint-of-mice

Index

Crow and Walshaw's Manual of Clinical Procedures in Dogs, Cats, Rabbits, and Rodents, Fourth Edition. Edited by Jennifer E. Boyle.

Published 2016 by John Wiley & Sons, Inc.
Companion Website: www.wiley.com/go/boyle/manual4e